COSMETIC SURGERY

Cosmetic Surgery

A Feminist Primer

Edited by

CRESSIDA J. HEYES
University of Alberta, Canada

MEREDITH JONES
University of Technology, Sydney, Australia

Routledge
Taylor & Francis Group
LONDON AND NEW YORK

First published 2009 by Ashgate Publishing

Published 2016 by Routledge
2 Park Square, Milton Park, Abingdon, Oxfordshire OX14 4RN
711 Third Avenue, New York, NY 10017, USA

First issued in paperback 2016

Routledge is an imprint of the Taylor & Francis Group, an informa business

British Library Cataloguing in Publication Data
Cosmetic surgery : a feminist primer.
1. Surgery, Plastic--Social aspects. 2. Body image in women. 3. Feminist ethics.
I. Heyes, Cressida J. II. Jones, Meredith (Meredith Rachael), 1965-
306.4'613-dc22

Library of Congress Cataloging-in-Publication Data
Cosmetic surgery : a feminist primer / [edited] by Cressida J. Heyes and Meredith Jones.
p. cm.
Includes bibliographical references and index.
ISBN 978-0-7546-7699-7 (hbk. : alk. paper) -- ISBN 978-0-7546-9399-4 (ebook) 1. Surgery, Plastic--Social aspects. 2. Surgery, Plastic--Psychological aspects. 3. Feminine beauty (Aesthetics) 4. Body image in women. 5. Feminist theory. I. Heyes, Cressida J. II. Jones, Meredith (Meredith Rachael), 1965-
RD119.C682 2009
362.197'95--dc22

2009016279

ISBN 13: 978-1-138-25309-4 (pbk)
ISBN 13: 978-0-7546-7699-7 (hbk)

Contents

List of Illustrations *vii*
Notes on Contributors *ix*
Acknowledgments *xiii*

1 Cosmetic Surgery in the Age of Gender 1
Cressida J. Heyes and Meredith Jones

PART 1: REVISITING FEMINIST CRITIQUE

2 Twenty Years in the Twilight Zone 21
Susan Bordo

3 Revisiting Feminist Debates on Cosmetic Surgery:
Some Reflections on Suffering, Agency, and Embodied Difference 35
Kathy Davis

4 Women and the Knife: Cosmetic Surgery and the Colonization of Women's Bodies 49
Kathryn Pauly Morgan

5 Scary Women: Cinema, Surgery, and Special Effects 79
Vivian Sobchack

PART 2: REPRESENTING COSMETIC SURGERY

6 Agency Made Over? Cosmetic Surgery and Femininity in Women's Magazines and Makeover Television 99
Suzanne Fraser

7 The "Natural Look": Extreme Makeovers and the Limits of Self-Fashioning 117
Dennis Weiss and Rebecca Kukla

8 Selling the "Perfect" Vulva 133
Virginia Braun

PART 3: BOUNDARIES AND NETWORKS

9 "Engineering the Erotic": Aesthetic Medicine and Modernization in Brazil 153
Alexander Edmonds

10 Pygmalion's Many Faces 171
Meredith Jones

11 All Cosmetic Surgery is "Ethnic": Asian Eyelids, Feminist Indignation, and the Politics of Whiteness 191
Cressida J. Heyes

PART 4: AMBIVALENT VOICES

12 In Your Face 209
Cindy Patton and John Liesch

13 Crossing the Cosmetic/Reconstructive Divide: The Instructive Situation of Breast Reduction Surgery 225
Diane Naugler

14 Farewell My Lovelies 239
Diana Sweeney

Index *249*

List of Illustrations

1.1	"Finally, a gift you can both enjoy"	xvi
2.1	"Never too Early?"	20
3.1	"Plastic People No. 2"	34
4.1	"Nip/Tuck"	48
4.2	Various scalpels	51
5.1	"Dorothy" 2006	78
6.1	"Modular Face" 2007	98
7.1	"Hook and Eyes" 2007	116
8.1	"Anatomy Lesson" 2007	132
9.1	"Rio de Janeiro plastic surgery clinic" 2006	152
10.1	"Botox Happy Hour" 2006, photo taken in Franklin Lakes, New Jersey, USA	170
11.1	"Eyelid Tape" 2006, photo taken in Hong Kong	190
12.1	"Untitled No. 12" from the series "Meditations on Mortality" 2004	208
13.1	"DIY Cosmetic Surgery/Breast Reduction" 2006	224
14.1	"Untitled 1" from the series "Plastic Surgery" 2004	238

Notes on Contributors

Susan Bordo holds the Otis A. Singletary Endowed Chair in the Humanities and is a professor of English and Gender Studies at the University of Kentucky. She is the author of *Unbearable Weight: Feminism, Western Culture and the Body* (University of California Press, 1993), *The Male Body: A New Look at Men in Public and in Private* (Farrar, Straus and Giroux, 1999), and other influential books and articles. She is currently writing a book about Anne Boleyn.

Virginia Braun is a Senior Lecturer in Psychology at The University of Auckland. Her research is located within feminist and critical psychology, and focuses on topics related to sex, sexual health, and female genital cosmetic surgery. She is currently writing a textbook on qualitative methods in psychology (for Sage) with Victoria Clarke (The University of the West of England), and is co-editor, with Nicola Gavey (The University of Auckland), of the journal *Feminism & Psychology*.

Kathy Davis is Senior Researcher at the Institute of History and Culture at Utrecht University in the Netherlands. Her books include *Reshaping the Female Body* (Routledge, 1995), *Dubious Equalities and Embodied Differences* (Rowman & Littlefield, 2003) and *The Making of Our Bodies, Ourselves: How Feminism Travels Across Borders* (Duke, 2007) as well as several anthologies, including *Embodied Practices: Feminist Perspectives on the Body* (Sage, 1997) and *The Handbook of Gender and Women's Studies* (Sage, 2006).

Alexander Edmonds is a cultural and medical anthropologist specializing in urban Brazil. Drawing on ethnographic fieldwork, his current research focuses on beauty and body culture in capitalist peripheries. He is Assistant Professor in the Department of Anthropology at the University of Amsterdam. He has a book forthcoming with Duke University Press tentatively entitled *Pretty Modern: Plastic Surgery and Beauty in Brazil*.

Suzanne Fraser is Senior Lecturer in the Centre for Women's Studies and Gender Research, School of Political and Social Inquiry, Faculty of Arts, Monash University. Her research focuses on intersections between the body, technology, and gender, and explores areas as diverse and connected as drug use, obesity, gambling, and blood-borne viruses. She is the author of two books, *Cosmetic Surgery, Gender and Culture* (Palgrave, 2003) and, with Kylie Valentine, *Substance and Substitution: Methadone Subjects in Liberal Societies* (Palgrave, 2008).

Cressida Heyes is Canada Research Chair in Philosophy of Gender and Sexuality at the University of Alberta, Canada, where she writes and teaches in feminist and political philosophy, queer theory, and theories of embodiment. She is the author of *Line Drawings: Defining Women through Feminist Practice* (Cornell University Press, 2000) and *Self-Transformations: Foucault, Ethics, and Normalized Bodies* (Oxford University Press, 2007).

Meredith Jones is a media and cultural studies scholar based at the University of Technology, Sydney. She is the author of *Skintight: An Anatomy of Cosmetic Surgery* (Berg, 2008) and has written extensively about cosmetic surgery with articles appearing in *Space and Culture*, *Continuum*, and *Body and Society*. She is the co-founder of TRUNK books, which is publishing an anthology about hair in 2009. Her current research is about cosmetic surgery tourism in Thailand and medical tourism in India.

Rebecca Kukla is Professor of Philosophy and of Obstetrics and Gynecology at the University of South Florida, where she is also affiliated with the Department of Women's Studies and the graduate program in Medical Humanities and Bioethics. She is the current co-coordinator of the Feminist Approaches to Bioethics Network. Her recent books include *Mass Hysteria: Medicine, Culture, and Mothers' Bodies* (Rowman & Littlefield, 2005) and, with Mark Lance, *"Yo!" and "Lo!": The Pragmatic Topography of the Space of Reasons* (Harvard University Press, 2009).

John Liesch is a community-based researcher, a long time activist and volunteer in gay and HIV/AIDS related issues, and is the Data Manager at the Health Research Methods and Training Facility at Simon Fraser University, Vancouver. He is also an avid choral singer and challenge level square dancer.

Kathryn Pauly Morgan received her philosophy Ph.D. from Johns Hopkins University. She is Professor of Philosophy at the University of Toronto where she is cross-appointed to the Women and Gender Studies Institute. She has published extensively in the areas of feminist ethics and feminist bioethics (on such topics as cosmetic surgery, sexuality, reproductive technologies, and weight loss surgery), philosophy of the body, feminist technoscience, medicalization politics and Foucault, and feminist pedagogy. She is a co-author of *The Gender Question in Education: Theory, Pedagogy, and Politics* and recently published "Gender Police" in *Foucault and the Government of Disability*, ed. Shelley Tremain.

Diane Naugler has a Ph.D. in Women's Studies from York University in Toronto. She currently teaches in the Sociology Department at Kwantlen Polytechnic University in Surrey, British Columbia. Her primary research interests include feminist theories of embodiment and the construction of gendered social norms through discourses of sexism and homophobia.

Cindy Patton holds the Canada Research Chair in Community, Culture and Health in the Department of Sociology at Simon Fraser University. She is also Professor of Women's Studies. Her research has dealt extensively with cultural and social aspects of the AIDS epidemic, as well as works on race and gender in the media. She currently directs a qualitative research lab, which is involved in many community-based projects, including the one from which this work is drawn.

Vivian Sobchack is Professor Emerita in the Department of Film, Television, and Digital Media at UCLA. Her essays have appeared in *Film Quarterly, Film Comment, camera obscura*, and the *Journal of Visual Culture* and her books include *The Address Of The Eye: A Phenomenology Of Film Experience* (Princeton, 1992), *Screening Space: The American Science Fiction Film* (Rutgers University Press, 1997), and *Carnal Thoughts: Embodiment And Moving Image Culture* (University of California Press, 2004). She has also edited *The Persistence Of History: Cinema, Television and The Modern Event* (Routledge, 1996) and *Meta-Morphing: Visual Transformation and The Culture Of Quick Change* (University of Minnesota Press, 2000).

Diana Sweeney modeled from 1975 until 1990. As one of Australia's top fashion models she worked for national and international designers, appeared in all the major fashion magazines, and was on the covers of *Cosmopolitan, Cleo, Women's Weekly, Woman's Day*, and *New Idea*. In 1990 she quit modeling and changed direction, enrolling in university in 1994. She completed her Ph.D. in 2007. Her thesis explored white/ness and racism within the Australian women's magazine genre. She returned to modeling in 2005.

Dennis Weiss is Professor of Philosophy in the English and Humanities Department at York College of Pennsylvania. He is the editor of *Interpreting Man* and has published articles on philosophical anthropology, philosophy of technology, and the posthuman. He is currently at work on a project exploring the philosophical implications of human enhancement technologies.

Acknowledgments

Putting this volume together has been a long process, and I would like to thank all the contributors for their patience and willingness to work with our pace (whether slow or fast) and editorial demands. My own editorial and authorial contributions to the project were made possible in part through the support of the Canada Research Chairs program of the Social Sciences and Humanities Research Council of Canada, and I am grateful for the luxuries of time and money that this program affords its chairholders. My excellent students at the University of Alberta are always willing to debate the feminist intricacies of the cosmetic surgical world (which, increasingly even in this unassuming Canadian city, are the intricacies of their own lives). I am particularly grateful to all those people (students, colleagues, friends) who have taken the risk of sharing with me their own encounters—positive or negative, direct or indirect, transitory or life-long—with cosmetic surgery. Most of all I would like to thank my co-editor, Meredith Jones, whose phenomenally clever and deep engagement with cosmetic surgery as a feminist problematic in its own right, as well as a gateway to a rich intellectual and political terrain has been a model of scholarly excellence and creativity for me. Her good humor, comradeship, lightness of touch, and commitment to doing it right have made the project more than worthwhile.

Cressida J. Heyes

I wish to extend warm thanks to the anonymous peer-reviewers who gave us such thoughtful advice and insightful suggestions about an earlier version of this anthology. Each of the contributors to the volume has borne patiently with us through the protracted process of editing and compilation—for that I am deeply grateful. I would not be able to write and research as I do without the support of my colleagues at the University of Technology, Sydney and my wider circle of academic friends—I would particularly like to thank Jo McKenzie and Zoë Sofoulis for their unflagging enthusiasm and interest. Compiling a co-edited volume is logistically, intellectually, and sometimes emotionally difficult; further, long-distance co-editing has its own special challenges that are only partly overcome by email and Skype. However, I could not have asked for a more excellent co-editor. Cressida Heyes, whose insights into contemporary transformative bodily practices are never short of remarkable, has been an absolute pleasure to work with. Her collegial generosity and her academic rigor combined with her deep sensitivity inspire me as both feminist and academic. Although I'm older than Cressida I hope to grow up to be just like her.

Meredith Jones

Chapter 2, "Twenty Years in the Twilight Zone" is excerpted with permission from Susan Bordo, *Unbearable Weight: Feminism, Western Culture, and the Body* © 1993, 2004 and *Twilight Zones: The Hidden Life of Cultural Images from Plato to O.J.* © 1997 Regents of the University of California. Published by the University of California Press.

Chapter 3, "Revisiting Feminist Debates on Cosmetic Surgery: Some Reflections on Suffering, Agency, and Embodied Difference" is excerpted with permission from Kathy Davis, *Dubious Equalities and Embodied Differences: Cultural Studies on Cosmetic Surgery*. Lanham, MD: Rowman and Littlefield, 2003.

Chapter 4, "Women and the Knife: Cosmetic Surgery and the Colonization of Women's Bodies," was first published in *Hypatia* 6:2, copyright © Kathryn Pauly Morgan 1991. Reproduced with permission of John Wiley & Sons, Inc.

Chapter 5, "Scary Women: Cinema, Surgery, and Special Effects" is reprinted with permission from Vivian Sobchack, *Carnal Images: Embodiment and Moving Image Culture* © 2004 Regents of the University of California. Published by the University of California Press.

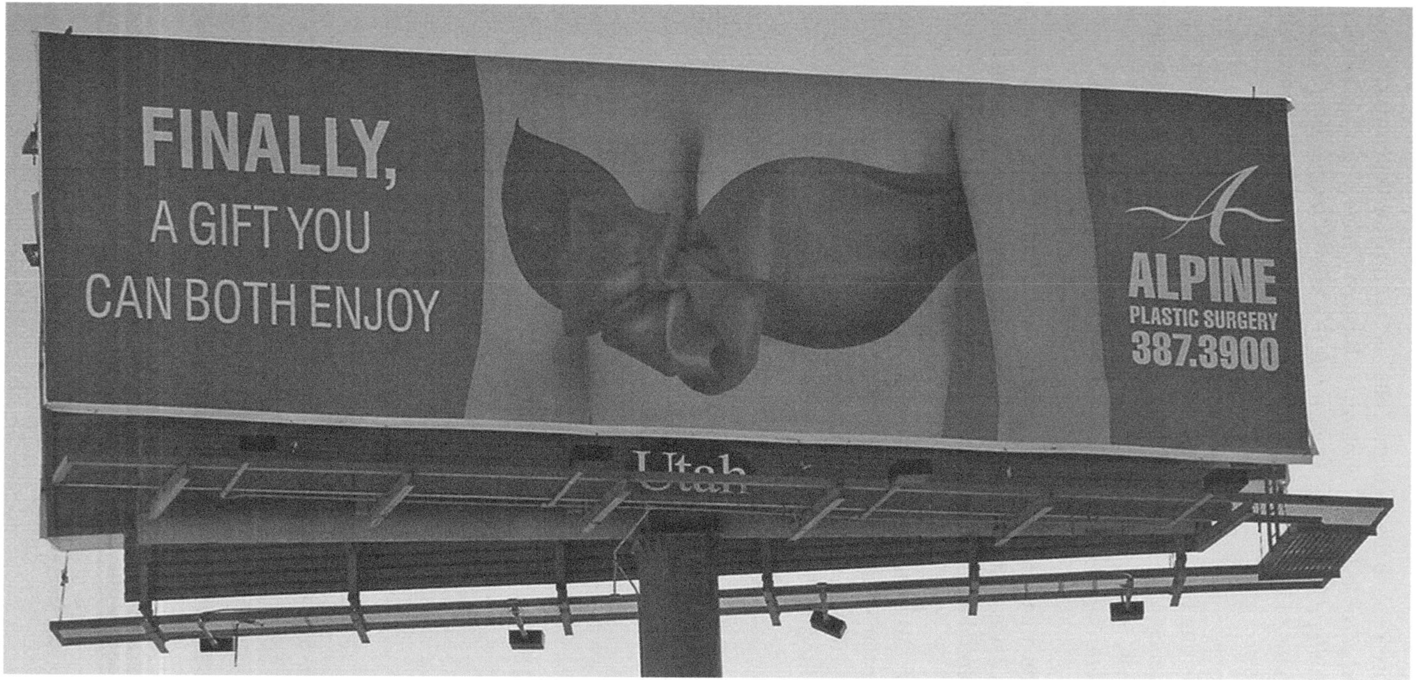

Figure 1.1 “Finally, a gift you can both enjoy”

Chapter 1
Cosmetic Surgery in the Age of Gender

Cressida J. Heyes and Meredith Jones

We're watching a clip from a TV documentary about cosmetic surgery on YouTube.[1] It introduces Toni Wildish, 28-year-old mother of four, part-time shop assistant, and aspiring glamour model. Toni went to Prague as a cosmetic surgery tourist after determining that she couldn't afford breast implants in the UK. The majority of the YouTube clip is a hand-held video diary made by Toni and her friend Claire, who accompanies her for moral support. They shriek and joke to camera, and Toni flashes her pre-op B-cup breasts; they seem to be having an exciting time, albeit that the shots of their cheap hotel room reveal it to be "very dark and dingy and a bit spooky." Visiting the Czech surgeon, it's immediately clear that he and Toni are not on the same page about the size and shape of her proposed implants. Toni rejects the first implant she's shown, saying "oh that's too natural, oh I don't want *them* ... Let me show you, I've brought my pictures ... I want them so they're really *round*." She pulls out a file of images of Jordan (Katie Price)—the C-grade British celebrity well known for her huge augmented bosom—and the surgeon tries to suggest that her breasts' very spherical look is created by an uplift bra. But Toni is one step ahead of him. She whips out her mobile phone, on which she has a photo of Jordan, topless—the massive breasts clearly standing independent of a bra. The surgeon is appalled, and declares in awkward English, "Oh, that's horrible! I refuse to do something like that!" Later, in a talking head for the documentary, Toni says, "He was standing his ground, not giving me what I wanted. And I'd been told [by the medical tourism company that organized the trip] I could have what I wanted. And, well, I was just extremely let down." Toni and the surgeon eventually compromise, but Toni still gets F-cup breasts, round and high on her chest, with nothing "too natural" about them. After the surgery she jumps up and down in her hotel room, hamming for the camcorder, declaring triumphantly, "They don't move!"

When feminists first began thinking and writing about cosmetic surgery some twenty years ago, the state of affairs they confronted was dramatically different to the one described above. The conglomeration of global, media, technological, and aesthetic conditions that forms the backdrop to Toni Wildish's story was the stuff of science fiction. Cosmetic surgery recipients were patients, not consumers; their desires were pathologized and people seeking cosmetic surgery were often

1 The clip was from "Pete Burns' Cosmetic Surgery Nightmares," and it has since been removed from the site.

secretive and ashamed. Talking about one's surgery—let alone videoing it for global access—would have been both technically impossible and socially deviant. So Toni's video story is a new kind of narrative, told via a new kind of medium in a new set of global circumstances, and it demonstrates significant changes in how cosmetic surgery is now chosen, undertaken and received.

In contrast, Carole Spitzack's classic 1988 article "The Confession Mirror" (the first feminist publication on cosmetic surgery in English we know of) describes a very different visit to a cosmetic surgeon. Spitzack is asked to account for her "disease" to an expert who is completely authoritative, and who aspires to make her look more "natural." It is imperative that her surgical outcome be subtle—even undetectable—as having been achieved through surgery. She is made abject, and must rely on the surgeon as her sole source of information about the technical and aesthetic possibilities for her body. Her experience is localized not only within her own country of residence, but even within the sanctum of the clinic and the context of her relationship with the surgeon.

The differences between Spitzack's 1980's foray into the secret world of "the confession mirror" and Wildish's 2007 highly public surgical holiday highlight two issues that have been key to the formation of this volume: first, the landscape for feminists concerned to articulate cultural critique of cosmetic surgery has changed radically during the last twenty years, and political commitments or research methodologies that might have been a good match for the cosmetic surgical scene in 1988 may not suffice in 2008. Second, cosmetic surgery is far from being a parochial topic of limited political and ethical significance. There is increasing scholarly interest in it accompanied by intense popular fascination. It occurs at and highlights the intersection of tremendously complex and significant social trends concerning the body, gender, psyche, medical practice and ethics, globalization, aesthetic ideologies, and both communication and medical technologies. Indeed, cosmetic surgery is among the most interdisciplinary of topics and thus feminist analysis needs to start from a variety of disciplinary perspectives. So, represented in this volume are philosophers, sociologists, film studies theorists, cultural studies theorists, anthropologists, and those working in medical humanities.

Landscapes of cosmetic surgery are undergoing rapid change. For every newly touted technique (from silicone buttock implants to "combo packages" of Botox, Restylane, and laser resurfacing), and for every newly created media product (from shock-horror documentaries to award-winning television dramas like *Nip/Tuck*) there could be a corresponding new feminist examination and approach. This is perhaps all the more reason to gather together the best "early" feminist writing about cosmetic surgery. We reprint excerpts from the work of four well-known feminist critics of cosmetic surgery—Susan Bordo (1993 and 1997), Kathy Davis (the earliest work she draws upon for this piece is from 1995), Kathryn Pauly Morgan (1991), and Vivian Sobchack (1999). We wanted to reproduce these "classics" while also recognizing that the world of cosmetic surgery has changed since they were first published, so we asked each author to revisit her original analysis to revise or comment upon her earlier perspective. While these chapters may be familiar to readers who have followed feminist critique of cosmetic surgery for some time (although the authors' updates may provide some surprises), they provide vital orientation for readers beginning to look at the worlds of cosmetic surgery and the ways in which feminist scholarship has approached them. They are a tacit background against which more recent writing can be understood. The majority of the volume consists of newly commissioned work that takes on the feminist challenge of understanding the very complex shifting landscape of cosmetic surgery in its contemporary modes. The feminist literature on cosmetic surgery is not yet large and is dispersed among very diverse journals or contained in books oriented around other topics, and so feminists have been relatively disconnected from an ongoing scholarly conversation on the topic. This volume thus seeks to gather together and represent the existing field while also starting new feminist dialogues about cosmetic surgery.

Cosmetic Surgery in "the Age of Gender"

Medical techniques on which much cosmetic surgery is based emerged in the years following World War I, as male soldiers returned from the front with new kinds of injury (Haiken 1997: esp. 29–43, Gilman 1999a: esp. 157–68). The contemporary field of "plastic" surgery—intervention aimed at restoring the normal configuration of the body's soft tissues—made its most rapid progress in response to these burns and wounds (perhaps especially of the face, as artist Paddy Hartley has demonstrated with his moving *Project Façade*[2]). Thus the distinction between reconstructive and cosmetic surgery emerged—the former, as the name suggests, *restoring* a body's "normal" appearance or functioning after injury or so-called congenital defect, with the latter *enhancing* a body already taken to fall within "normal" parameters. Feminists have by and large accepted this distinction, and have limited their political critique to cosmetic procedures while implicitly accepting that reconstructive surgery—including that aimed solely at improving appearance (such as birthmark or scar revision)—is fully justified. However, a number of essays in this volume question these distinctions and examine the blurry boundaries between them.

In the modern history of cosmetic surgery, the first written account of a face-lift is dated 1901; breast augmentation dates back to risky injections of—briefly—paraffin, followed by a longer postwar period of experimentation with liquid silicone (Haiken 1997: 235–55); liposuction was invented in 1974 and has become increasingly popular since the 1980s. Since at least the 1950s, women have overwhelmingly been the target consumers for cosmetic surgery, while men have practiced it: in 2007, 91 percent of all cosmetic surgical procedures in North America were performed on women, while eight out of nine cosmetic surgeons are men. Furthermore, these women have been mostly white: in 2007,

2 http://www.projectfacade.com. [Last accessed June 15, 2008.]

76 percent of cosmetic surgical procedures in North America were performed on "Caucasian" patients.[3] Historically speaking, this feminization of cosmetic surgery will probably be short-lived: in the *longue durée* cosmetic surgery may be, as Sander Gilman (1999a: esp. 31–6) has argued, more implicated with ethnicity and national belonging than with gender, while statistical trends indicate that a steadily increasing proportion of recipients are men as well as non-white. New procedures continue to be developed, and there has been an explosive growth in the number and type of cosmetic surgeries performed, in new national markets and among more diverse class, gender, ethnic, and age groups.

The work in this volume thus responds to the "age of gender" in cosmetic surgery—our play between gender and chronology is intentional here—while at the same time illustrating a more general trajectory in feminist attitudes to bodies. Thus it demonstrates how a big picture analysis in which body-transforming practices are understood as top-down pressures on women to conform to patriarchal ideals is giving way to the more fine-grained and multi-factoral analyses that are required to understand contemporary constraints and incitements. Recent feminist research on cosmetic surgery (Davis's work is a notable older exception) has begun to interview and engage with a wide range of cosmetic surgery recipients through interviews and participant observation, deploying empirically grounded ethnographic methods: Debra Gimlin, for example, has found that, far from working on "body projects" in voluntarily self-conscious ways, women use cosmetic surgery as a way of dealing with the unwanted intrusion of the body into consciousness (2006), and that narrative tactics for explaining and justifying the decision to have cosmetic surgery vary by national context (2007).

---

3 In 2007, 91 percent of cosmetic surgical procedures (excluding "minimally invasive" procedures such as Botox) performed by a member of the American Society for Plastic Surgeons (in both the US and Canada) were performed on women. See http://www.plasticsurgery.org > media > statistics. No reliable statistics are available for Australasia or other markets. Kathy Davis (2003: 41) cites the statistic for the gender distribution of plastic surgeons. A March 25, 2008 press release entitled "Cosmetic Plastic Surgery Procedures for Ethnic Patients Up 13 Percent in 2007" claims that: "Almost a quarter (2,626,700) of cosmetic plastic surgery procedures were performed on ethnic patients in 2007, up 13 percent from last year, including Hispanics, African Americans and Asian Americans, according to statistics released today by the American Society of Plastic Surgeons (ASPS)." President Richard D'Amico remarks that "A key take-away from this data is that the plastic surgery patient profile is changing … The majority of patients remain Caucasian women, but it is noteworthy that cosmetic plastic surgery procedures were performed on almost as many Hispanic patients as male patients." Available on-line at http://www.plasticsurgery.org/media/press_releases/Cosmetic-Plastic-Surgery-Procedures-for-Ethnic-Patients-Up-13-Percent-in-2007.cfm. Last accessed June 15, 2008.

Since 2006, cosmetic plastic surgery procedures increased in the following demographic categories: up 8 percent (1,011,000) in Hispanics, up 8 percent (847,800) in African Americans, and up 26 percent (767,800) in Asian Americans.

The epistemic and ethical challenge of interpreting these self-justifications is, however, enormous. Cosmetic surgery has always had a complex relationship to psychology: since it cannot be justified on the basis of physical medical need, it must be justified in relation to the patient's own desires. Elizabeth Haiken argues that in the US cosmetic surgery finds an early rationale in the "inferiority complex"—a syndrome first mooted by Austrian psychologist Alfred Adler in the 1910s (Haiken 1997: esp. 108–30; see also Gilman 1997: 263–65).[4] Most Americans, Haiken implies, needed little more than a label to invoke the inferiority complex as a justification for numerous practices of self-improvement, and it enjoyed a significant vogue in media and advertising—and in selling the services of cosmetic surgeons (Haiken 1997: 111–23). Because the concept was vague and relative to the patient's perception of her own psychology, surgeons could more easily justify intervention on the basis of psychic need. The individual stipulated of herself that she had an inferiority complex (a claim that could not be disproved), which she attributed (if she hoped to get cosmetic surgery) to a bodily defect. Thus, cosmetic surgery advertising both called forth the self-diagnosis while at the same time surgeons were quick to deny any psychiatric expertise that might actually necessitate psychological selection procedures. Against this background it is a short distance to justifying cosmetic surgical intervention whenever the patient makes a convincing enough case, and the surgeon believes that risk of a negative outcome (whether physical, psychological, or legal) is low enough.

This dynamic continues today, although the language of the inferiority complex has fallen away. As Cressida Heyes (2007a) has pointed out, the growing body of literature on the sequelae of cosmetic surgery is far from showing that recipients consistently experience positive, long-term psychological benefits. As we might expect, some people are very happy with surgical results and have no regrets, while others are deeply disappointed (even with a technically "good" outcome) and feel more damaged by surgery than by their initial dissatisfaction. Some return for more surgeries—a practice both encouraged by surgeons (who, like any businessmen, need repeat customers), and treated with some suspicion as evidence of addiction or dysmorphia (not least because the returning cosmetic surgery patient may be more likely to complain or sue) (see Kuczynski 2006, Pitts-Taylor 2007). Toni Wildish had a life-threatening experience with post-surgical infection, yet in a follow-up cameo she says that she plans to have even larger, rounder breast implants to achieve the "Jordan" look, as well as facial cosmetic surgeries. Here

4 On Adler's view, a central developmental task for all humans is to transform the inevitable powerlessness of the young child into a sense of capability and self-sufficiency. Adequate parenting is clearly central to this task, and the parent who is not "good enough" (to borrow Winnicott's later phrase) will create a child who is insecure or timorous, and will need to compensate for their perceived inadequacy. Whatever personality style this results in, Adler suggested, a failure to adapt to the possibilities of independence and mastery in adult life as contrasted with the early sense of vulnerability and impotence will result in an "inferiority complex."

again, many surgeons' expectations of the compliant, normalized "patient" who wants a so-called natural, feminine appearance achieved through a conservative procedure may be thwarted by contemporary clients who want extreme results, total transformation, and who treat their surgeon as a service provider whom they expect to acquiesce to their demands. This new psychology and the way it transforms client–surgeon relations reaches its limit in the extreme cosmetic surgery practitioner—those public figures who use surgery to make statements far removed from any conventional presentation of a beautiful body. Whether, as in Orlan's case, the surgeries are used to make philosophical and visual aesthetic statements,[5] or, as for Michael Jackson or Jocelyn Wildenstein, they produce a kind of mythical, monstrous cyborg (Jones 2008) whose political or aesthetic values are opaque, these celebrities disrupt the historical stereotype of the normatively feminine cosmetic surgery recipient who has any kind of "inferiority complex."

There is another limit in the practice of "rogue" cosmetic procedures—those undertaken without medical supervision (and sometimes outside the law) by individuals who could not afford or would not be permitted access to medically sanctioned procedures. For example, Don Kulick describes how Brazilian transgendered prostitutes inject liters of liquid silicone into their bodies to achieve a normative form (Kulick 1998). Since his fieldwork the number of "minimally invasive" procedures available and their increasing popularity has spurred a global black market of unlicensed or unqualified practitioners offering cheap and quick "salon" services, sometimes using knock-off or non-medical injectables, while some are willing to undertake more invasive surgeries such as liposuction (see Singer 2006). This emergent market has barely been explored by any researchers, including feminists.

Part 1: Revisiting Feminist Critique

Understanding why so many people—most of them women—are attracted to cosmetic surgery to alter their "normal" appearance is a key question for feminists, who have not long had serious scholarship on the personal narratives of diverse constituencies of cosmetic surgery recipients to draw on. When we started work on this volume we imagined we would find an early feminist literature that was quick to see women who have cosmetic surgery as either vain social strivers, or as victims of a patriarchal beauty system. These attitudes may indeed have had a heyday in unpublished feminist conversations—and in the anomalous but persistent feminist moments that surface in popular representations of cosmetic

5 The French performance artist Orlan is famous for making art of a series of radical and public cosmetic surgeries in the early 1990s. Orlan's audacious literalization of the body-as-text metaphor has itself birthed a large devoted literature, including two recent monographs. See O'Bryan 2005 and Ince 2000; also see Jones 2008 (esp. 151–78), Brand 2000, Goodall 1999, and Augsburg 1998.

surgery. Certainly when Kathy Davis describes this dominant perspective—in which cosmetic surgery is "unanimously regarded as not only dangerous to women's health, but demeaning and disempowering"—she identifies a common belief, one held not only by self-described feminists. However, we have found that the feminist literature, on review, has actually *always* evinced a certain flexibility and curiosity about what cosmetic surgery might mean to individuals, and how that meaning might be understood as informing and being informed by a larger social context. Although different feminist theoretical models and disciplinary styles place different epistemic emphasis on women's narratives (and use different interpretive strategies to theorize them), feminist scholarship is marked by a consistent interest in the reasons that cosmetic surgery recipients give for their surgeries.

Here in Part 1 Susan Bordo's "Twenty Years in the Twilight Zone" comprises parts of her germinal essays "Material Girl" (1993) and "Braveheart, Babe, and the Contemporary Body" (1997), together with a brief 2008 update. Bordo is, recall, critical of the "postmodern imagination of human freedom from bodily determination"—especially in its pop cultural moments—for the way it denies the materiality of the flesh and levels political critique. In these selections she reminds us of how defect is not only corrected but also created by the economic and technological engine that carries us along, generating ever more impossible images. In her update, Bordo is pessimistic about the possibility that cultural critique can have any impact on this process; this is an important reminder from a commentator with a long perspective on cosmetic surgery that (viewed from a certain angle) things have become dramatically worse.

In "Revisiting Feminist Debates on Cosmetic Surgery: Some Reflections on Suffering, Agency, and Embodied Difference," Kathy Davis reintroduces her more recent work on cosmetic surgery as a critical response to feminist interpretations that represent women as cultural dopes, taken in by a beauty system hungry for profit and control. Instead, her well-known argument runs, the women she interviewed and observed wanted to become "normal" and wished to overcome a degree of psychosocial suffering they found intolerable that could not be assuaged by any other means. Stressing choice (albeit choices made under conditions of constraint) and agency, Davis continues to charge that critics like Bordo are too quick to see themselves as offering a privileged epistemic perspective on women's reasons for opting for cosmetic surgery.

The debate between Bordo and Davis centers around the question of whether women can be said to choose cosmetic surgery, or whether that "choice" is overdetermined by a larger patriarchal structure that makes cosmetic surgery seem like the only option for psychological survival in a world hostile to women's bodies.[6] How should feminist viewers categorize Toni Wildish, for example? Is she a victim of a beauty myth? Of global consumer culture? Or is she a canny and

6 Davis is critical of Bordo in her 1995 book *Reshaping the Female Body*, and Bordo responds to this critique in her essay "Braveheart, Babe, and the Contemporary Body."

resourceful heroine, who after enduring some trials and setbacks finally got what she wanted?

Kathryn Morgan's classic "Women and the Knife," (1991, reprinted here in abbreviated form) is clearly strongly informed by radical feminism, as when she argues that

> For virtually all women as women, success is defined in terms of interlocking patterns of compulsion: compulsory attractiveness, compulsory motherhood, and compulsory heterosexuality, patterns that determine the legitimate limits of attraction and motherhood. Rather than aspiring to self-determined and woman-centered ideals of health or integrity, women's attractiveness is defined as attractive-to-men; women's eroticism is defined as either nonexistent, pathological, or peripheral when it is not directed to phallic goals; and motherhood is defined in terms of legally sanctioned and constrained reproductive service to particular men and to institutions such as the nation, the race, the owner, and the class—institutions that are, more often than not, male-dominated.

But the text also includes a section called "listening to the women," and Morgan reflects on the forms of subjectivity that this institutional backdrop cultivates (see the critique of her method in Davis 1995: 164–72). Her update, "All of me … Why Don't You Nip/Tuck/Suck/Inject/Laser ALL of me?" is a creative, not-so-dystopic look at medical tourism, cosmetic surgery as fashionable commodity, and class issues in what she calls an "exciting, brave and frightening transnational world."

Vivian Sobchack's "Scary Women: Cinema, Surgery, and Special Effects" (1999) with its "(Not Quite) Post-Mortem" rounds off the first section. Foregrounding later work by scholars on relations between media images and real bodies (see Part 2), Sobchack insists that "insofar as we subjectively live both our bodies and our images, each not only informs the other, but they also often become significantly confused." Looking at the "horrors" of aging women in film she demonstrates how cosmetic surgery is a "sort of magic" akin to cinema's special effects. Finally, after making it clear that "middle-aged women … are demonized and made monstrous in our present culture" Sobchack describes her own self-image, at 67, as positively and confidently glowing. She writes inspiringly: "today, I am kinder to both myself and others and accept those sags, wrinkles, and imperfect bodies as—and because of—what they are; signs of life and not the stuff of images."

Part 2: Representing Cosmetic Surgery

Cosmetic surgery is no longer represented as a distant possibility reserved for the Hollywood celebrity or the wealthy socialite. It is increasingly marketed as

---

Davis revisits the debate in the introduction to her later book *Dubious Equalities and Embodied Differences*, on which her essay here is based.

an everyday option for ordinary women (and men), and its recipients cross lines of class, age, occupation, gender, and national context. Part 2, "Representing Cosmetic Surgery," contains chapters that examine surgeons' websites, makeover television, and women's magazines. As cosmetic surgery has entered the ambit of more and more people, the popular cultural discussion of its merits and drawbacks has also proliferated. This discussion tends to follow certain well-trodden paths, as Suzanne Fraser points out in her chapter, "Agency Made Over? Cosmetic Surgery and Femininity in Women's Magazines and Makeover Television." Fraser identifies repertoires of nature, agency, and vanity—patterns of discourse production that individuals can tap into in order to make sense of their desires and actions. These repertoires function, she suggests, to recreate an imaginary that both undermines and reinforces gender stereotypes. Further, the repertoire of naturalness serves a particularly important but ambivalent role, as Dennis Weiss and Rebecca Kukla illustrate in their chapter "The Natural Look: Extreme Makeovers and the Limits of Self-Fashioning." They provide an analysis of the deployment of the concept of the "natural" in TV makeovers—and, by extension, throughout popular representations of cosmetic surgery. They show that, as our own reading of Toni Wildish's case suggests, "the natural" is neither the limit against which possibilities for change are defined, nor an irrelevant fiction in the face of individual choice. Such repertoires serve to educate, inform, and create the context within which cosmetic surgery is received; perhaps the greatest conceit of those who contribute to the representational world of cosmetic surgery is that they are only responding to consumer demand and do not themselves construct our desires, fears, and possibilities. This last point is well illustrated by Virginia Braun's chapter, "Selling the 'Perfect' Vulva," in which she analyzes surgeons' websites promoting female genital cosmetic surgeries, which, she argues, contribute "to the ongoing construction of experiential as well as material bodies, to the production of desires, and practices around these desires." Specifically, the websites function to demarcate and pathologize the "abnormal" vulva or vagina, generating dissatisfaction and anxiety among women about body parts that they may previously never have subjected to this kind of aesthetic or functional evaluation.

Part 3: Boundaries and Networks

The chapters in Part 3, "Boundaries and Networks," attempt to explore cosmetic surgery in ways that redefine its borders. Alex Edmonds's "'Engineering the Erotic': Aesthetic Medicine and Modernization in Brazil" is a brilliant ethnographic intervention into a national case study. Brazil has gripped the sociological imagination for the drama of its huge cosmetic surgical industry, which is part of the national health care system of a country with tremendous social inequalities. Edmonds argues that the availability of "*plástica*" to the Brazilian poor shows how shifting economic and cultural context invites a reconceptualization of the shared feminist premise that "more extreme beauty practices function as a means for the social control of the female body within patriarchy." Convincingly situating Brazilian cosmetic surgery in a global context, Edmonds argues that *plástica* is "a 'localized' form, produced by the encounter of global medicine and media with Brazil's particular bureaucratic rationality of the health system, political economy of reproduction, and cultural notions of sexuality and beauty." His chapter therefore exemplifies the larger point that what cosmetic surgery means for feminists may now need to be worked through where local contexts meet the emerging and rapidly transforming global picture, and without taking patriarchy as the sole or even key theoretical axis of analysis.

Meredith Jones argues in her chapter, "Pygmalion's Many Faces" that despite the deep significance to feminist scholarship of narrative and testimony, to see cosmetic surgery's political meaning as residing in the minds of its recipients is to fail to grasp the full range of actors and relationships that shape it. We suspect that feminists have to some extent focused on the women who have cosmetic surgery because they constitute a relatively accessible (even vulnerable) research target. It is much harder to inquire into the self-understandings of cosmetic surgeons, for example, because they protect their professional territory in ways that explicitly foreclose the possibility that their motives, beliefs, and desires are ethically or psychologically suspect. It is even harder to grasp how the roles of other institutional structures (such as health care bureaucracies) and non-human actors (such as implant technologies) might inform the subjectivities of human agents. Jones begins by documenting the established dynamics of surgeon as expert, lover, and artist, working on the female body—his "raw material"—to transform it in the image he chooses. She argues, however, that the exclusivity of the male surgeon/female patient dyad may be challenged by the emergence of new actors (her example is Botox) and by consumer expectations.

Cressida Heyes's chapter, "All Cosmetic Surgery is 'Ethnic': Asian Eyelids, Feminist Indignation, and the Politics of Whiteness" explores so-called "ethnic" cosmetic surgery. Heyes examines the dominant feminist critique of, which constructs racially inflected surgeries (the most obvious example being Asian double eyelid surgery) as seeking solely to "whiten" recipients and erase embodied ethnic difference, and thus reflecting internalized racism on the part of their recipients. When ethnic cosmetic surgery is typically justified by surgeons (and to some extent by recipients) by using a rhetoric of objective, race-transcendent bodily flaws (Dull and West 1991: 58–9), or, more recently, one of making ethnic bodies more normative without erasing their distinctive features (Heyes 2007b: 23), this emphasis is understandable. The persistent popular tendency to see cosmetic surgery as outside history (especially the histories of ethnocentrism and assimilationism), unconnected to normative whiteness, and an expression of freedom of choice and upward mobility clearly requires a feminist counter. Nonetheless, Heyes suggests that, following an existing hermeneutic trajectory, feminist critics have implied that those women of color who deny (or challenge) a univocal reading of the larger institutional picture behind their choices bear the double burden of collusion with racist norms. The foregrounding of certain key examples of ethnic cosmetic surgery, she argues, also distracts attention from the surgical whitening of white people, perpetuating the invisibility of the construction of whiteness and the neutrality of white people's cosmetic aspirations.

Part 4: Ambivalent Voices

As the case of the surgeons' promotional websites analyzed by Braun in Part 2 makes clear, our access to new technologies transforms possibilities for the representation and interpretation of bodies. Furthermore, new medical technologies and pharmaceuticals used in cosmetic surgery itself increase the range and consequences of aesthetic interventions on the flesh: the advent of Botox, Restylane and other "fillers," for example, has opened the way for less physically consequential and less risky "minimally invasive procedures." More and more procedures can be undertaken more and more often. And some of these are even prophylactic: start Botox in your twenties, and your frown lines may never appear.

These new possibilities for materiality and representation extend cosmetic surgery to new constituencies, where procedures may be used in ways that do not sit easily with dominant feminist interpretations. For example, Cindy Patton and John Liesch's chapter, "In Your Face," examines the use of facial fillers by gay men living with HIV/AIDS to counteract facial wasting—an increasingly legible marker of positive HIV status. As Patton and Liesch remark, the feminist literature on cosmetic surgery has been until quite recently unconcerned with men's experience—and not only because men have until recently formed the small minority of cosmetic surgery recipients. As Diana Dull and Candace West argue, cosmetic surgery narratives by both recipients and surgeons *accomplish* gender, representing surgery for women as normal and natural, but for men as extrinsic to their gender identity and hard to justify unless related to employment or health (1991: esp. 64–7). If cosmetic surgery is understood as undertaken to conform within a patriarchal beauty system acting through the bodies of women, it then follows that the men who have it are making almost unintelligible choices. Existing feminist scholarship (including the work of Davis and Morgan), as Ruth Holliday and Allie Cairnie (2007) argue, tends to simply exclude men from analysis *ad hoc*, treating them as aberrant exceptions to a gendered system. Examining the motivations of a small group of white British men who elected to have aesthetic procedures ranging from hair transplants, to scar revision, to tattoo removal, to liposuction, they conclude that their

> participants are active investors in their bodies, spending large sums of money on consuming surgery now in the hope of eliciting future success (in different fields). The investments they make may be normative, but outcomes enable them to gain distinction, to distinguish themselves from the aging, balding,

> spreading men around them. Consuming better bodies, in one sense, reinforces highly masculine notions of competition, yet it should not be reduced to this simple logic. (74–5)

This interpretive weakness has a currency in the clinical literature, too, where male prospective patients have historically been viewed with a certain amount of suspicion due to their alleged psychopathology as well as their greater tendency to assert their preferences and complain about outcomes. The old message is that men who seek cosmetic surgery are either neurotic or gay (or both, where the latter necessarily includes the former)—in contrast to women, whose dissatisfaction with their appearance is seen as a normal feature of heterosexual femininity.[7] This model—in both its feminist and clinical forms—could only explain men's choices as pathologically mimetic or tangential to a dominant understanding of femininity, but has yet to be fully supplanted by more nuanced, less reductive contemporary paradigms. Michael Atkinson remarks on the paucity of literature on men and aesthetic bodywork, and suggests that

> the lack of theoretically innovative research symbolizes … a general tendency to view masculinity as a singularly constructed and unproblematic gender identity. Masculinity still tends to be framed by gender researchers along very narrow conceptual lines … Dominant constructions of masculinity are either interpreted as rigidly hegemonic/traditional or drastically alternative and deeply marginalized. Neither of these polar positions accurately captures how clusters of men often wrestle with and negotiate established constructions of masculinity in novel ways. (Atkinson 2008: 68)

Atkinson argues that for the Canadian men he interviewed cosmetic surgery enabled the construction of a "male-feminine" identity, which re-establishes "a sense of empowered masculine identity in figurational settings that they perceive to be saturated by gender doubt, anxiety and contest" (73). Their narratives use mechanisms of neutralization that meet the charge of participating in an effeminate practice: for example, "their willingness to endure painfully invasive surgeries re-establishes their ability to meet social threats with 'modern' masculine resolve" (80). Within the rapidly changing context of the cultural and socio-economic crisis of masculinities, the men's narratives can be understood as reinstalling their bodies as "texts of strength, authority, and power;" having cosmetic surgery became a practice in which masculine aggression and risk-taking are turned inward rather than enacted intersubjectively; and the men appropriated traditionally feminine terrain for the purpose of gaining power (83–4). They were still, however, reticent

7 For a summary of this history with references see Davis 2003: 117–31 esp. 123–6; Haiken 1997: 155–61. For a more recent study that references the older literature on men and psychopathology as well as offering a more contemporary psychological model, see Pertschuk et al. 1998.

in talking about their decisions and experiences (83), reflecting perhaps that men are still rewriting scripts of cosmetic surgery in a time of tremendous ideological and material flux but have not yet normalized the kind of stigma that confronted women twenty years ago.

Atkinson makes no reference to the sexualities of his interviewees—a surprising omission in light of the troubled association of cosmetic surgery with effeminacy (and hence a stereotyped homosexuality). Rather than seeing their participants as using cosmetic surgery to "improve" their masculinity, Patton and Liesch in this volume show how they seek "to decrease their legibility as persons living with AIDS." However, they aver, "this too is complex because to acknowledge a desire to diminish the signs of long-term survivorship risks altering their connections with their community." This work is, we hope, at the beginning of a new generation of research on men, masculinities, and cosmetic surgeries.[8]

Diane Naugler's chapter "Crossing the Cosmetic/Reconstructive Divide: The Instructive Situation of Breast Reduction Surgery" challenges the view that there are inherent (and some would argue, moral) differences between reconstructive and cosmetic surgeries. Naugler shows that breast reduction occupies an instructively ambiguous place on the continuum between such categories and argues that "the conceptual hegemony of the cosmetic/reconstructive divide participates in the naturalization of feminine aesthetic norms which produce women as available sexual surfaces and subjects." Further, she references the vagaries of different national health care contexts; for example, her respondents are negotiating breast reduction in the Canadian system where a medical rationale will get the procedure paid for by provincial health care.

We complete the volume with "Farewell My Lovelies," Diana Sweeney's poignant and compelling reflection on the cosmetic surgery she undertook. Sweeney describes her breast augmentation and subsequent implant removal and eyelift surgery. Her essay makes excellent sense of the aesthetic, ethical, and political dilemmas that feminists face while also exemplifying how women can write from *within* the practice of cosmetic surgery. It highlights the challenges, dilemmas, moments of choice and moments of lack of choice, opacity of consciousness and clarity both after and before the fact about the meanings of surgery. Like Toni Wildish, Sweeney "wasn't shopping for an opinion, but a technician; someone I could trust to do the job." She was also made to "see" that parts of her body she wasn't seeking surgery for were also defective: during a consultation for breast enlargement a surgeon pointed out her drooping nipples, and "the strength of his comment was such that it caused me to view my nipples as failures." She sensitively narrates the culturally condoned desire to possess large breasts and looks back nostalgically on her "seven sweet years" of having them before her silicone implants began to encapsulate, precipitating their removal. This is an intimate and at times funny analysis of a life journey partly accompanied by cosmetic surgery, demonstrating aptly and honestly its pleasures as well as its horrors.

8 In addition to works already cited, see Atkinson 2006 and Gill et al. 2005.

Future Directions

There are many more under-examined aspects of contemporary cosmetic surgery that cry out for feminist attention. Cosmetic surgery is increasingly globalized, and little published feminist work explores the emerging relations between, for example, ethnically or nationally defined communities in their countries of origin and their diasporic locations (Zane 1998, Gilman 1999b). How do neoliberalism and globalization function to encourage the export of cosmetic surgeries developed in Western countries to the rest of the world, as well as to foster the emergence of new cosmetic surgical markets for currency-advantaged medical tourists? In her analysis of *Around the World with Oprah*, for example, a show that focused on women and global cosmetic surgical practices, Sharon Heijin Lee argues that Oprah unequally deploys a neoliberal rhetoric of individual choice. Echoing the dynamics described in Heyes's chapter in this volume with regard to ethnic cosmetic surgeries, only this time on a global scale, Lee suggests that popular eyelid surgeries (*sangapul*) among South Korean women are represented by Oprah in a very different way than the medical tourism of American women (Lee 2008: 27). South Korean women are depicted as the victims of internalized racism, which places an artificial constraint on their ability to exercise unfettered freedom of choice (30), whereas Oprah lauds the choices of Western women surgical tourists, who go to Brazil (the "Mecca" of cosmetic surgery), when she implicitly notes "American women's cost-effective choice to undergo cosmetic surgery and vacation at the same time." Lee argues that Oprah thus highlights

> American women's abilities to "optimize choices, efficiency, and competitiveness in turbulent market conditions." Not only does this failure highlight American women's capacity for neoliberal rationality but it also animates liberal assumptions that Western subjects, guided by their individuality, are able to make choices in ways that non-Western subjects cannot. In other words, Americans electing plastic surgery in Brazil are not only choosing to do so for somehow "better" reasons than their Korean counterparts, but smart enough to do it for cheap, and in a tropical location at that. (Lee 2008: 30)

Much more feminist work is needed on cosmetic surgery tourism, as well as on non-Western national contexts where cosmetic surgery is emerging as a commodity both for visitors and for the new middle classes. Brazil is the most studied example of such a mixed market (see Edmonds this volume and 2007), but various Asian markets (India, Thailand, Singapore, Malaysia) as well as South Africa and Costa Rica are increasingly significant players (see O'Connell 2003, Connell 2006, Kuczynski 2006: 18–32). Countries where cosmetic surgery has little history have developed distinctive practices and preoccupations, as Susan Brownell's (2005) work on China exemplifies; a final topic for future feminist investigation is the growth of cosmetic surgical markets as a result of the impact of neoliberal ideals on non-capitalist economies such as China (Xu and Feiner 2007).

Neoliberal incitements and pressures work at both global and local levels, and there is clearly much more to be said about each of these, as well as about their interaction. Feminist economic analysis of how and why cosmetic surgery is marketed with increasing success to more and more lower income people, the impact of credit schemes and surgery loans, the roles of different consumers in shaping services and pricing, and the different practices and aesthetics that characterize different market sectors is overdue. Morgan's ambivalently dystopic update to her classic "Women and the Knife" (this volume) flags these issues. More prosaically, Vicki Mayer's acerbic comment on the politics of the TV makeover is apropos: randomly seated next to a semi-finalist on a plane, she meets "Sue Ellen," who hopes that *Extreme Makeover* can save her smile. The show's website "promises to make every woman's 'fairy-tale fantasies come true.'" However, "for Sue Ellen, this was basic health care. In the age of primary coverage cutbacks, medical mismanagements, and shrinking access to specialists in rural America, *Extreme Makeover* was her last hope. 'I got to do this show now or I'm going to lose them,' she explained. 'I don't want to lose my teeth ...'" (2005). If here over-glamorized cosmetic surgery substitutes for basic health care, we might also ask whether the reverse is true: does cosmetic surgery divert the resources invested in medical education or the time and expertise of surgeons away from other, arguably more pressing, health care needs?

An utterly comprehensive look at feminism and cosmetic surgery would include detailed work on breast reconstructions after mastectomy, cosmetic dental work, the many trans surgeries available in various countries, intersex genital surgeries on infants undertaken in the name of sexual normativity, the increasingly popular "non-surgical" options such as "injectables" of Botox and Restylane, and procedures that blur the beauty salon/medical clinic line such as microdermabrasion and laser treatments. While this volume can only address a fraction of these issues, it demonstrates that the study of cosmetic surgery is a rich and complicated area. The challenge for feminist scholars when approaching the myriad of topics it covers includes coming to terms with our own implicated roles in a globalized and media-saturated world in which bodies play increasingly complex roles. We hope that while this volume provides a solid introduction to the important feminist work already done on cosmetic surgery, it will also offer inspiration to feminist researchers and scholars to tackle some of these new, fascinating, and deeply important questions.

References

Atkinson, Michael. 2006. "Masks of Masculinity: Cosmetic Surgery and (Sur)passing Strategies," in *Body/Embodiment: Symbolic Interaction and the Sociology of the Body*, edited by P. Vanni and D. Waskul. London: Ashgate.

Atkinson, Michael. 2008. "Exploring Male Femininity in the 'Crisis': Men and Cosmetic Surgery." *Body and Society*, 14(1), 67–87.

Augsburg, Tanya. 1998. "Orlan's Performative Transformations of Subjectivity," in *The Ends of Performance*, edited by Peggy Phelan and Jill Lane. New York: New York University Press.

Brand, Peg Zeglin. 2000. "Bound to Beauty: An Interview with Orlan," in *Beauty Matters*. Bloomington: Indiana University Press.

Brownell, Susan. 2005. "China Reconstructs: Cosmetic Surgery and Nationalism in the Reform Era," in *Asian Medicine and Globalization*, edited by Joseph Alter. Philadelphia: University of Pennsylvania Press.

Connell, John. 2006. "Medical Tourism: Sea, Sun, Sand and … Surgery." *Tourism Management*, 27(6), 1093–1100.

Davis, Kathy. 1995. *Reshaping the Female Body: The Dilemma of Cosmetic Surgery*. New York: Routledge.

Davis, Kathy. 2003. *Dubious Equalities and Embodied Differences: Cultural Studies on Cosmetic Surgery*. Lanham, MD: Rowman and Littlefield.

Dull, Diana and West, Candace. 1991. "Accounting for Cosmetic Surgery: The Accomplishment of Gender." *Social Problems*, 38(1), 54–70.

Edmonds, Alexander. 2007. "'The Poor Have the Right to be Beautiful': Cosmetic Surgery in Neoliberal Brazil." *Journal of the Royal Anthropological Institute*, 13(2), 363–81.

Gill, Rosalind, Henwood, Karen and McLean, Carl. 2005. "Body Projects and the Regulation of Normative Masculinity." *Body and Society*, 11(1), 37–62.

Gilman, Sander. 1997. *Creating Beauty to Cure the Soul: Race and Psychology in the Shaping of Aesthetic Surgery*. Durham, NC: Duke University Press.

Gilman, Sander. 1999a. *Making the Body Beautiful: A Cultural History of Aesthetic Surgery*. Princeton: Princeton University Press.

Gilman, Sander. 1999b. "By a Nose: On The Construction of 'Foreign Bodies.'" *Social Epistemology*, 13(1), 49–58.

Gimlin, Debra. 2006. "The Absent Body Project: Cosmetic Surgery as a Response to Bodily Dys-appearance." *Sociology*, 40(4), 699–716.

Gimlin, Debra. 2007. "Accounting for Cosmetic Surgery in the US and UK: A Cross-Cultural Analysis of Women's Narratives." *Body and Society*, 13(1), 43–62.

Goodall, Jane. 1999. "An Order of Pure Decision: Un-Natural Selection in the Work of Stelarc and Orlan." *Body and Society*, 5(2–3), 149–70.

Haiken, Elizabeth. 1997. *Venus Envy: A History of Cosmetic Surgery*. New York: Johns Hopkins University Press.

Holliday, Ruth, and Cairnie, Allie. 2007. "Man Made Plastic: Investigating Men's Consumption of Aesthetic Surgery." *Journal of Consumer Culture*, 7(1), 57–78.

Heyes, Cressida J. 2006. "Changing Race, Changing Sex: The Ethics of Self-Transformation." *Journal of Social Philosophy*, 37(2), 266–82.

Heyes, Cressida J. 2007a. "Normalisation and the Psychic Life of Cosmetic Surgery." *Australian Feminist Studies*, 22(52), 55–71.

Heyes, Cressida J. 2007b. "Cosmetic Surgery and the Televisual Makeover: A Foucauldian Feminist Reading." *Feminist Media Studies*, 7(1), 17–32.

Ince, Kate. 2000. *Orlan: Millennial Female*. Oxford: Berg.

Jeffreys, Sheila. 2005. *Beauty and Misogyny: Harmful Cultural Practices in the West*. London: Routledge.

Jones, Meredith. 2008. "Makeover Artists: Orlan and Michael Jackson," in *Skintight: An Anatomy of Cosmetic Surgery*. Oxford: Berg, 151–78.

Kuczynski, Alex. 2006. *Beauty Junkies: Inside our $15 Billion Obsession with Cosmetic Surgery*. New York: Doubleday.

Kulick, Don. 1998. *Travestis: Sex, Gender, and Culture Among Brazilian Transgendered Prostitutes*. Chicago: University of Chicago Press.

Lee, Sharon Heijin. 2008. "Lessons From 'Around the World with Oprah': Neoliberalism, Race, and the (Geo)politics of Beauty." *Women and Performance*, 18(1), 25–41.

Mayer, Vicki. 2005. "Extreme Health Care." *Flow: Journal of TV*, 2(4). Available at http://flowtv.org/?p=448 [accessed June 16, 2008].

O'Bryan, Jill C. 2005. *Carnal Art: Orlan's Refacing*. Minneapolis: University of Minnesota Press.

O'Connell, Brian. 2003. "Vanity Vacations." *Skin and Aging* 11(10), 48–53. Available at http://www.skinandaging.com/article/2099 [accessed: June 17, 2008].

Pertschuk, Michael J., Sarwer, David B., Wadden, Thomas A. and Whitaker Linton A. 1998. "Body Image Dissatisfaction in Male Cosmetic Surgery Patients." *Aesthetic Plastic Surgery*, 22, 20–24.

Pitts-Taylor, Victoria. 2007. *Surgery Junkies: Wellness and Pathology in Cosmetic Culture*. Rutgers University Press.

Singer, Natasha. 2006. "Beauty on the Black Market," *New York Times*, February 16. Available at http://www.nytimes.com/2006/02/16/fashion/thursdaystyles/16skin.html. [accessed June 16, 2008].

Sullivan, Nikki. 2004. "'It's as Plain as the Nose on His Face': Michael Jackson, Modificatory Practices, and the Question of Ethics." *Scan Journal* 1(3), November. Available at: http://www.scan.net.au/scan/journal/display.php?journal_id=44 [accessed: June 16, 2008].

Xu, Gary and Feiner, Susan. 2007. "*Meinü Jingji*/China's Beauty Economy: Buying Looks, Shifting Value, and Changing Place." *Feminist Economics*, 13(3–4), 307–23.

Zane, Kathleen. 1998. "Reflections on a Yellow Eye: Asian I(\Eye/)Cons and Cosmetic Surgery," in *Talking Visions: Multicultural Feminism in a Transnational Age*, edited by Ella Shohat. Cambridge, MA: MIT Press.

PART 1
Revisiting Feminist Critique

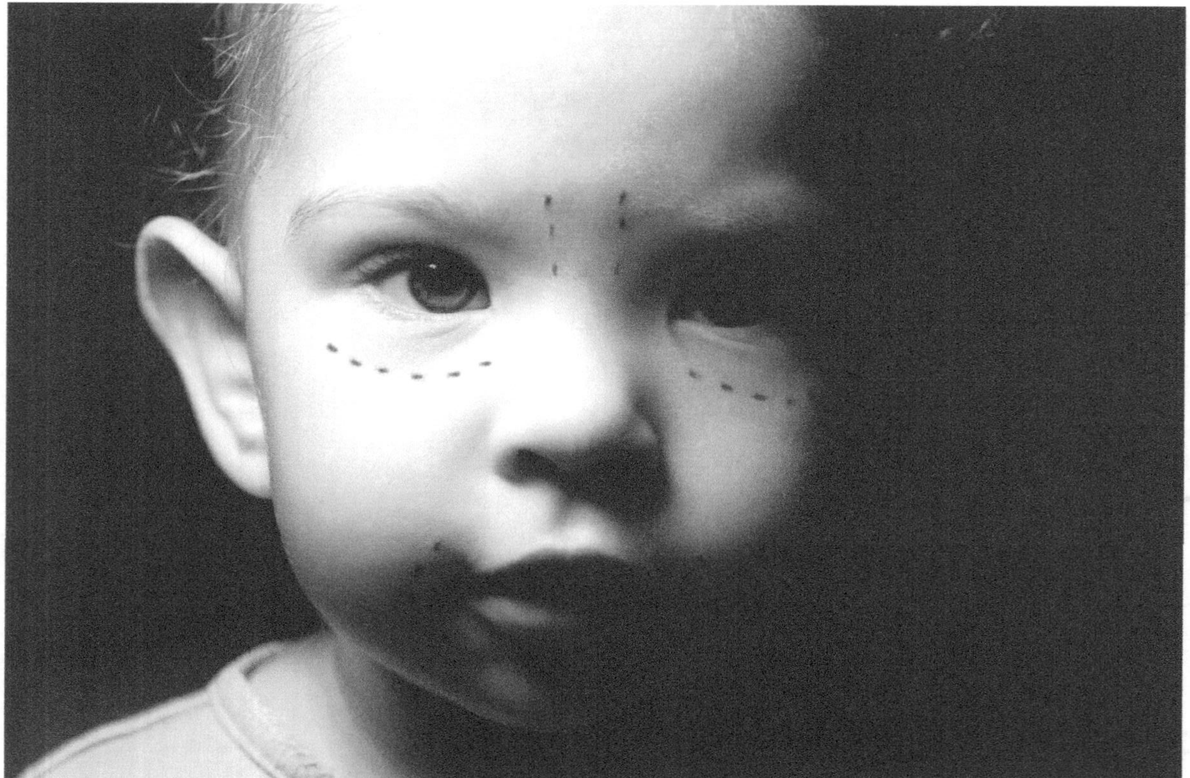

Figure 2.1 "Never too Early?"

Source: © Clara Gonzalez

Chapter 2
Twenty Years in the Twilight Zone

Susan Bordo

Plasticity and Normalization (1988)[1]

In a culture in which organ transplants, life-extension machinery, microsurgery, and artificial organs have entered everyday medicine, we seem on the verge of practical realization of the seventeenth-century imagination of body as machine. But if we have technically and technologically realized that conception, it can also be argued that metaphysically we have deconstructed it. In the early modern era, machine imagery helped to articulate a totally determined human body whose basic functionings the human being was helpless to alter. The then-dominant metaphors for this body—clocks, watches, collections of springs—imagined a system that is set, wound up, whether by nature or by God the watchmaker, ticking away in predictable, orderly manner, regulated by laws over which the human being has no control. Understanding the system, we can help it to perform efficiently, and we can intervene when it malfunctions. But we cannot radically alter its configuration.

Pursuing this modern, determinist fantasy to its limits, fed by the currents of consumer capitalism, modern ideologies of the self, and their crystallization in the dominance of United States mass culture, Western science and technology have now arrived, paradoxically but predictably (for it was an element, though submerged and illicit, in the mechanist conception all along), at a new, postmodern imagination of human freedom from bodily determination. Gradually and surely, a technology that was first aimed at the replacement of malfunctioning parts has generated an industry and an ideology fueled by fantasies of rearranging, transforming, and correcting, an ideology of limitless improvement and change, defying the historicity, the mortality, and, indeed, the very materiality of the body.

In place of that materiality, we now have what I will call cultural plastic. In place of God the watchmaker, we now have ourselves, the master sculptors of that plastic.

"Create a masterpiece, sculpt your body into a work of art," urges *Fit* magazine. "You visualize what you want to look like, and then you create the form." (quoted in Rosen 1983: 72, 61). The precision technology of body-sculpting, once the secret of Arnold Schwarzeneggers and Rachel McLishes of the professional body-building world, has now become available to anyone who can afford the price

1 Excerpted from "Material Girl: The Effacements of Postmodern Culture," originally printed in *Michigan Quarterly Review* (Fall 1990) and reprinted in Bordo 1993.

of membership in a gym. "I now look at bodies," says John Travolta, after training for the movie *Staying Alive*, "almost like a piece of clay that can be molded."[2] On the medical front, plastic surgery, whose repeated and purely cosmetic employment has been legitimized by Michael Jackson, Cher, and others, has become a fabulously expanding industry, extending its domain from nose jobs, face-lifts, tummy tucks, and breast augmentations to collagen-pumped lips and liposuction-shaped ankles, calves, and buttocks. The trendy *Details* magazine describes "surgical stretching, tucking and sucking" as "another fabulous [fashion] accessory" and invites readers to share their cosmetic-surgery experiences in their monthly column "Knife-styles of the Rich and Famous." In that column, the transportation of fat from one part of the body to another is described as breezily as changing hats might be:

> Dr. Brown is an artist. He doesn't just pull and tuck and forget about you. … He did liposuction on my neck, did the nose job and tightened up my forehead to give it a better line. Then he took some fat from the side of my waist and injected it into my hands. It goes in as a lump, and then he smooths it out with his hands to where it looks good. I'll tell you something, the nose and neck made a big change, but nothing in comparison to how fabulous my hands look. The fat just smoothed out all the lines, the veins don't stick up anymore, the skin actually looks soft and great. [But] you have to be careful not to bang your hands. (Lizardi and Frankel 1990: 38)

Popular culture does not apply any brakes to these fantasies of rearrangement and self-transformation. Rather, we are constantly told that we can "choose" our own bodies. "The proper diet, the right amount of exercise and you can have, pretty much, any body you desire," claims an ad for Evian [water]. But the rhetoric of choice and self-determination and the breezy analogies comparing cosmetic surgery to fashion accessorizing are deeply mystifying. They efface, not only the inequalities of privilege, money, and time that prohibit most people from indulging in these practices, but [the reality that] despite the claims of the Evian ad, one cannot have *any* body that one wants—for not every body will *do* ... Does anyone in this culture have his or her nose reshaped to look more 'African' or 'Jewish'? The answer, of course, is no. Given our history of racism—a history in which bodies that look "too black" or obviously Jewish have been refused admittance to public places and even marked for death—how can we regard these choices as merely "individual preferences"? In Japan it has become increasingly common for job-seeking female college graduates to have their eyes surgically altered to appear more occidental. Such a "Western" appearance, it is widely acknowledged, gives a woman the edge in job interviews. But capitulating to this requirement—although it may be highly understandable from the point of view of the individual's economic survival and advancement—is to participate in a process of racial normalization and to make it

2 "Travolta: 'You Really Can Make Yourself Over,'" *Syracuse Herald-American*, Jan. 13, 1985.

harder for others to refuse to participate. The more established the new norm, the higher the costs of resisting. And while some might celebrate being able to "choose" one's features as part of a "melting pot" society, as eradicating racial differences that we don't need and that have only caused pain and suffering, we should face the fact that only certain ingredients in the pot are being encouraged to "melt" here.

Recognizing that normalizing cultural forms exist does not entail, as some writers have argued, the view that women are "cultural dopes," blindly submitting to oppressive regimes of beauty ... People know the routes to success in this culture—they are advertised widely enough—and they are not "dopes" to pursue them. Often, given the racism, sexism, and ageism of the culture, their personal happiness and economic security may depend on it. When I lost 25 pounds through a national weight-loss program, some of my colleagues viewed it as inconsistent and even hypocritical, given my work. But in my view, feminist cultural criticism is not a blueprint for the conduct of personal life (or political action, for that matter) and does not empower or require individuals to "rise above" their culture or to become martyrs to feminist ideals. It does not tell us what to *do*—whether to lose weight or not, wear makeup or not, lift weights or not. Its goal is edification and understanding, enhanced *consciousness* of the power, complexity, and systemic nature of culture, the interconnected webs of its functioning. It's up to the reader to decide how, when, and where (or whether) to put that understanding to further use, in the particular, complicated, and ever-changing context that is his or her life and no one else's.

"Agency," Consumer Culture, and the Proliferation of Defect (1997)[3]

It's become clear to me, from the protests of audience members at my talks, from popular cultural discourse, and from contemporary "postmodern" theory, that there is a great deal of resistance nowadays to acknowledging the power of social norms. Women who have had or are contemplating cosmetic surgery consistently deny the influence of media images (see Goodman 1994). "I'm doing it for me," they insist. This has become the mantra of the television talk show, and I would gladly accept it if "for me" meant "in order to feel better about myself in this culture that has made me feel inadequate as I am." But people rarely mean this. Most often on these shows, the "for me" answer is produced in defiant refutation of some cultural "argument" (talk-show style, of course) on topics such as "Are Our Beauty Ideals Racist?" or "Are We Obsessed with Youth?" "No, I'm not having my nose (straightened) (narrowed) in order to look less ethnic. I'm doing it *for me*." "No, I haven't had my breasts enlarged to a 38D in order to be more attractive to men. I did *it for me*." In these constructions "me" is imagined as a pure and precious inner space, an "authentic" and personal reference point untouched by external values and demands. A place where we live free and won't be pushed around.

3 Excerpted From "Braveheart, Babe, and the Contemporary Body," in Bordo 1997.

Postmodern feminist theorists of beauty, on their part, keen to distinguish themselves from "old-fashioned" critics of the beauty "system," emphasize the honor, integrity, and creativity of women's choices—a corrective I would applaud, if it didn't so often sound like a scholarly version of the talk-show mantra. It seems to me, for example, that feminist theory has taken a very strange turn indeed when plastic surgery can be described, as it has been by Kathy Davis, as "*first and foremost* ... about taking one's life into one's own hands." Now, I agree with Davis that as an individual choice that seeks to make life as livable and enjoyable as possible within certain cultural constraints and directives, of course such surgery can be experienced as liberating. But "*first and foremost* ... about taking one's life into one's own hands"?

Unlike Davis, I do not view the choice for cosmetic surgery as being first and foremost "about" self-determination *or* self-deception. Rather, my focus is on the complexly and densely institutionalized values and practices within which a high level of physical modification is continually presented as a prerequisite for romantic success and very often demanded by employers as well. This does not imply, as Davis has suggested, that I fail to endow individuals with "agency." But unlike many theorists who consider themselves "postmodern," the word "agency" doesn't carry any glamour for me, and certainly doesn't bear the critical weight that those who use it to critique others seem to think. No feminist theorist, as far as I can tell (certainly not myself) has ever denied that human beings are continually making choices. Few would deny, either, that these choices are exercised within both constraints and opportunities, material and cultural. As a cultural critic of a Marxist/Foucauldian bent, I am most interested in understanding the configuration and direction of constraints and opportunities; others are more interested in describing how people exercise creativity, purpose, and choice within them. I don't see these different projects as in competition or mutually negating. Indeed, they ought to be viewed as demanding integration rather than as a contest.

In fact, where the power of cultural images is concerned, Davis and I actually have very little quarrel with each other. We both see cultural images as central elements in women's lives and we see them as contributing to a pedagogy of defect, in which women learn that various parts of their bodies are faulty, unacceptable. Neither of us views women as passive sponges in this process but (as I put it in *Unbearable Weight*) as engaged "in a process of making meaning, of 'labor on the body.'" We both recognize that there is ambiguity and contradiction, multiple meanings and consequences, in human motivations and choices.

Where Davis and I most differ is over that magic word "agency." I don't see the word as adding very much beyond rhetorical cheerleading concerning how *we*, not the images are "in charge." More important, I believe that the cheers of "agency" create a diversionary din that drowns out the orchestra that is always playing in the background, the consumer culture we live in and need to take responsibility for. For cosmetic surgery is more than an individual choice; it is a burgeoning industry and an increasingly normative cultural practice. As such, it is a significant contributory *cause* of women's suffering by continually upping the ante on what counts as an acceptable face and body.

To make this point clear, I need to look a bit more closely at what I find wrong with Davis's arguments. Advertisements, fashion photos, cosmetic instructions, she points out (drawing on the work of eminent sociologist Dorothy Smith) all require "specialized knowledge" and "complex and skilled interpretive activities on the part of the female agent" who must "plan a course of action, making a series of on-the-spot calculations about whether the rigorous discipline required by the techniques of body improvement will actually improve her appearance given the specifics of her particular body." By showing her how to correct various defects in her appearance ("Lose those unsightly bags under your eyes," "Turn your flabby rear-end into buns of steel," "Have a firm, sexy bosom for the first time in your life!") the ads and instructions transform the woman into an agent of her own destiny, providing concrete objectives, goals, strategies, a plan of action. Davis quotes Smith here: "The text instructs her that her breasts are too small/too big; she reads of a remedy; her too small breasts become remediable. She enters into the discursive organization of desire; now she has an objective where before she had only a defect." … In other words, it is precisely our instruction in learning to see ourselves as defective and lacking, needful of improvement and remedy … that mobilizes us, put us in charge of our lives!

By this logic it would be a sorry day indeed if women were to become content with the way they look. Without all those defects to correct we would lose an important arena for the enactment of our creative agency! There doesn't seem to be much chance of that happening though. Instead, the sites of defect have multiplied. Consider breast augmentation, now increasingly widespread, and its role in establishing new norms against which smaller or less firm breasts are seen as *defective.* Micromastia is the clinical term, among plastic surgeons, for "too small" breasts. Such "disorders" are, of course, entirely aesthetic and completely socially "constructed." Anyone who doubts this should recall the 1920s, when women were binding their breasts to look more boyish. Today, with artificial implants the norm among movie stars and models, an adolescent boy who has grown up learning what a woman's body looks like from movies, cable television, and magazines may wonder what's wrong when his girlfriend lies down and her breasts flop off to the side instead of standing straight up in the air. (Will we soon see a clinical term for "too floppy" breasts?) No wonder breast enhancement is one of the most common surgical procedures for teenagers. These girls are not superficial creatures who won't be satisfied unless they look like goddesses. Rather, as the augmented breast becomes the norm, the decision to have one's breasts surgically enhanced becomes what the psychiatrist Peter Kramer has called "free choice under pressure." We can choose not to have such surgery. No one is holding a gun to our heads. But those who don't—for example, those who cannot afford the surgery—are at an increasingly significant professional and personal disadvantage.

Men, too, have increasingly been given more of their own wonderful opportunities for "agency," as magazines and products devoted to the enhancement and "correction" of their appearance have multiplied … Men used to be relatively exempt, for example, from the requirement to look young; gray hair and wrinkles were (and still mostly are) a code for experience, maturity, and wisdom. But in a "Just Do It" culture that now equates youth and fitness with energy and competence—the "right stuff—fortyish businessmen are feeling increasing pressure to dye their hair, get liposuction on their spare tires, and have face-lifts in order to compete with younger, fitter-looking men and women. In 1980 men accounted for only 10 percent of plastic surgery patients. In 1994 they were 26 percent [but in 2007 only 13 percent] (Spindler 1996). These numbers will undoubtedly rise, as plastic surgeons develop specialized angles to attract men ("penile enhancement" is now advertised in the sports sections of major newspapers) and disinfect surgery of its associations with feminine vanity.

Thanks also to the efforts of surgeons, who now argue that one should start "preventive" procedures while the skin is still elastic, younger and younger people are having surgery. Here is an advertisement I came across recently in the local (Lexington, Kentucky) paper:

> Picture this scenario. You're between the ages of thirty-five and fifty. You feel like you are just hitting your stride. But the face in the mirror is sending out a different message. Your morning facial puffiness hangs around all day. You're beginning to resemble your parents at a point when they began looking old to you. If you prefer a more harmonic relationship between your self-perception and outer image, you may prefer to tackle these concerns before they become too obvious. You may benefit from a face-lift performed at an earlier age. There is no carved-in-stone perfect time or age to undergo a face-lift. For those who place a high priority on maintaining a youthful appearance, any visual disharmony between body and soul can be tackled earlier when cosmetic surgical goals tend to be less aggressive and it is easier to obtain more natural-looking results. The reason is: Younger skin and tissues have more elasticity so smoothness can be achieved with surgery.

What this ad obscures is that the "disharmonies" between body and soul that 35- and 40-year-old (!!) women may be experiencing are not "carved-in-stone" either but are in large part the product of our *cultural* horror of wrinkles and lines—a horror, of course, that surgeons are fueling. Why should a few lines around our eyes be experienced as "disharmonious" with the energy and vitality that we feel "inside," *unless* they are coded as a sign of decrepitude (looking like our parents—good heavens, what a fate!).

Most plastic surgeons have no ethical problem with constantly promoting new procedures for ever-growing populations of people. "I'm not here to play philosopher king," says Dr. Randal Haworth in *Vogue* interview; "I don't have a problem with women who already look good who want to look perfect." … What Haworth isn't saying (besides the fact that "perfection" seems an odd ideal for a human body) is that the bar of what we considered "perfection" is constantly being raised—by cultural imagery and by the surgeon's own recommendations. The slippery slope of "perfection" is also made more treacherous by eyes that have become habituated to interpreting every deviation as "defect." … "Plastic surgery sharpens your eyesight," admits a more honest surgeon, "You get something done, suddenly you're looking in the mirror every five minutes—at imperfections nobody else can see."

Situating "personal" choices in social, cultural, and economic contexts such as these raises certain issues for the thoughtful individual … Not that many years ago parents who smoked never thought twice about the instructional effect this might be having on their children, in legitimizing smoking, making it seem adult and empowering. A cultural perspective on augmentation, face-lifts, cosmetic "ethnic cleansing" of Jewish and black noses, Asian eyes, and so on similarly might make parents think twice about the messages they are sending their children, might make them less comfortable with viewing their decisions as purely "personal" or "individual" ones. And they *should* think twice. We are all culture makers as well as culture consumers, and if we wish to be considered "agents" in our lives—and have it mean more than just a titular honor—we need to take responsibility for that role.

To act consciously and responsibly means understanding the culture we live in, even if it requires acknowledging that we are not always "in charge." That we are not always in charge does not mean that we are "dopes." In fact, I think the *really* dopey thing is living with the illusion that we are "in control," just because some commercial (or ad for surgery) tells us so. In the culture we live in, individuals are caught between two contradictory injunctions. On the one hand, an ideology of triumphant individualism and mind-over-matter heroism urges us to "Just Do It" and tries to convince us that we *can* "Just do it," whatever our sex, race, or circumstances. This is a mystification. We are not runners on a level field but one that is pocked with historical inequities that make it much harder for some folks to lace up their Nikes and speed to the finish line—until the lane in which they are running has been made less rocky and the hidden mines excavated and removed. A few of us, if we are very, very lucky (circumstances still do count, willpower isn't everything, despite what the commercials tell us), do have our moments of triumph. But it is often after years of struggle in which we have drawn on many resources other than our own talent, resolve, and courage. We have been helped by our friends and our communities, by social movements, legal and political reform, and sheer good fortune. And many, of course, don't make it.

But on the other hand, while consumerism assures us that we can (and should) "just do it," it continually sends the contradictory message that we are defective, lacking, inadequate. This is the … essence of advertising and the fuel of consumer capitalism, which cannot allow equilibrium or stasis in human desire. Thus, we are not permitted to feel satisfied with ourselves and we are "empowered" only and always through fantasies of what we *could* be. This is not a plot; it's just the way the system works. Capitalism adores proliferation and excess; it abhors moderation. One moment the culture begins talking about greater health consciousness, which is surely a good thing that no one would deny. But the next moment we've got commercials on at every hour for every imaginable exercise and diet product, and people are spending huge quantities of their time trying to achieve a level of "fitness" that goes way beyond health and straight into obsession. Technological possibilities emerge that allow surgeons to make corrective repairs of serious facial conditions;

before long our surgeons have become Pygmalions of total self-transformation, advertising the slightest deviation from the cultural "norm" as a problem needing to be solved, an impediment to happiness. Drugs like Prozac are developed to treat serious clinical depressions; the next moment college clinics are dispensing these pills to help students with test anxiety.

The multiplication of human "defect" is aided by factors other than economic. Drug companies may be focused on profits, but those folks at the university clinic are genuinely concerned about students and want to make their lives easier. Cosmetic surgeons, while fabulously paid, are rarely in it for the money alone. Often, they are carried to excess not by dreams of yachts but by savior fantasies and by pure excitement about the technological possibilities. Nowadays, those can be pretty fantastic, as fat is suctioned from thighs and injected into lips, breast implants inserted through the bellybutton, penises enlarged through "phalloplasty," and nipples repositioned.

Under these cultural conditions the desire to be "normal" or "ordinary," which Kathy Davis, criticizing feminist critics of the female cultural imperative to be beautiful, claims is the motivation for most cosmetic surgeries, is much more slippery than she makes it out to be. Davis makes the point that none of her subjects describe their surgeries as having been done for the sake of "beauty" but insist they only wanted to feel "ordinary." But in a culture that proliferates defect and in which the surgically perfected body ("perfect" according to certain standards, of course) has become the model of the "normal," even the ordinary body becomes the defective body. This continual upping of the ante of physical acceptability is cloaked by ads and features that represent the cosmetic surgeon as a blessed savior, offering miraculous technology to end long-standing pain. This indeed used to be their primary function. Nowadays, however, many women who are basically satisfied with their appearance begin to question their self-image on the basis of images and advice presented in magazine features, or—even more authoritatively—dispensed to them by their doctors. Writing for *New York* magazine, 28-year-old, 5-foot 6-inch, and 118-pound Lily Burana (1996) describes how a series of interviews with plastic surgeons—the majority of whom had recommended rhinoplasty, lip augmentation, implants, liposuction, and eyelid work—changed her perception of herself from "a hardy young sapling that could do with some pruning … to a gnarled thing that begs to be torn down to the root and rebuilt limb by limb."

Aging in the Empire of Images (2003)

They carded me until I was 35. Even when I was 45, people were shocked to hear my age. Young men flirted with me, even at 50. Having hated my face as a child—bushy red hair, freckles, Jewish nose—I was surprised to find myself fairly pleased with it as an adult. Then, suddenly, it all changed. The women at the makeup counter no longer compliment me on my skin. Men don't catch my eye with playful promise in theirs.

I'm 56. The magazines tell me that at this age, a woman can still be beautiful. But they don't mean me. They mean Cher, Goldie, Faye, Candace. Women whose jowls have disappeared as they've aged, whose eyes have become less droopy, lips grown plumper, foreheads smoother with the passing years. They mean Susan Sarandon, who looked older in 1991's *Thelma and Louise* than she does in her movies today. "Aging beautifully" used to mean wearing one's years with style, confidence, and vitality. Today, it means not appearing to age at all. And—like breasts that defy gravity—it's becoming a new bodily norm.

Greta Van Susterin: former CNN legal analyst, 47 years old. When she had a face-lift, it was a real escalation in the stakes for ordinary women. She had a signature style: no bullshit, down-to-earth lack of pretense. (During the O.J. trial, she was the only white reporter many Blacks trusted.) Always stylishly dressed and coiffed, she wasn't really pretty. No one could argue that her career was built on her looks. Perhaps quite the opposite. She sent out a subversive message: brains and personality still count, even on television.

When Greta had her face lifted, another source of inspiration and hope bit the dust. The story was on the cover of *People*, and folks tuned in to her new show on Fox just to see the change—which was significant. But at least she was open about it. The beauties never admit they've had "work." Or if they do, it's vague, nonspecific, minimizing of the extent. Cher: "If I'd had as much plastic surgery as people say, there'd be another whole person left over!" (reported in Smith 2002) Okay, so how much have you had? The interviewers accept the silences and evasions. They even embellish the lie. How many interviews have you read which began: "She came into the restaurant looking at least twenty years younger than she is, fresh and relaxed without a speck of make-up."

This collusion, this myth, that Cher or Goldie or Faye Dunaway, unaltered, is "what fifty-something looks like today" has altered my face, however—and without benefit of surgery. By comparison with theirs, it has become much older than it is.

My expression now appears more serious, too (just what a feminist needs), thanks to the widespread use of Botox. "It's now rare in certain social circles," a *New York Times* reporter observed, "to see a woman over the age of 35 with the ability to look angry" (Kuczynski 2002: A1). This has frustrated some film directors, like Baz Luhrman (who did *Moulin Rouge*). "Their faces can't really move properly," Luhrman complained (Kuczynski 2002: A26). Last week I saw a sign in the beauty parlor where I get my hair cut. "Botox Party! Sign Up!" So my 56-year-old forehead will now be judged against my neighbor's, not just Goldie's, Cher's, and Faye's. On television, a commercial describes the product (which really is a toxin, a dilution of botulism) as "Botox cosmetic." No different from mascara and blush, it's just stuck in with a needle and makes your forehead numb. To add insult to injury, the rhetoric of feminism has been picked up to help advance and justify the industries in anti-aging and body alteration. Face-lifts, implants, and liposuction are advertised as empowerment, "taking charge" of one's life. "I'm doing it for me"—the mantra of the talk shows. "Defy your age!"—Melanie Griffith, for Revlon. We're making a revolution, girls. Get your injection and pick up a sign!

Am I immune? Of course not. My bathroom shelves are cluttered with the ridiculously expensive age-defying lotions and potions that constantly beckon to me at the Lancôme and Dior counters. I want my lines, bags, and sags to disappear, and so do the women who can only afford to buy their alpha-hydroxies at K-Mart. There's a limit, though, to what fruit acids can do. As surgeons develop ever more extensive and fine-tuned procedures to correct gravity and erase history from the faces of their patients, the difference between the cosmetically altered and the rest of us grows more and more dramatic.

"The rest of us" includes not only those who resist or are afraid of surgery but the many people who cannot afford basic health care, let alone aesthetic tinkering—not even of the K-Mart variety. As celebrity faces become increasingly more surreal in their wide-eyed, ever-bright agelessness, as *Time* and *Newsweek* (and *Discover* and *Psychology Today*) proclaim that we can now all "stay young forever," the poor continue to sag and wrinkle and lose their teeth.[4] But in the empire of images, where even people in the news for stock scandals or producing septuplets are given instant digital dental work for magazine covers,[5] this is a well-guarded secret. The celebrity testimonials, the advertisements, the beauty columns all participate in the fiction that the required time, money, and technologies are available to all.[6]

Postscript: Looking Back (2007)

For the first few years, I was a second-wave throwback, a paranoid scold vastly overestimating the power of popular culture. "Why don't you just turn off your television and throw away your glossy magazines?" they challenged me at conferences. Or: "Aren't you just talking about a handful of rich, over-privileged white people?"

The next few years brought the feminist protests. Now I was not only "totalizing" but also unsisterly. "What about women's agency in all this? Do you think we're all just 'cultural dopes'?" Or: "How about all the women whose lives have been

4 Fitness is class-biased, too, of course. Oprah presents each new diet and exercise program she embarks on as an inspiration for her fans. But how many of them have the money for a gym membership, let alone a personal trainer? How many even have the *time* to go to the gym? Magazines engage in debates about high-protein versus low-fat diets, as though our nation's "epidemic of obesity" can be solved by nutritional science. But high-quality, low-fat protein is expensive. So are fresh fruits and vegetables, and, unless you have the time to shop frequently, they are highly perishable. Millions of Americans exist on fatty, fried, carb-loaded fast food because it's the cheapest way to feed their families.

5 For those who were attentive, an unintentional visual exposé was provided when *Newsweek* decided to "fix" the crooked teeth of Bobbi McCaughey (mother of the McCaughey septuplets) for their cover—while *Time* neglected to.

6 See "*Braveheart*, *Babe*, and the Contemporary Body," in Bordo 1997, for extended discussions of cosmetic surgery and other forms of body alteration.

empowered by surgery?" Or: "Women who haven't had surgery shouldn't be so quick to criticize those who have."

From the postmodernists came the celebrations of the mutable, cyborg subject, and charges that I was secretly "nostalgic" for "authenticity" and the myth of a "natural" body that was not "discursively produced."

It was exhausting to be constantly arguing, explaining, clarifying. After I adopted a baby, I became particular impatient with positions that seemed to me to be oblivious to what I saw as the biological and material realities that my little daughter continually reminded me of. I stopped giving interviews. I snapped at my PoMo colleagues. I had to rev myself up before my talks, to convince myself that any of what I had to say mattered.

Never before had I felt such a personal stake in it all, with a young daughter to worry about, while still trying to "gracefully" accept my own transformation from an older babe with whom very young men still flirted to a lady they passed on the street. And never before had cultural criticism seemed so useless to me. Everything was coming true—indisputably, horrifically, round-the-bend true, with statistics to blow the mind, and televised makeover madness to seriously upset the digestion. In barely twenty years, we'd gone from cosmetic surgery as a "lifestyle of the rich and famous" to breast implants as middle-class graduation gifts. But no one seemed to care. Not really. Sure, there would be the occasional tabloid eruption about botched surgeries, the occasional *People* magazine cover story on *Extreme Makeover* or *The Swan:* "Have We Gone Too Far?" The answer always was: Do what makes you happy, but be sure to go to a board-certified surgeon.

When a tenth anniversary edition of *Unbearable Weight* was in the planning stages, I was asked to write a new preface, an update. I agreed, feeling very much that it was the last gasp of the cultural critic in me. *The Chronicle of Higher Education* reprinted a large chunk of it, and I got many appreciative emails. I was thankful for every one of them, but the issue, for me, was no longer about being "right" as an individual writer. It was about the failure—or perhaps, more accurately, impotence—of the enterprise in which I'd invested most of my life. Cultural critique. Pissing in the wind.

I've become convinced that nothing I or anyone else writes or says will stop this creeping science fiction-turned-normalcy. It's too lucrative, too technologically fascinating, and too personally gratifying for those who dispense it. And too perceptually and emotionally powerful for those who "elect" to have it. So when Cressida and Meredith asked me to contribute to this collection, my first reaction was a shudder. But they were charmingly and sympathetically persistent, and I finally agreed to a chronologically arranged compilation of excerpts from my writings on cosmetic surgery and how it has crept, slyly, multiplicitously, and seemingly inexorably, into the stuff of the everyday.

I thought a compilation was the most I could muster, but as I was considering what I would include, I received the following email, after a phone message:

> I am calling on behalf of a major international healthcare company regarding a project on *Aesthetic Anthropology: Beauty across Cultures*, and because of your

> research and publications, as well as your prestigious position, credentials and expertise, was hoping to connect with you.
>
> The study represents one of the largest international surveys ever conducted into the beauty and grooming habits of 10,000 women and men across the U.S., U.K., Italy, France, Spain, and Germany. The research was conducted online by a well regarded company—International Research—and was designed to assess how women and men across cultures perceive beauty, how beauty affects their self-esteem, what motivates them to practice beauty regimens, what kind of beauty regimes do they do, what their partners think about their beauty, how much they spend on beauty regimes, and more.
>
> We are currently looking for an expert to help us take the data and add a cultural perspective to the findings. Because of your expertise, we thought you might be an ideal professional with whom to connect. It will be an exciting and rewarding opportunity and one that will attract international media attention.

The woman who called me was energetic and infectiously enthusiastic. The cultural differences were fascinating, she told me. And truth be told, I was less interested in appearing on *The Today Show* than in seeing the results of the survey. I knew from experience how these interviews get nipped and tucked—and besides, I'd have to lose at least 30 pounds before I put myself in front of a camera again. But being the first to see—and interpret!!!—such magnificent data wasn't something I could easily refuse. We spoke for about a half-hour and I got more and more interested.

"It sounds great, but before we go on, could you tell me exactly what organization you represent?" I asked.

Her gulp was audible. The "major healthcare company," she finally admitted, was a manufacturer of Botox.

My mouth and eyes gaped wide for the benefit of my husband, who was standing at the sink, listening in on the conversation. But I was determined not to say anything predictably p.c. "Will I have complete autonomy in my interpretation and reporting of the data?"

A pause. "Well, of course, we don't want someone who is going to *trash* Botox …"

I told her my concerns (which, had she really been familiar with my "expertise," would already have been known to her) and that I probably wasn't the person for the job. The remainder of the conversation consisted largely in her trying to convince me that I should withhold my judgment until I had tried Botox myself. "Millions of women's lives have been changed because of it!" She'd had several injections herself, and was a devoted convert. I asked her if she'd seen "The Real Housewives of Orange County," a *Bravo* reality show that might more accurately have been called "The Stepford Breasts." The only housewife whose face ever changed expression in that show was 23 years old. (She'd had implants—they all had—but she alone was pre-Botox.)

She hadn't seen the show, but apparently my reaction was not entirely unexpected. Or unprecedented. "This is the problem with finding an academic to do this," she said wearily, and I wondered how many of us she'd gone through. Not wanting to seem rude or utterly dogmatic—and still salivating over the data—I said I would think about it. A week later, however, I got a second email.

> At the moment, we have a social scientist who seems quite interested, and we are talking to him this week. If things do not work out, I would welcome a chance to reconnect with you again and revisit this project. I hear your concerns, so I think this approach may be best and hope it works for you as well.

I guess that "things" with the social scientist (wonder if she urged him to try Botox, too?) *did* "work out," because I didn't hear from her again. But she did provide me with a fitting, concluding anecdote to this piece—and the opportunity for a tiny, sweet dollop of revenge. Despite everything, I still believe that knowledge is power. And someday, when you hear Matt Lauer's voice on television, introducing a social science "expert" to talk about the results of the largest international beauty survey ever to be conducted, you'll *know* …

Acknowledgments

Thanks to my writing group—Janet Eldred, Kathi Kern, and Ellen Rosenman—for helping me to pick out the themes and selections from my published work, and providing their (always astute) feedback on my introductory "update." Thanks also to Cressida Heyes for pushing me (gently) and Meredith Jones for inspiration for the title.

References

Bordo, Susan. 1993. *Unbearable Weight: Feminism, Western Culture, and the Body*. Berkeley: University of California Press.

Bordo, Susan. 1997. *Twilight Zones*. Berkeley: University of California Press.

Burana, Lily. 1996. "Bend Me, Shape Me." *New York*, July 15, 30–34.

Goodman, Marcene. 1994. "Social, Psychological, and Developmental Factors in Women's Receptivity to Cosmetic Surgery." *Journal of Aging Studies*, 8(4), 375–96.

Kuczynski, Alex. 2002. "Frowns Are Victims of Progress in Quest for Wrinkle-Free Look." *New York Times*, Feb. 7.

Lizardi, Tina and Frankel, Martha. 1990. "Hand Job." *Details*, Feb. 1990: 38.

Rosen, Trix. 1983. *Strong and Sexy*. New York: Putnam.

Smith, Liz. 2002. "What Cher Wants." *Good Housekeeping*, Nov. 2002, p. 112, p. A1.

Spindler, Amy. 1996. "It's a Face-Lifted Tummy-Tucked Jungle out There." *New York Times*, Sunday, June 9, 6–10.

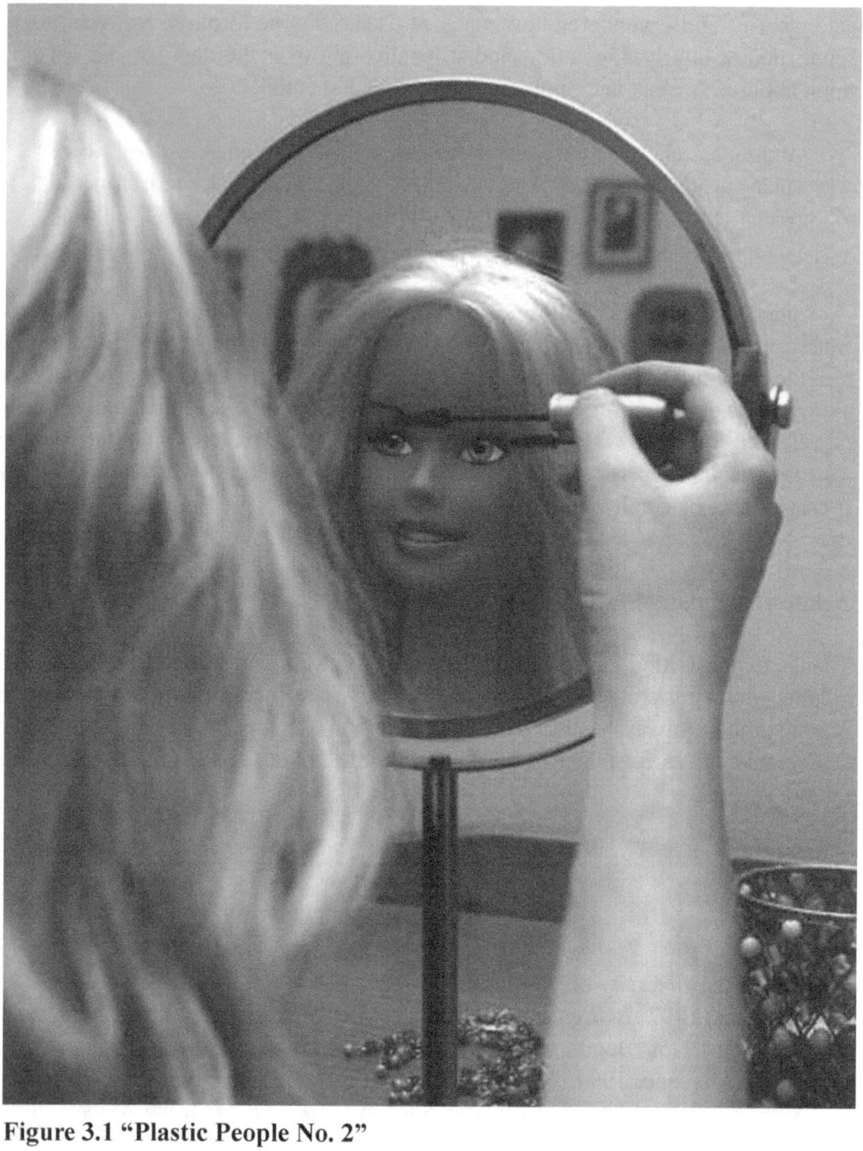

Figure 3.1 "Plastic People No. 2"

Source: © Pennie Naylor

Chapter 3
Revisiting Feminist Debates on Cosmetic Surgery: Some Reflections on Suffering, Agency, and Embodied Difference

Kathy Davis

In 1995 I published *Reshaping the Female Body*, in which I provided a feminist reading of cosmetic surgery.[1] The book was grounded in the specific histories of suffering of those women who undergo cosmetic surgery as well as in a critique of the culture that compels them to view surgical alteration of bodies as a viable solution for their suffering. While this study was one of the first of its kind,[2] it was written against the backdrop of the long-standing feminist critique of the cultural system in which beauty was analyzed as one of the central ways Western femininity is produced and regulated (MacCannell and MacCannell 1987, Bartky 1990, Young 1990a, 1990b, Morgan 1991, Wolf 1991, Bordo 1993). Beauty practices (including everything from everyday procedures like leg-waxing and putting on makeup to hair straightening, starvation diets, and brutal exercise regimes) were viewed as a way to channel women's energies into the hopeless race for a perfect body—a body that is always different than the one they have. If feminists had reason to be skeptical of the more mundane practices of the beauty system, they were even more critical of cosmetic surgery, which was unanimously regarded as not only dangerous to women's health, but demeaning and disempowering. Cosmetic surgery was regarded as—literally—a way to "cut women down to size." It is not surprising, therefore, that for many feminists, any woman who would willingly put her body under the surgeon's knife was unaware of the risks or had been manipulated by profit-hungry surgeons, pressured by her sexist boyfriend or probably blinded by the false promises of the media. In short, she was the "cultural dope"[3] of the feminine beauty system.

1 This chapter is a revised and abridged version of the Introduction of Davis 2003.

2 Later studies include Haiken 1997, Gilman 1999, Jacobson 2000, Gimlin 2002, Negrin 2002, and Blum 2005.

3 This term was initially coined by Garfinkel 1967 and taken up later by Giddens 1976 and other sociologists. It was intended as a criticism of functionalist as well as Marxist conceptions of agency where the human actor has so completely "internalized" the norms and values of her society that her activities become limited to acting out a predetermined script. The Marxist variant refers to "internalized oppression."

While I shared this critical assessment of the feminine beauty system and the cultural discourses and practices that make the female body inferior, I was also uneasy about the tendency among feminist critics to view women who have cosmetic surgery as frivolous, mistaken, or manipulated. The conflation of cosmetic surgery with other more mundane beauty practices allowed even well-intentioned feminists to treat women's struggles with their appearance as the outcome of their ideological mystification or an expression of their unquestioning acquiescence to the cultural ideals of feminine beauty.

I began my inquiry with the assumption that the specific particularities of women's embodied experiences should be the starting point for understanding why women alter their bodies surgically as well as for a critical exploration of the historical, social, and cultural circumstances that enable and constrain their decisions to embark upon the "surgical fix." Based on my interviews with women who had actually undergone cosmetic surgery, I discovered that their stories told a somewhat different tale than the standard feminist narrative about women's involvement in cosmetic surgery. To begin with, they told me that they had not had cosmetic surgery first and foremost because they wanted to become beautiful. Rather they explained that they were different or abnormal and wanted to become ordinary, normal, "just like everyone else." Their decisions were often the outcome of long and painful struggles in which they weighed the—admittedly inadequate—information about the risks and dangers of operations against their specific histories of suffering and the potential benefits they hoped to achieve from having surgery. Their choices were invariably difficult and always ambivalent. They presented cosmetic surgery not as a perfect solution, but as the only way they saw to alleviate suffering which had gone beyond the point of what they felt a woman should "normally" have to endure. In other words, they presented cosmetic surgery as a choice—not a choice in the absolute sense of being free from constraint, but rather in the more everyday sense of choices as messy and contradictory affairs, invariably taken under less than perfect circumstances.

Based on women's accounts of their experiences with their appearance and how they decided to have cosmetic surgery, I found myself having to take what was, at that time—in feminist circles, at least—a somewhat dissident standpoint. I argued that cosmetic surgery should best be viewed as a dilemma: disempowering and empowering, problem and solution all in one. This meant trying to understand how cosmetic surgery might be the best course of action for a particular woman at a particular moment in her life, while, at the same time, problematizing the situational, social, and cultural constraints which make cosmetic surgery an option in the first place. It meant critically engaging with the technologies, practices, and discourses that define women's bodies as deficient and in need of change, and producing a sociological understanding of why women might view cosmetic surgery as their best, and, in some cases, only option for alleviating unbearable suffering. This position left feminist critics (including myself, of course), without the comfort of a "just say no" approach to cosmetic surgery. However, I argued that as feminist critics of cosmetic surgery, we cannot afford the comforts of such a position. Instead we need to embrace our uneasiness about women's involvement in cosmetic surgery and continue to explore what makes it both fervently desired by and yet invariably problematic for women.

My dissident approach resonated with and in some cases encouraged other feminist scholars to explore women's agency in other bodily practices—ranging from makeup use (Dellinger and Williams 1997) to the training regimes of classical ballet (Aalten 1997), hormone replacement therapy (Klinge 1997), pornography (Chancer 1998), beauty pageants (Banet-Weiser 1999), tattooing practices (Atkinson 2002) and hymen reconstructions (Saharso 2003). These scholars also engaged in "balancing acts" in which they combined a critical analysis of potentially problematic feminine body practices with a respectful reading of women's experiences and reasons for doing them.

However, other feminist scholars have been less sanguine about my focus on the experiences of individual women as well as my emphasis on women's agency in the context of cosmetic surgery. In their view, such a stance is not only theoretically misguided, but it can be politically dangerous. I want to return to some of the arguments I made in *Reshaping the Female Body* in light of these critiques, and in particular to the issue of choice and what constitutes an appropriate feminist response to cosmetic surgery. I will then turn to the issue of bodily difference and what it means to have a body that is defined as falling outside the realm of what is considered "normal." In view of recent developments in the field of cosmetic surgery, I will argue that the issue of difference has complicated my earlier arguments and required me to rethink what is at stake with cosmetic surgery and what would constitute an adequate feminist response.

Critiques

The most sustained and well-argued critique of my approach is by the well-known feminist philosopher Susan Bordo (1993, 1997). Bordo has provided a penetrating analysis of the current cultural obsession with slenderness, including eating disorders, the fitness craze, and cosmetic surgery. Much of her work entails a critical deconstruction of representations of women's bodies in popular culture (advertisements, television, films). Drawing upon Foucauldian notions of power, she shows how processes of normalization (measuring women's bodies against contemporary ideals of femininity) and homogenization (the containment of disturbing bodily differences) are integral to contemporary body culture. A central feature of this culture, she suggests, is the pernicious discourse of choice and the mentality of personal empowerment. In Bordo's view, this discourse is not only employed in the anti-feminist media, or echoed by women who defend their decisions to have their faces "lifted" or their tummies "tucked." It is also modeled by post feminists like Naomi Wolf (1993) or Katie Roiphe (1993), who criticize "old feminists" for viewing women as victims and refusing to respect their choices. However, even their more "moderate, sober, scholarly sisters" who, under the influence of poststructuralist theory, "celebrate" women's agency, are guilty of jumping on the freedom bandwagon (Bordo 1997: 35). It is to this latter brand of feminism, which Bordo calls "agency feminism," that my work on cosmetic surgery belongs.

According to Bordo, I have gone overboard in taking women who have cosmetic surgery at their word (Bordo 1997: 35–6). Just because they claim that cosmetic surgery is their best option under the circumstances, doesn't mean that I should take their words at face value. By directing my attention to individual women's experiences with their bodies and their decisions to have cosmetic surgery in *Reshaping the Female Body*, I have missed the bigger picture. I have not only *denied* the systematic constraints that operate on women and compel them to have their bodies altered surgically, but am guilty of *condoning* cosmetic surgery and the beauty industry by suggesting that it "in fact plays an important role in *empowering* women" (Bordo 1997: 35–6, my emphasis).

Bordo claims that *Reshaping the Female Body* is "dominated" by metaphors of choice and freedom—of women "taking their life into their own hands" (1997: 35). Structural constraints like sexism and racism are nothing more than "hurdles to be jumped" or "personal challenges to be overcome" (34). Since the same metaphors of choice and freedom can be found in contemporary advertising campaigns, Bordo concludes that my analysis unwittingly supports the pernicious discourse of individualism and personal empowerment, which is endemic in contemporary Western culture. She does not deny that I—or feminists like me—are aware of the power of cultural images and their contribution to women's viewing their bodies as defective and unacceptable. However, by focusing "*first and foremost* on women's agency" and by describing their decisions as a "locus of creativity, power, and self-definition," *Reshaping the Female Body* has failed to give sufficient attention to the systematic constraints that operate on women and compel them to have cosmetic surgery (Bordo 1993: 20, emphasis in original; Bordo 1997: 36, 42). A critical cultural analysis of cosmetic surgery would put the systematic and institutional features of the beauty culture at the forefront of the analysis rather than only exploring and giving credence to individual's women's experiences and choices.

Bordo assumes that one of the primary problems of contemporary culture is that its workings are not obvious to most of us. In fact, we are continually "tricked" by false promises of individual freedom, choice, and the possibility of controlling our lives by manipulating our bodies. It is difficult for most of us to see structures of inequality based on sexism or racism, when they are constantly being obscured by discourses of individualism and the primacy of "mind" over "matter." Bordo, therefore, sees it as her task to become a "diagnostician" of culture. She situates herself as someone who must "excavate and explore" the "hidden and unquestioned aspects" of Western culture which treat women and other marginalized individuals as abhorrent or inferior and deny systematic structures of domination under the guise of individual freedom (Bordo 1997: 174). In her view, any cultural analysis worth its salt has to provide a "picture of the landscape" and not just "individual snapshots" (43). Focusing on individual women's narratives (as I do) runs the risk of obscuring the bigger picture—a picture that is essential for cultural critique. While I agree with Bordo's insistence that we need to take a critical view of the culture which makes cosmetic surgery seem like a viable option to so many women, I disagree with her dismissal of the particularities of individual women's experiences and practices as well as the concrete contexts in which they are embedded as mere "snap shots." It is my contention that despite the similarities in our normative agenda (i.e. the need for a feminist cultural critique of cosmetic surgery), we differ in our theoretical approach toward women's "agency" as well as in our conception of what a "good" feminist cultural critique should entail. As both are central to understanding the cultural significance of cosmetic surgery and, consequently, to the present inquiry, I will provide a brief rejoinder.

The Problem of Agency

"Agency" as a sociological concept plays a central role in my inquiry into women's involvement in cosmetic surgery. I drew upon it to help me understand how women could view cosmetic surgery—a costly, painful, dangerous, and demeaning practice—as their best, and, in some cases, only option under the circumstances. Bordo conflates my use of "agency" with the discourses of "choice" and "freedom," which she finds in the media and in popular culture. "Agency" as a term is rarely found in the media, however, let alone in advertising jargon. It is a sociological concept and refers to the active participation of individuals in the constitution of social life. It does not represent "free choice," although individuals generally have some degree of freedom in their actions in the sense of in most cases being able to act otherwise. Individual agency is always situated in relations of power, which provide the conditions of enablement and constraint under which all social action takes place. There is no "free space" where individuals exercise "choice" in any absolute sense of the word. "Choices" are always messy affairs, rarely undertaken with perfect knowledge of circumstances, let alone certain or predictable outcomes.

The relationship between agency and structure has been the subject of one of the most long-standing and important debates within social sciences during the past century.[4] What is at stake in the sociological use of agency is how to understand the ways that social action and social structures are mutually constitutive and sustaining without falling into the twin traps of methodological individualism, on the one hand, and structural determinism, on the other. Agency is invariably linked to social structures and yet never entirely reducible to them. It is always multilayered, involving a complicated mix of intentionality, practical knowledge, and unconscious motives.

It is in this context that my focus on women's agency (including my use of another sociological notion, "cultural dope") should be seen: as a needed

4 See McNay 2000 for an excellent account of the implications of these debates for feminist gender theory.

corrective of overly deterministic accounts of social action, which I perceived in some feminist scholarship on women's involvement in the "beauty system." Given the pervasiveness of the constraints upon women to meet the cultural ideals of feminine appearance, it almost goes without saying that feminists will be inclined to view women who have cosmetic surgery—the most dramatic beauty practice of all—as victims of ideological manipulation. This was also my initial response as a feminist (Davis 1995: 1–5). However, it was a response that also seemed too easy. As Anthony Giddens has pointed out: "every competent actor has a wide-ranging, but intimate and subtle, knowledge of the society of which he or she is a member" (1976: 73). By underlining this knowledge ability, social action does not suddenly become a matter of "doing one's own thing." But neither can it be reduced to a simple knee-jerk reflex of social forces, imposed upon unwitting or deluded individuals. A focus on agency opens the door to a sociological exploration of how people draw upon their knowledge of themselves and their circumstances as they negotiate their everyday lives.

Following Giddens's strategy, I tried to avoid what would have been relatively easy for me, as a feminist, to do—namely, to treat women as deluded by the false promises of the feminine beauty system, as "cultural dopes." Instead I tried to make sense of what—at least initially—did not make sense to me. Against my own inclination to view women who have cosmetic surgery as "cultural dopes," I positioned them as "competent actors" with an "intimate and subtle knowledge of society," including the dominant discourses and practices of feminine beauty. This approach enabled me to understand what I had not been able to understand before—namely, why, given their specific experiences with their bodies and the possibilities available to them for alleviating their suffering, cosmetic surgery could be an action of choice, solution and problem, empowering and disempowering, all at once.

However, even if Bordo and I were to agree that the problem of "agency" is a theoretical difference of opinion or even a misunderstanding resulting from our disciplinary backgrounds, I believe that more is at stake in her critique of my work than agency. The question of whether a consideration of individual women's stories is relevant for a feminist cultural critique of cosmetic surgery may be even more salient and, more generally, what a cultural critique of ethically or politically problematic practices like cosmetic surgery should entail.

Cultural Critique

In *Reshaping the Female Body*, I chose to explore what Bordo has called "individual snapshots"—that is, women's stories of suffering and their attempts to overcome their suffering through cosmetic surgery—because these stories tend to get lost in debates about the ethical and political implications of cosmetic surgery. This is hardly a new research strategy and, as most feminist scholars would agree, women's voices have often required some "retrieval" as they tend to get lost between the cracks. Bordo has herself admitted that it was a good thing to "listen to those women."[5] However, the problems begin when I not only "listen" to what they say, but treat what they have to say as consequential for a critical feminist perspective on cosmetic surgery. Based on "these women's" accounts, I came to appreciate that women often have "good"—that is, credible and justifiable—reasons for wanting to have cosmetic surgery. This does not mean that I "condone" the practice, let alone the cultural norms that make women hate their bodies and long to have them altered. Indeed, I discovered that most of the women I spoke with don't condone cosmetic surgery either, but are, typically, highly critical of it, arguing that it is only defensible in specific cases (notably, their own) to relieve suffering that has passed the point of what a person should have to endure.

But taking women at their word is not simply a matter of "honoring their choices." It is precisely my concern about the continued popularity of cosmetic surgery—even in the face of increased media coverage of the risks and drawbacks—that made it seem imperative for me to understand why individual women were so determined to undertake it. Cosmetic surgery is not just popular; it is also controversial. Recipients struggle with the side effects and dangers of the surgery, welfare bureaucrats and insurance companies worry about the costs, and even surgeons express objections about whether surgery should be performed on otherwise healthy bodies just "for looks." While these concerns do not necessarily result in a refusal of the practice, the hesitations, which participants express and which are embedded in public debates about cosmetic surgery, provide insight into what makes cosmetic surgery not only desirable, but also problematic. Looking at the ambivalences that are already present can not only help us understand what is at stake with cosmetic surgery, it can enable us to see how, under different circumstances, another course of action might have been possible. If we can understand the circumstances which made it seem impossible for a woman to live with her body as it is, we can imagine what might need to be changed so that she would not need to look to cosmetic surgery as a solution to her problem.

In contrast to Bordo, I do not see feminist cultural critique as a matter of "excavation," nor do I position myself as an excavator, who unearths hitherto unknown truths about culture. The assumption of this privileged position presents some rather obvious difficulties. On what ground am I to discover the hidden truth of the culture to which I belong, while others are doomed to muddling along, blinded by their culture and, unlike me, unable to make sense of it? And even if I were able to justify taking such a privileged position, my conception of what constitutes critical cultural analysis differs from Bordo's.

In *Reshaping the Female Body*, I described myself as engaged in a "feminist balancing act"—on a "razor's edge"

---

5 In a discussion at the Hastings Center where we were both present, Bordo acknowledged, for example, that "of course, it's a good thing that you talked to those women," but then went on to emphasize the necessity of focusing on structures rather than the words of individual women.

> between a feminist critique of the cosmetic surgery craze (along with the ideologies of feminine inferiority which sustain it) and an equally feminist desire to treat women as agents who negotiate their bodies and their lives within the cultural and structural constraints of a gendered social order. This has meant exploring cosmetic surgery as one of the most pernicious expressions of the Western beauty culture without relegating women who have it to the position of "cultural dope." It has involved understanding how cosmetic surgery might be the best possible course of action for a particular woman, while, at the same time, problematizing the situational constraints which make cosmetic surgery an option. (Davis 1995: 5)

In order to engage in this balancing act, I had to draw upon my own "intimate and subtle knowledge of society." My membership in the very culture I was criticizing was an indispensable resource, which helped me to recognize the dilemmas confronting women who have cosmetic surgery as well as the cultural discourses they used to explain, criticize, but also justify or defend the practice. If I had anything special to offer as a critic, it was not the truth, let alone a higher moral ground. Rather, I demonstrated a willingness to entertain the unease and—at times—outright discomfort that cosmetic surgery evokes, particularly among feminists, and to do so long enough to unravel what might be at stake in some of its dilemmas.

Cosmetic surgery evokes deep-seated apprehension and ambivalence. As a feminist cultural critic, I have engaged with those aspects of cosmetic surgery that are puzzling, troubling, or, quite simply, don't make sense to me, and used them as an occasion for further exploration. I have taken up women's reasons for having cosmetic surgery precisely because they expressed sentiments that were different and sometimes even antithetical to my own. While this often made me uncomfortable, it also provided an opportunity to understand aspects of "our" cultural obsession with the makeability of the body, which might otherwise have been unavailable to me. But, more importantly, it allowed me to keep a discussion open in what the philosopher Paul Ricoeur (1999) in his ethics of conflict has called "reasonable disagreement."[6] I concluded *Reshaping the Female Body* with the claim that as feminist critics of cosmetic surgery, "we simply cannot afford the comfort of the correct line." Given the visibility and impact of cosmetic surgery in our contemporary cultural landscape, I believe that—if anything—it is even more essential as cultural critics to find ways to keep the discussion about cosmetic surgery open, so that we can explore what makes it both popular and problematic.

---

6 Ricoeur draws on Karl Jaspers's notion of "loving conflict" to describe the dangers of consensus ("if we miss consensus, we think we have failed"), the impossibility of a common or identical history, and the importance of assuming and living conflicts as a kind of practical wisdom (Ricoeur 1999: 12).

Equality and Embodied Differences

Cosmetic surgery is predicated upon definitions of physical normality. It was developed to alleviate deviations in normal appearance and, indeed, the recent "revolution" in cosmetic surgery attests to plastic surgeons' increasing authority to distinguish between normal and abnormal bodies. In Western culture, the white, propertied, male has enjoyed the normative position against which all others—women, the working classes or the ethnically marginalized—are measured and found wanting. It is hardly surprising that women have been the particular targets of cosmetic surgery. Although many cosmetic surgical techniques were not originally developed as interventions in femininity, in a sexist, racist or class society, certain groups (women, the ethnically marginalized, elderly people, homosexuals, disabled or fat people) are defined as "ugly, fearful or loathsome" through a process that Iris Marion Young refers to as the "aesthetic scaling of bodies" (1990a: 123–4). Individuals who represent groups falling outside white, Western, middle-class norms are defined through their bodily characteristics and constructed as different, as "Other." They find themselves under pressure to at least appear "normal" and, consequently, may be prepared to go to extreme lengths to achieve a normal-looking body. In a culture where feminine beauty is idealized, the "aesthetic scaling of bodies" specifically structures the dynamics of gender oppression, rendering ordinary-looking women ugly and deficient and trapping them into the hopeless race for a perfect body. Or, as Bernice Hausman somewhat ironically notes: "If women can't be normal because of their sex, they might as well be perfect" (1995: 65).

In *Reshaping the Female Body*, I showed how the categories of "normality" and "abnormality" are drawn upon in both medical discourse on cosmetic surgery (as cosmetic surgeons justify their professional practice, setting the parameters for debates about professional, technical, and ethical implications of cosmetic surgery) and in individuals' accounts of their surgical experiences (how they made sense of their suffering with their appearance or justified their decisions to have their bodies altered surgically). Cosmetic surgery becomes a legitimate reaction to the desire to appear normal ("just like everyone else"). Surgeons have had to defend cosmetic surgery against accusations of quackery (operating on healthy bodies), triviality (pampering their patient's vanity) and need (cosmetic surgery as luxury). To this end, they have argued that cosmetic surgery is necessary in a culture where appearance is important to a person's happiness and well-being; it is a requirement for a patient's welfare (Davis 1998).

Since the mid 1990s, however, cosmetic surgery has not only been taken up increasingly by the media and in popular culture. Cultural discourses about bodies and embodiment have shifted, altering the way cosmetic surgery is represented as well. Difference has become a "commodity," with none of the negative associations with which "abnormality" is imbued. Differences in color, sex and sexuality, or nation are celebrated (Lury 2000). Multiculturalism is the ostensible ideal in morphed images like the SimEve gracing the cover of *Time* magazine (Haraway 1997). It presents "race" or "sex," once markers of inequality, as matters of stylistic choice, to be mixed and matched like putting on different outfits. The body is treated as nothing more than a vehicle for recognizing our individual desires and projects. In short, the Benetton ideal reigns supreme.

In this cultural context, cosmetic surgery is increasingly presented as neutral technology, ideally suited to altering the body in accordance with an individual's personal preferences. This can include enhancing femininity or eradicating physical features associated with ethnicity or "race." After all, why are pectoral implants on a man any different than silicone implants for a woman? And what is the difference between dreadlocks on a white teenager and the widespread practice of hair straightening among Afro-American women (Rooks 1996, Banks 2000)? The discourse of "we are all different," along with individual choice and neutral technology, seem to have taken cosmetic surgery out of the "old" discourse of normality and abnormality and allowed it to transcend such categories altogether. Cosmetic surgery promises a different body; but this time, a body that has nothing to do with normative constraints associated with gender or "race" or nationality. Indeed, it seems to promise a society where problematic differences—differences that are associated with structured or systematic social inequalities—have been smoothed out or "homogenized." Once invisible, they will ostensibly cease to exist. Or, as Michael Jackson, one of the most vocal recipients of cosmetic surgery, has noted, "Black or white? I'm tired of being a color" (quoted in Davis 2003: 96).

The ideological celebration of individuality and the simultaneous erasure of embodied difference seem to suggest a desirable kind of equality (we are all individuals, the same no matter how we look or what the particular circumstances of our lives are). This focus on equality is, however, not without problems, as various feminist cultural critics have convincingly demonstrated.[7] Applied to the current cultural phenomenon of cosmetic surgery, I see, in particular, three problems with equality discourse.

The first problem is that equality discourse downplays the significance of cosmetic surgery, trivializing its dangers and transforming it into a neutral technology which can be deployed by any individual in the interests of his or her personal "identity project." As long as cosmetic surgery was viewed as a solution for "abnormal" appearance (however spurious that category has been in the past), it could be treated as an exceptional solution for an exceptional problem. However, if all individuals are "different" to the same degree, that is, different in "equal" measure, then anyone can be a potential candidate for surgical intervention. Cosmetic surgery—like any other consumer good—is a matter of personal preference and the means to afford it. Thus, the threshold to the surgeon's office is lowered, making cosmetic surgery an option for individuals who might not have considered it before.

The second problem with equality discourse is that it deflects attention from structural inequalities based on gender, ethnicity, nationality, age, or other categories

7 In addition to Bordo's work, I have particularly benefited from Wiegman 1995, Haraway 1997, and Lury 2000.

of difference. It ignores specific histories and current conditions of inequality, which give body practices different meanings. Cher's rumored decision to have her belly button tucked or her bottom rib removed is not the same as an Asian American teenager choosing to have her eyes Westernized. Treating these interventions as commensurate—both a matter of individual choice, both equally responsive to the current beauty ideals—depoliticizes cosmetic surgery. It discounts the universality of white, Western norms of appearance, which shape individuals' perceptions of what they consider to be desirable appearance as well as the kinds of interventions that are deemed acceptable. Not every body will do; nor are all differences the same in Western culture. Eyes are rarely made more "oriental"-looking, any more than noses are made to look more "Jewish." Thus, one ideal—a white, Western model—becomes the norm to which everyone, explicitly or implicitly, aspires. Cosmetic surgery becomes decontextualized and depoliticized when changes in appearance are seen as having the same cultural meaning and the same political (or normative) valence. In effect, this means that cosmetic surgery has *no* cultural meaning and *no* political valence (Bordo 1993: 253).

The third problem with equality discourse is that it ignores the individual's interactions with her/his material, fleshy body and, through this body, with the outside world. Bodies are not like pieces of clothing, to be donned or taken off at will. Individuals have specific histories of suffering with their bodies, born of their interactions with others. Their embodiment takes shape within specific cultural constraints, which require ongoing negotiation. When the media proclaims that men have become the "new" victims of the beauty craze (Davis 2002), women's long-standing tradition of suffering "for the sake of beauty" is not only downplayed, but men's specific experiences with *their* bodies in the context of culturally specific discourses and practices of masculinity are ignored as well. Equality discourse erases the specificity that would allow us to understand the lived experience of embodiment within concrete historical, social, and cultural contexts.

In conclusion, equality discourses seem to stand in the way of a critical understanding of cosmetic surgery precisely because they ignore embodied difference. Cosmetic surgery on differently embodied individuals is quickly becoming an unproblematic road toward equality—an acceptable avenue for the physically disadvantaged to have a shot at the "good life." In the face of the enormous expansion of technologies for eradicating differences of all kinds, it may not only be our *ability* to feel compassion, concern, or shock, which is at stake. Our *inability* to sympathize, our lack of concern, or our numbness toward any individual or group embarking on the "surgical fix" may be equally worthy of our critical attention.

This does not mean that I am advocating a surgery-free future. In this respect, my position has changed very little since 1995. However, it is my contention that a future that contains cosmetic surgery to eliminate visible markers of embodied difference should make us deeply uneasy. We need to continue to treat it as controversial and always requiring ongoing public debate. It is my contention that the first and most important question, which we ongoingly need to ask, is not whether individuals should have cosmetic surgery or whether surgeons should perform it or even whether the media should promote it. The first question facing each of us should be why the world we live in prefers to disguise difference rather than to confront it in everyday life and whether this is the kind of world we really want to live in.

References

Aalten, Anna. 1997. "Performing the Body, Creating Culture," in *Embodied Practices: Feminist Perspectives on the Body*, edited by K. Davis. London: Sage, 41–58.

Atkinson, Michael. 2002. "Pretty in Ink: Conformity, Resistance, and Negotiation in Women's Tattooing." *Sex Roles*, 47(5–6), 219–35.

Banet-Weiser, Sarah. 1999. *The Most Beautiful Girl in the World: Beauty Pageants and National Identity*. Berkeley: University of California Press.

Banks, Ingrid. 2000. *Hair Matters: Beauty, Power, and Black Women's Consciousness*. New York: New York University Press.

Bartky, Sandra. 1990. *Femininity and Domination: Studies in the Phenomenology of Oppression*. New York: Routledge.

Blum, Virginia L. 2005. *Flesh Wounds: The Culture of Cosmetic Surgery*. Berkeley: University of California Press.

Bordo, Susan. 1993. *Unbearable Weight: Feminism, Western Culture, and the Body*. Berkeley, Los Angeles, London: University of California Press.

Bordo, Susan. 1997. *Twilight Zones: The Hidden Life of Cultural Images from Plato to O.J.* Berkeley, Los Angeles, London: University of California Press.

Chancer, Lynn S. 1998. *Reconcilable Differences: Confronting Beauty, Pornography, and the Future of Feminism*. Berkeley: University of California Press.

Davis, Kathy. 1995. *Reshaping the Female Body: The Dilemma of Cosmetic Surgery*. New York and London: Routledge.

Davis, Kathy. 1998. "The Rhetoric of Cosmetic Surgery: Luxury or Welfare?" in *Enhancing Human Traits. Ethical and Social Implications*, E. Parens. Washington, DC: Georgetown University Press, 12–134.

Davis, Kathy. 2002. "'A Dubious Equality': Men, Women, and Cosmetic Surgery." *Body & Society*, 8(1), 49–66.

Davis, Kathy. 2003. *Dubious Equalities and Embodied Differences: Cultural Studies on Cosmetic Surgery*. Lanham, MD: Rowman & Littlefield.

Dellinger, Kirsten and Williams, Christine L. 1997. "Makeup at Work. Negotiating Appearance Rules in the Workplace." *Gender & Society*, 11(2), 151–77.

Garfinkel, Harold. 1967. *Studies in Ethnomethodology*. Englewood Cliffs, NJ: Prentice-Hall/Cambridge: Polity.

Giddens, Anthony. 1976. *New Rules of Sociological Method*. London: Hutchinson.

Gilman, Sander. 1999. *Making the Body Beautiful*. Princeton: Princeton University Press.

Gimlin, Debra L. 2002. *Body Work: Beauty and Self-Image in American Culture*. Berkeley: University of California Press.

Haiken, Elizabeth. 1997. *Venus Envy: A History of Cosmetic Surgery*. Baltimore and London: The Johns Hopkins University Press.
Haraway, Donna J. 1997. *Modest Witness@Second_Millennium.FemaleMan_Meets-OncoMouse: feminism and technoscience*. New York: Routledge.
Hausman , Bernice L. 1995. *Changing Sex: Transsexualism, Technology, and the Idea of Gender*. Durham, NC: Duke University Press.
Jacobson , Nora. 2000. *Cleavage: Technology, Controversy and the Ironies of the Man-made Breast*. New Brunswick, NJ: Rutgers University Press.
Klinge, Ineke. 1997. "Female Bodies and Brittle Bones: Medical Interventions in Osteoporosis," in *Embodied Practices. Feminist Perspectives on the Body*, edited by K. Davis. London: Sage, 59–72.
Lury, Celia. 2000. "The United Colors of Diversity: Essential and Inessential Culture," in *Global Nature, Global Culture*, edited by S. Franklin, C. Lury, and J. Stacey. London: Sage, 146–87.
MacCannell, Dean and MacCannell, Juliet Flower. "The beauty system," in *The Ideology of Conduct*, edited by N. Armstrong and L. Tennenhouse. New York: Methuen, 206–38.
McNay, Lois. 2000. *Gender and Agency: Reconfiguring the Subject in Feminist and Social Theory*. Cambridge: Polity.
Morgan, Kathryn Pauly. 1991. "Women and the Knife: Cosmetic Surgery and the Colonization of Women's Bodies." *Hypatia*, 6(3), 25–53.
Negrin, Llewellyn. 2002. "Cosmetic Surgery and the Eclipse of Identity." *Body & Society*, 8(4), 21–42.
Ricoeur, Paul (with Brian Cosgrave, Gayle Freyne, David Scott, Imelda McCarthy, Redmond O'Hanlon, Brian Garvey, John Cleary, Margaret Kelleher, Dermot Moran, and Maeve Cooke). 1999. "Imagination, testimony and trust: a dialogue with Paul Ricoeur," in *Questioning Ethics. Contemporary Debates in Philosophy*, edited by R. Kearney and M. Dooley. London: Routledge, 12–17.
Roiphe, Katie. 1993. *The Morning After: Sex, Fear, and Feminism*. Boston: Little, Brown and Company.
Rooks, Noliwe M. 1996. *Hair Raising: Beauty, Culture, and African American Women*. New Brunswick: Rutgers University Press.
Saharso, Sawitri. 2003. "Culture, Toleration and Gender: A Contribution from the Netherlands." *The European Journal of Women's Studies*, 10(1), 7–28.
Wiegman, Robyn. 1995. *American Anatomies. Theorizing Race and Gender*. Durham, NC: Duke University Press.
Wolf, Naomi. 1991. *The Beauty Myth*. New York: William Morrow and Company, Inc.
Wolf, Naomi. 1993. *Fire With Fire*. New York: Random House.
Young, Iris Marion. 1990a. *Justice and the Politics of Difference*. Princeton: Princeton University Press.
Young, Iris Marion. 1990b. *Throwing Like a Girl and Other Essays in Feminist Philosophy and Social Theory*. Bloomington and Indianapolis: Indiana University Press.

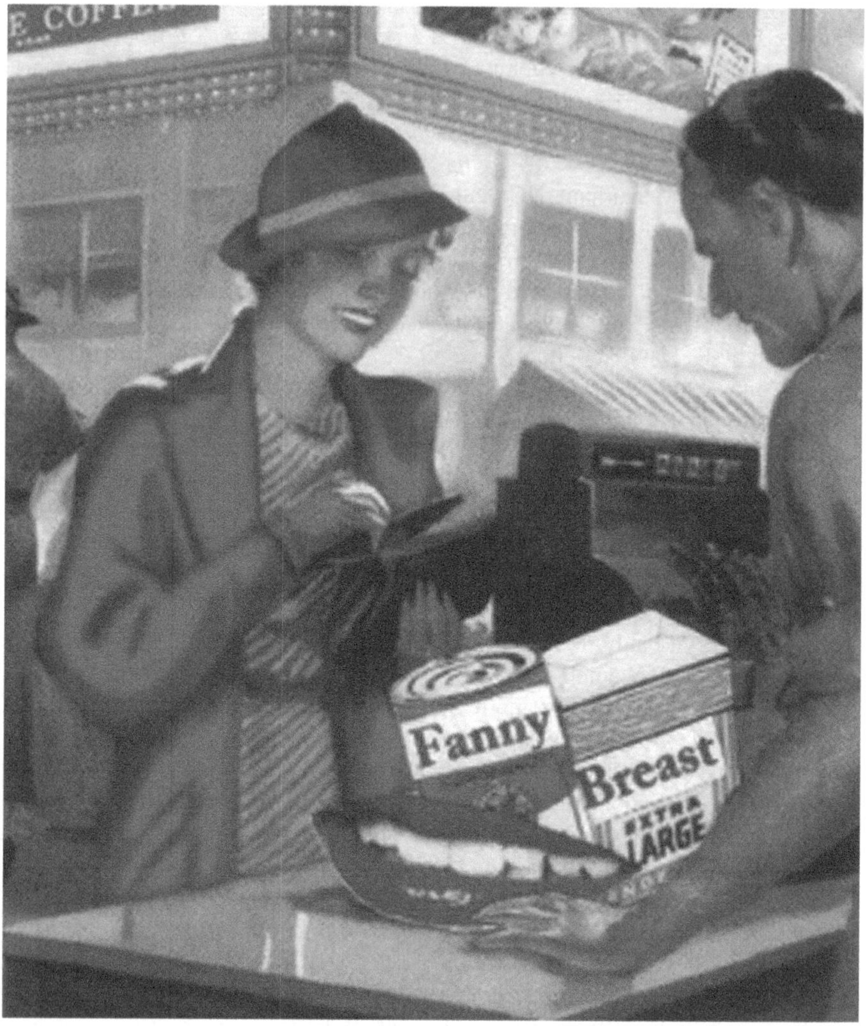

Figure 4.1 "Nip/Tuck"

Source: © Michelle Lanter, Dadadreams

Chapter 4
Women and the Knife: Cosmetic Surgery and the Colonization of Women's Bodies

Kathryn Pauly Morgan

Introduction

Consider the following passages:

> If you want to wear a Maidenform Viking Queen bra like Madonna, be warned: A body like this doesn't just happen. … Madonna's kind of fitness training takes time. The rock star *whose muscled body was recently on tour* spends a minimum of three hours a day working out. ("Madonna Passionate About Fitness" 1990; italics added)

> A lot of the contestants [in the Miss America Pageant] do not owe their beauty to their Maker but to their Re-Maker. Miss Florida's nose came courtesy of her surgeon. So did Miss Alaska's. And Miss Oregon's breasts came from the manufacturers of silicone. (Goodman 1989)

> Jacobs [a plastic surgeon in Manhattan] constantly answers the call, for cleavage. "Women need it for their holiday ball gowns." ("Cosmetic Surgery for the Holidays" 1985)

> We hadn't seen or heard from each other for 28 years. … Then he suggested it would be nice if we could meet. I was very nervous about it. How much had I changed? I wanted a facelift, tummy tuck and liposuction, all in one week. (A woman, age forty-nine, being interviewed for an article on "older couples" falling in love; "Falling in Love Again" 1990)

> It's hard to say why one person will have cosmetic surgery done and another won't consider it, but generally I think people who go for surgery are more aggressive, they are the doers of the world. It's like makeup. You see some women who might be greatly improved by wearing make-up, but they're, I don't know, granola-heads or something, and they just refuse. (Dr. Ronald Levine, director of plastic surgery education at the University of Toronto and

> vice-chairman of the plastic surgery section of the Ontario Medical Association; "The Quest to Be a Perfect 10" 1990)

> Another comparable limitation [of the women's liberation movement] is a tendency to reject certain good things only in order to punish men. ... There is no reason why a women's liberation activist should not try to look pretty and attractive. (Markovic 1976)

Now imagine the needles and knives of the cosmetic surgeon. Look at this picture of surgical tools (Figure 4.2) . Look at the tools for a long time. *Imagine them cutting into your skin.* Imagine that you have been given [cosmetic] surgery as a gift from your loved one who read a persuasive and engaging press release from Drs. John and Jim Williams that ends by saying, "The next morning the limo will chauffeur your loved one back home again with a gift of beauty that will last a lifetime" (Williams and Williams 1990). Imagine the beauty that you have been promised.

We need a feminist analysis to understand why actual, live women are reduced and reduce themselves to "potential women" and choose to participate in anatomizing and fetishizing their bodies as they buy "contoured bodies," "restored youth," and "permanent beauty." In the face of a growing market and demand for surgical interventions in women's bodies that can and do result in infection, bleeding, embolisms, pulmonary edema, facial nerve injury, unfavorable scar formation, skin loss, blindness, crippling, and death, our silence becomes a culpable one.

Not only is elective cosmetic surgery moving out of the domain of the sleazy, the suspicious, the secretively deviant, or the pathologically narcissistic, *it is becoming the norm*. This shift is leading to a predictable inversion of the domains of the deviant and the pathological, so that women who contemplate *not using* cosmetic surgery will increasingly be stigmatized and seen as deviant. Cosmetic surgery entails the ultimate envelopment of the lived temporal *reality* of the human subject by technologically created appearances that are then regarded as "the real." Youthful appearance triumphs over aged reality.

I. "Just the Facts in America, Ma'am"

As of 1990, the most frequently performed kind of cosmetic surgery is liposuction, which involves sucking fat cells out from underneath our skin with a vacuum device. This is viewed as the most suitable procedure for removing specific bulges around the hips, thighs, belly, buttocks, or chin. It is most appropriately done on thin people who want to get rid of certain bulges, and surgeons guarantee that even if there is weight gain, the bulges won't reappear since the fat cells have been permanently removed. At least twelve deaths are known to have resulted from complications such as hemorrhages and embolisms. "All we know is there was a complication and that complication was death," said the partner of Toni Sullivan, age 43 ("hardworking mother of two teenage children" says the press; "Woman, 43, Dies After Cosmetic Surgery" 1989). Cost: $1,000–7,500.

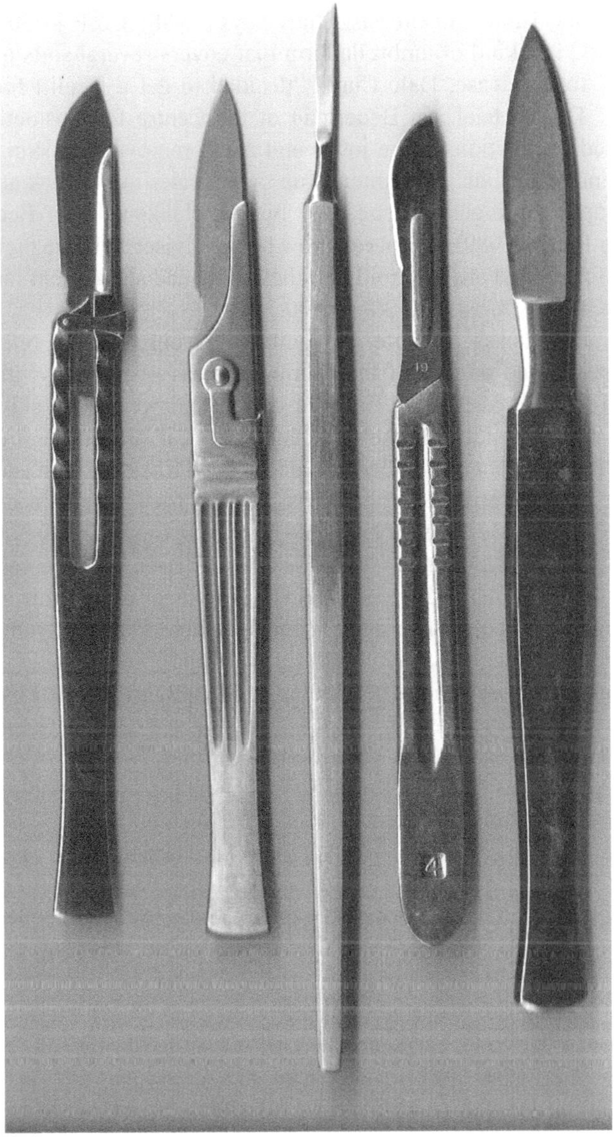

Figure 4.2 Various scalpels

The second most frequently performed kind of cosmetic surgery is breast augmentation, which involves an implant, usually of silicone. Often the silicone implant hardens over time and must be removed surgically. Over one million women in the United States are known to have had breast augmentation surgery. Two recent studies have shown that breast implants block X-rays and cast a shadow on surrounding tissue, making mammograms difficult to interpret, and that there appears to be a much higher incidence of cancerous lumps in "augmented women" ("Implants Hide Tumors in Breasts, Study Says" 1988). Cost: $1,500–3,000.

"Face-lift" is a kind of umbrella term that covers several sorts of procedures. In a recent Toronto case, Dale Curtis "decided to get a facelift for her fortieth birthday … Dr. Michael Jon Bederman of the Centre for Cosmetic Surgery in Toronto used liposuction on the jowls and neck, removed the skin and fat from her upper and lower lids and tightened up the muscles in the neck and cheeks. … 'She was supposed to get a forehead lift but she chickened out,' Bederman says" ("Changing Faces" 1989). Clients are now being advised to begin their face-lifts in their early forties and are also told that they will need subsequent face-lifts every five to fifteen years. Cost: $2,500–10,500.

"Nips" and "tucks" are cute, camouflaging labels used to refer to surgical reduction performed on any of the following areas of the body: hips, buttocks, thighs, belly, and breasts. They involve cutting out wedges of skin and fat and sewing up the two sides. These are major surgical procedures that cannot be performed in outpatient clinics because of the need for anesthesia and the severity of possible postoperative complications. Hence, they require access to costly operating rooms and services in hospitals or clinics. Cost: $3,000–7,000.

The number of "rhinoplasties," or nose jobs, has risen by 34 percent since 1981. Some clients are coming in for second and third nose jobs. Nose jobs involve either the inserting of a piece of bone taken from elsewhere in the body or the whittling down of the nose. Various styles of noses go in and out of fashion, and various cosmetic surgeons describe the noses they create in terms of their own surnames, such as "the Diamond nose" or "the Goldman nose" ("Cosmetic Surgery for the Holidays" 1985). Cost: $2,000–3,000.

More recent types of cosmetic surgery, such as the use of skin-expanders and suction lipectomy, involve inserting tools, probes, and balloons *under* the skin either for purposes of expansion or reduction (Hirshson 1987).

Lest one think that women (who represent between 60 and 70 percent of all cosmetic surgery patients) choose only one of these procedures, heed the words of Dr. Bederman:

> We see working girls, dental technicians, middle-class women who are unhappy with their looks or are aging prematurely. And we see executives—both male and female. … Where before someone would have a tummy tuck and not have anything else done for a year, frequently we will do liposuction and tummy tuck and then the next day a facelift, upper and lower lids, rhinoplasty *and other*

> *things.* The recovery time is the same whether a person has one procedure or *the works*, generally about two weeks. ("Changing Faces" 1989; italics added)

In principle, there is no area of the body that is not accessible to the interventions and metamorphoses performed by cosmetic surgeons intent on creating twentieth-century versions of "femina perfecta."

II. From Artifice to Artifact: The Creation of Robo Woman?

Today, what is designated as "the natural" functions primarily as a frontier rather than as a barrier. While genetics, human sexuality, reproductive outcome, and death were previously regarded as open to variation primarily in evolutionary terms, they are now seen by biotechnologists as domains of creation and control. Cosmetic surgeons claim a role here too. For them, human bodies are the locus of challenge. As one plastic surgeon remarks, "Patients sometimes misunderstand the nature of cosmetic surgery. It's not a shortcut for diet or exercise. *It's a way to override the genetic code*" ("Retouching Nature's Way": 1990; italics added).

The beauty culture is coming to be dominated by a variety of experts, and consumers of youth and beauty are likely to find themselves dependent not only on cosmetic surgeons but on anesthetists, nurses, aestheticians, nail technicians, manicurists, dietitians, hairstylists, cosmetologists, masseuses, aromatherapists, trainers, pedicurists, electrolysists, pharmacologists, and dermatologists. All these experts provide services that can be bought; all these experts are perceived as administering and transforming the human body into an increasingly artificial and ever more perfect object.

For virtually all women as women, success is defined in terms of interlocking patterns of compulsion: compulsory attractiveness, compulsory motherhood, and compulsory heterosexuality, patterns that determine the legitimate limits of attraction and motherhood.[1] Rather than aspiring to self-determined and woman-centered ideals of health or integrity, women's attractiveness is defined as attractive-to-men; women's eroticism is defined as either nonexistent, pathological, or peripheral when it is not directed to phallic goals; and motherhood is defined in terms of legally sanctioned and constrained reproductive service to particular men and to institutions such as the nation, the race, the owner, and the class—institutions that are, more often than not, male-dominated. Biotechnology is now

---

1 I say "virtually all women" because there is now a nascent literature on the subject of fat oppression and body image as it affects lesbians. For a perceptive article on this subject, see Dworkin (1989). I am, of course, not suggesting that compulsory heterosexuality and obligatory maternity affect all women equally. Clearly, women who are regarded as "deviant" in some respect or other—because they are lesbian or women with disabilities or "too old" or poor or of the "wrong race"—are under enormous pressure from the dominant culture *not* to bear children, but this, too, is an aspect of patriarchal pro-natalism.

making beauty, fertility, the appearance of heterosexuality through surgery, and the appearance of youthfulness accessible to virtually all women who can afford that technology—and growing numbers of women are making other sacrifices in their lives in order to buy access to the technical expertise.

In Western industrialized societies, women have also become increasingly socialized into an acceptance of technical knives. We know about knives that can heal: the knife that saves the life of a baby in distress, the knife that cuts out the cancerous growths in our breasts, the knife that straightens our spines, the knife that liberates our arthritic fingers so that we may once again gesture, once again touch, once again hold. But we also know about other knives: the knife that cuts off our toes so that our feet will fit into elegant shoes, the knife that cuts out ribs to fit our bodies into corsets, the knife that slices through our labia in episiotomies and other forms of genital mutilation, the knife that cuts into our abdomens to remove our ovaries to cure our "deviant tendencies" (Barker-Benfield 1976), the knife that removes our breasts in prophylactic or unnecessary radical mastectomies, the knife that cuts out our "useless bag" (the womb) if we're the wrong color and poor or if we've "outlived our fertility," the knife that makes the "bikini cut" across our pregnant bellies to facilitate the cesarean section that will allow the obstetrician to go on holiday. We know these knives well.

And now we are coming to know the knives and needles of the cosmetic surgeons—the knives that promise to sculpt our bodies, to restore our youth, to create beauty out of what was ugly and ordinary. What kind of knives are these? Magic knives. Magic knives in a patriarchal context. Magic knives in a Eurocentric context. Magic knives in a white supremacist context. What do they mean? I am afraid of these knives.

III. Listening to the Women

In order to give a feminist reading of any ethical situation we must listen to the women's own reasons for their actions (Sherwin 1984–85; 1989). It is only once we have listened to the voices of women who have elected to undergo cosmetic surgery that we can try to assess the extent to which the conditions for genuine choice have been met and look at the consequences of these choices for the position of women. Here are some of those voices:

> ***Voice* 1** (*a woman looking forward to attending a prestigious charity ball*): "There will be a lot of new faces at the Brazilian Ball" ("Changing Faces" 1989). [Class/status symbol]
>
> ***Voice* 2**: "You can keep yourself trim. … But you have no control over the way you wrinkle, or the fat on your hips, or the skin of your lower abdomen. If you are *hereditarily predestined* to stretch out or wrinkle in your face, you will. If your parents had puffy eyelids and saggy jowls, you're going to have puffy eyelids and

saggy jowls" ("Changing Faces" 1989). [Regaining a sense of control; liberation from parents; transcending hereditary predestination]
***Voice* 3**: "Now we want a nose that makes a statement, with tip definition and a strong bridge line" ("Changing Faces" 1989). [Domination; strength]
***Voice* 4**: "I decided to get a facelift for my fortieth birthday after ten years of living and working in the tropics had taken its toll" ("Changing Faces" 1989). [Gift to the self; erasure of a decade of hard work and exposure]
***Voice* 5**: "I've gotten my breasts augmented. I can use it as a tax write-off" ("Changing Faces" 1989). [Professional advancement; economic benefits]
***Voice* 6**: "I'm a teacher and kids let schoolteachers know how we look and they aren't nice about it. A teacher who looks like an old bat or has a big nose will get a nickname" ("Retouching Nature's Way: Is Cosmetic Surgery Worth It?" 1990). [Avoidance of cruelty; avoidance of ageist bias]
***Voice* 7**: "I'll admit to a boob job." (Susan Akin, Miss America of 1986 quoted in Goodman, 1989). [Prestige; status; competitive accomplishments in beauty contest]
***Voice* 8** (*45-year-old grandmother and proprietor of a business*): "In my business, the customers expect you to look as good as they do" (Hirshson 1987). [Business asset; economic gain; possible denial of grandmother status]
***Voice* 9**: "People in business see something like this as showing an overall aggressiveness and go-forwardness. *The trend is to, you know, be all that you can be"* ("Cosmetic Surgery for the Holidays" 1985). [Success; personal fulfillment]
***Voice* 10** (*paraphrase*): "I do it to fight holiday depression" ("Cosmetic Surgery for the Holidays" 1985). [Emotional control; happiness]
***Voice* 11**: "I came to see Dr. X for the holiday season. I have important business parties, and the man I'm trying to get to marry me is coming in from Paris" ("Cosmetic Surgery for the Holidays" 1985). [Economic gain; heterosexual affiliation]

Women have traditionally regarded (and been taught to regard) their bodies, particularly if they are young, beautiful, and fertile, *as a locus of power* to be enhanced through artifice and, now, through artifact. In 1792, in *A Vindication of the Rights of Woman*, Mary Wollstonecraft remarked: "Taught from infancy that beauty is woman's scepter, the mind shapes itself to the body and roaming round its gilt cage, only seeks to adorn its prison." How ironic that the mother of the creator of *Frankenstein* should be the source of that quote. We need to ask ourselves whether today, involved as we are in the modern inversion of "our bodies shaping themselves to our minds," we are creating a new species of woman-monster with new artifactual bodies that function as prisons or whether cosmetic surgery for women does represent a potentially liberating field of choice.

When Snow White's stepmother asks the mirror "Who is fairest of all?" she is not asking simply an empirical question. In wanting to continue to be "the fairest of all," she is striving, in a clearly competitive context, for a prize, for a position, for power. The affirmation of her beauty brings with it privileged heterosexual affiliation, privileged access to forms of power unavailable to the plain, the ugly, the aged, and the barren.

The voices are seductive—they speak the language of gaining access to transcendence, achievement, liberation, and power. And they speak to a kind of reality. First, electing to undergo the surgery necessary to create youth and beauty artificially not only appears to but often actually does give a woman a sense of identity that, to some extent, she has chosen herself. Second, it offers her the potential to raise her status both socially and economically by increasing her opportunities for heterosexual affiliation (especially with white men). Third, by committing herself to the pursuit of beauty, a woman integrates her life with a consistent set of values and choices that bring her widespread approval and a resulting sense of increased self-esteem. Fourth, the pursuit of beauty often gives a woman access to a range of individuals who administer to her body in a caring way, an experience often sadly lacking in the day-to-day lives of many women. As a result, a woman's pursuit of beauty through transformation is often associated with lived experiences of self-creation, self-fulfillment, self-transcendence, and being cared for. The power of these experiences must not be underestimated.

While I acknowledge that these choices can confer a kind of integrity on a woman's life, I also believe that they are likely to embroil her in a set of interrelated contradictions. I refer to these as "Paradoxes of Choice."

IV. Three Paradoxes of Choice

In exploring these paradoxes, I appropriate Foucault's analysis of the diffusion of power in order to understand forms of power that are potentially more personally invasive than are more obvious, publicly identifiable aspects of power. In the chapter, "Docile Bodies" in *Discipline and Punish*, Foucault (1979: 136–7) highlights three features of what he calls disciplinary power:

1. The *scale* of the control. In disciplinary power the body is treated individually and in a coercive way because the body itself is the *active* and hence apparently free body that is being controlled through movements, gestures, attitudes, and degrees of rapidity.
2. The *object* of the control, which involves meticulous control over the efficiency of movements and forces.
3. The *modality* of the control, which involves constant, uninterrupted coercion.

Foucault argues that the outcome of disciplinary power is the docile body, a body "that may be subjected, used, transformed, and improved" (Foucault 1979, 136). Foucault is discussing this model of power in the context of prisons and armies, but we can adapt the central insights of this notion to see how women's bodies are entering "a machinery of power that explores it, breaks it down, and rearranges it" through a recognizably political metamorphosis of embodiment (Foucault 1979: 138).[2] What is important about this notion in relation to cosmetic surgery is the extent to which it makes it possible to speak about the diffusion of power throughout Western industrialized cultures that are increasingly committed to a technological beauty imperative. It also makes it possible to refer to a set of experts—cosmetic surgeons—whose explicit power mandate is to explore, break down, and rearrange women's bodies.

Paradox One: The Choice of Conformity—Understanding the Number 10

While the technology of cosmetic surgery could clearly be used to create and celebrate idiosyncrasy, eccentricity, and uniqueness, it is obvious that this is not how it is presently being used. Cosmetic surgeons report that legions of women appear in their offices demanding "Bo Derek" breasts ("Cosmetic Surgery for the Holidays" 1985). Jewish women demand reductions of their noses so as to be able to "pass" as one of their Aryan sisters who form the dominant ethnic group (Lakoff and Scherr 1984). Adolescent Asian girls who bring in pictures of Elizabeth Taylor and of Japanese movie actresses (whose faces have already been reconstructed) demand the "Westernizing" of their own eyes and the creation of higher noses in hopes of better job and marital prospects ("New Bodies for Sale" 1985). Black women buy toxic bleaching agents in hopes of attaining lighter skin. What is being created in all of these instances is not simply beautiful bodies and faces but white, Western, Anglo-Saxon bodies in a racist, anti-Semitic context.

More often than not, what appear at first glance to be instances of choice turn out to be instances of conformity. The women who undergo cosmetic surgery in order to compete in various beauty pageants are clearly choosing to conform. So is the woman who wanted to undergo a face-lift, tummy tuck, and liposuction all in one week, in order to win heterosexual approval *from a man she had not seen in twenty-eight years* and whose individual preferences she could not possibly know. In some ways, it does not matter who the particular judges are. Actual men—brothers, fathers, male lovers, male beauty "experts"—and hypothetical men live in the aesthetic imaginations of women. Whether they are male employers, prospective male spouses, male judges in the beauty pageants, or male-identified women, these modern day Parises are generic and live sometimes ghostly but powerful lives in the reflective awareness of women (Berger 1972). A woman's makeup, dress, gestures, voice, degree of cleanliness, degree of muscularity, odors, degree of hirsuteness,

2 I view this as a recognizably *political* metamorphosis because forensic cosmetic surgeons and social archaeologists will be needed to determine the actual age and earlier appearance of women in cases where identification is called for on the basis of existing carnal data. See Griffin's (1978) poignant description in "The Anatomy Lesson" for a reconstruction of the life and circumstances of a dead mother from just such carnal evidence. As we more and more profoundly artifactualize our own bodies, we become more sophisticated archaeological repositories and records that both signify and symbolize our culture.

vocabulary, hands, feet, skin, hair, and vulva can all be evaluated, regulated, and disciplined in the light of the hypothetical often-white male viewer and the male viewer present in the assessing gaze of other women (Haug 1987). Men's appreciation and approval of achieved femininity becomes all the more invasive when it resides in the incisions, stitches, staples, and scar tissue of women's bodies as women choose to conform. And women's public conformity to the norms of beauty often signals a deeper conformity to the norms of compulsory heterosexuality along with an awareness of the violence that can result from violating those norms. Hence the first paradox: that what looks like an optimal situation of reflection, deliberation, and self-creating choice often signals conformity at a deeper level.

Paradox Two: Liberation into Colonization

As argued above, a woman's desire to create a permanently beautiful and youthful appearance that is not vulnerable to the threats of externally applied cosmetic artifice or to the aging process of the body must be understood as a deeply significant existential project. It deliberately involves the exploitation and transformation of the most intimately experienced domain of immanence, the body, in the name of transcendence: transcendence of hereditary predestination, of lived time, of one's given "limitations." What I see as particularly alarming in this project is that what comes to have primary significance is not the real given existing woman but her body viewed as a "primitive entity" that is seen only as potential, as a kind of raw material to be exploited in terms of appearance, eroticism, nurturance, and fertility as defined by the colonizing culture.[3]

But for whom is this exploitation and transformation taking place? Who exercises the power here? Sometimes the power is explicit. It is exercised by brothers, fathers, male lovers, male engineering students who taunt and harass their female counterparts, and by male cosmetic surgeons who offer "free advice" in social gatherings to women whose "deformities" and "severe problems" can all be cured through their healing needles and knives. And the colonizing power is transmitted through and by those women whose own bodies and disciplinary practices demonstrate the efficacy of "taking care of herself" in these culturally defined feminine ways. Sometimes, however, the power may be so diffused as to dominate the consciousness of a given woman with no other subject needing to be present.

In electing to undergo cosmetic surgery, women appear to be protesting against the constraints of the "given" in their embodied lives and seeking liberation from

3 I intend to use "given" here in a relative and political sense. I don't believe that the notion that biology is somehow "given" and culture is just "added on" is a tenable one. I believe that we are intimately and inextricably encultured and embodied, so that a reductionist move in either direction is doomed to failure. For a persuasive analysis of this thesis, see Lowe (1982) and Haraway (1978, 1989). For a variety of political analyses of the "given" as primitive, see Marge Piercy's poem "Right to Life" (1980), Morgan (1989), and Murphy (1984).

those constraints. But I believe they are in danger of retreating and becoming more vulnerable, at that very level of embodiment, to those colonizing forms of power that may have motivated the protest in the first place. Moreover, in seeking independence, they can become even more dependent on male assessment and on the services of all those experts they initially bought to render them independent.

Here we see a second paradox bound up with choice: that the rhetoric is that of liberation and care, of "making the most of yourself," but the reality is often the transformation of oneself as a woman for the eye, the hand, and the approval of the Other—the lover, the taunting students, the customers, the employers, the social peers. And the Other is almost always affected by the dominant culture, which is male-supremacist, racist, ageist, heterosexist, anti-Semitic, ableist, and class-biased.[4]

Paradox Three: Coerced Voluntariness and the Technological Imperative

Where is the coercion? At first glance, women who choose to undergo cosmetic surgery often seem to represent a paradigm case of the rational chooser. Drawn increasingly from wider and wider economic groups, these women clearly make a choice, often at significant economic cost to the rest of their life, to pay the large sums of money demanded by cosmetic surgeons (since American health insurance plans do not cover this elective cosmetic surgery).

Furthermore, they are often highly critical consumers of these services, demanding extensive consultation, information regarding the risks and benefits of various surgical procedures, and professional guarantees of expertise. Generally they are relatively young and in good health. Thus, in some important sense, they epitomize relatively invulnerable free agents making a decision under virtually optimal conditions.

Moreover, on the surface, women who undergo cosmetic surgery choose a set of procedures that are, by definition, "elective." This term is used, quite straightforwardly, to distinguish cosmetic surgery from surgical intervention for reconstructive or health-related reasons (e.g., following massive burns, cancer-related forms of mutilation, etc.). The term also appears to distinguish cosmetic surgery from apparently involuntary and more pathologically transforming forms of intervention in the bodies of young girls in the form of, for example, foot-

4 The extent to which ableist bias is at work in this area was brought home to me by two quotations cited by a woman with a disability. She discusses two guests on a television show. One was "a poised, intelligent young woman who'd been rejected as a contestant for the Miss Toronto title. She is a paraplegic. The organizers' excuse for disqualifying her: 'We couldn't fit the choreography around you.' Another guest was a former executive of the Miss Universe contest. He declared, 'Her participation in a beauty contest would be like having a blind man compete in a shooting match'" (Matthews 1985: 48).

binding or extensive genital mutilation.[5] But I believe that this does not exhaust the meaning of the term "elective" and that the term performs a seductive role in facilitating the ideological camouflage of the *absence of choice*. Similarly, I believe that the word "cosmetic" serves an ideological function in hiding the fact that the changes are *noncosmetic*: they involve lengthy periods of pain, are permanent, and result in irreversibly alienating metamorphoses such as the appearance of youth on an aging body.

There are two important ideological, choice-diminishing dynamics at work that affect women's choices in the area of cosmetic surgery. The first of these is the *pressure to achieve perfection through technology*. The second is the *double-pathologizing of women's bodies*. The history of Western science and Western medical practice is not altogether a positive one for women. As voluminous documentation has shown, cell biologists, endocrinologists, anatomists, sociobiologists, gynecologists, obstetricians, psychiatrists, surgeons, and other scientists have assumed, hypothesized, or "demonstrated" that women's bodies are generally inferior, deformed, imperfect, and/or infantile.

Now, women are being pressured to see plainness or being ugly as a form of pathology. Consequently, there is strong pressure to be beautiful in relation to the allegedly voluntary nature of "electing" to undergo cosmetic surgery. It is clear that pressure to use this technology is on the increase. Cosmetic surgeons report on the wide range of clients who buy their services, pitch their advertising to a large audience through the use of the media, and encourage women to think, metaphorically, in terms of the seemingly trivial "nips" and "tucks" that will transform their lives. As cosmetic surgery becomes increasingly normalized through the concept of the female "makeover" that is translated into columns and articles in the print media or made into nationwide television shows directed at female viewers, as the "success stories" are invited on to talk shows along with their "makers," and as surgically transformed women win the Miss America pageants, women who refuse to submit to the knives and to the needles, to the anesthetics and the bandages, will come to be seen as deviant in one way or another. Women who refuse to use these technologies are already becoming stigmatized as "unliberated," "not caring about their appearance" (a sign of disturbed gender identity and low self-esteem according to various health-care professionals), as "refusing to be all that they could be" or as "granola-heads."

And as more and more success comes to those who do "care about themselves" in this technological fashion, more coercive dimensions enter the scene. In the past, only those women who were perceived to be *naturally* beautiful (or rendered beautiful through relatively conservative superficial artifice) had access to forms of power and economic social mobility closed off to women regarded as plain or

5 It is important here to guard against facile and ethnocentric assumptions about beauty rituals and mutilation. See Lakoff and Scherr (1984) for an analysis of the relativity of these labels and for important insights about the fact that use of the term "mutilation" almost always signals a distancing from and reinforcement of a sense of cultural superiority in the speaker who uses it to denounce what other cultures do in contrast to "our culture."

ugly or old. But now womanly beauty is becoming technologically achievable, a commodity for which each and every woman can, in principle, sacrifice if she is to survive and succeed in the world, particularly in industrialized Western countries. Now technology is making obligatory the appearance of youth and the reality of "beauty" for every woman who can afford it. Natural destiny is being supplanted by technologically grounded coercion, and the coercion is camouflaged by the language of choice, fulfillment, and liberation.

Similarly, we find the dynamic of the double-pathologizing of the normal and of the ordinary at work here. In the technical and popular literature on cosmetic surgery, what have previously been described as *normal* variations of female bodily shapes or described in the relatively innocuous language of "problem areas," are increasingly being described as "deformities," "ugly protrusions," "inadequate breasts," and "unsightly concentrations of fat cells"—a litany of descriptions designed to intensify feelings of disgust, shame, and relief at the possibility of recourse for these "deformities." Cosmetic surgery promises virtually all women the creation of beautiful, youthful-appearing bodies. As a consequence, more and more women will be labeled "ugly" and "old" in relation to this more select population of surgically created beautiful faces and bodies that have been contoured and augmented, lifted and tucked into a state of achieved feminine excellence. I suspect that the naturally "given," so to speak, will increasingly come to be seen as the technologically "primitive"; the "ordinary" will come to be perceived and evaluated as the "ugly." Here, then, is the *third paradox*: that the technological beauty imperative and the pathological inversion of the normal are coercing more and more women to "choose" cosmetic surgery.

V. Are there any Politically Correct Feminist Responses to Cosmetic Surgery?

Attempting to answer this question is venturing forth into political quicksand. Nevertheless, I will discuss two very different sorts of responses that strike me as having certain plausibility: the response of refusal and the response of appropriation.[6] I regard both of these as utopian in nature.

---

6 One possible feminist response (that, thankfully, appears to go in *and* out of vogue) is that of feminist fascism, which insists on a certain particular and quite narrow range of embodiment and appearance as the only range that is politically correct for a feminist. Often feminist fascism sanctions the use of informal but very powerful feminist "embodiment police," who feel entitled to identify and denounce various deviations from this normative range. I find this feminist political stance incompatible with any movement I would regard as liberatory for women and here I admit that I side with feminist liberals who say that "the presumption must be on the side of freedom" (Warren, 1985) and see that as the lesser of two evils.

The Response of Refusal

In her witty and subversive parable, *The Life and Loves of a She-Devil*, Fay Weldon puts the following thoughts into the mind of the cosmetic surgeon whose services have been bought by the protagonist, "Miss Hunter," for her own plans for revenge:

> He was her Pygmalion, but she would not depend upon him, or admire him, or be grateful. He was accustomed to being loved by the women of his own construction. A soft sigh of adoration would follow him down the corridors as he paced them, visiting here, blessing there, promising a future, regretting a past: cushioning his footfall, and his image of himself. But no soft breathings came from Miss Hunter. [He adds, ominously,] … he would bring her to it. (Weldon 1983: 215–16)

But Miss Hunter continues to refuse, and so will many feminist women. The response of refusal can be recognizably feminist at both an individual and a collective level. It results from understanding the nature of the risks involved—those having to do with the surgical procedures and those related to a potential loss of embodied personal integrity in a patriarchal context. And it results from understanding the conceptual shifts involved in the political technologizing of women's bodies and contextualizing them so that their oppressive consequences are evident precisely as they open up more "choices" to women. "Understanding" and "contextualizing" here mean seeing clearly the ideological biases that frame the material and cultural world in which cosmetic surgeons practice, a world that contains racist, anti-Semitic, eugenicist, and ageist dimensions of oppression, forms of oppression to which current practices in cosmetic surgery often contribute.

The response of refusal also speaks to the collective power of women as consumers to affect market conditions. If refusal is practiced on a large scale, cosmetic surgeons who are busy producing new faces for the "holiday season" and new bellies for the "winter trips to the Caribbean" will find few buyers of their services. Cosmetic surgeons who consider themselves body designers and regard women's skin as a kind of magical fabric to be draped, cut, layered, and designer-labeled, may have to forgo the esthetician's ambitions that occasion the remark that "the sculpting of human flesh can never be an exact art" (Silver 1989). They may, instead, (re)turn their expertise to the victims in the intensive care burn unit and to the crippled limbs and joints of arthritic women. This might well have the consequence of (re)converting those surgeons into healers.

Although it may be relatively easy for some individual women to refuse cosmetic surgery even when they have access to the means, one deep, morally significant facet of the response of refusal is to try to understand and to care about individual women who do choose to undergo cosmetic surgery. It may well be that one explanation for why a woman is willing to subject herself to surgical procedures, anesthetics, postoperative drugs, predicted and lengthy pain, and possible "side effects" that might include her own death, is that her access to other forms of power and empowerment are or appear to be so limited that cosmetic surgery is the primary domain in which she can experience some semblance of self-determination. Choosing an artificial and technologically designed creation of youthful beauty may not only be necessary to an individual woman's material, economic, and social survival. It may also be the way that she is able to choose, to elect a kind of subjective transcendence against a backdrop of constraint, limitation, and immanence.

As a feminist response, individual and collective refusal may not be easy. As Bartky, I, and others have tried to argue, it is crucial to understand the central role that socially sanctioned and socially constructed femininity plays in a male supremacist, heterosexist society. And it is essential not to underestimate the gender-constituting and identity-confirming role that femininity plays in bringing woman-as-subject into existence while simultaneously creating her as patriarchally defined object (Bartky 1988; Morgan 1986). In these circumstances, refusal may be akin to a kind of death, to a kind of renunciation of the only kind of life-conferring choices and competencies to which a woman may have access. And, under those circumstances, it may not be possible for her to register her resistance in the form of refusal. The best one can hope for is a heightened sense of the nature of the multiple double-binds and compromises that permeate the lives of virtually all women and are accentuated by the cosmetic surgery culture. As a final comment, it is worth remarking that although the response of refusal has a kind of purity to recommend it, it is unlikely to have much impact in the current ideological and cultural climate.

The Response of Appropriation

Rather than viewing the womanly/technologized body as a site of political refusal, the response of appropriation views it as the site for feminist action through transformation, appropriation, parody, and protest. This response grows out of that historical and often radical feminist tradition that regards deliberate mimicry, alternative valorization, hyperbolic appropriation, street theater, counter-guerrilla tactics, destabilization, and redeployment as legitimate feminist politics. Here I am proposing a version of what Judith Butler regards as "Femininity Politics" and what she calls "Gender Performatives."

Rather than agreeing that participation in cosmetic surgery and its ruling ideology will necessarily result in further colonization and victimization of women, this feminist strategy advocates appropriating the expertise and technology for feminist ends. One advantage of the response of appropriation is that it does not recommend involvement in forms of technology that clearly have disabling and dire outcomes for the deeper feminist project of engaging "in the historical, political, and theoretical process of constituting ourselves as subjects as well as objects of history" (Hartsock 1990: 170).[7] Women who are increasingly immobilized bodily

7 In recommending various forms of appropriation of the practices and dominant ideology surrounding cosmetic surgery, I think it important to distinguish this set of disciplinary practices from those forms of simultaneous Retreat-and-Protest that Susan Bordo (1989, 20) so insightfully discusses in "The Body and the Reproduction of

through physical weakness, passivity, withdrawal, and domestic sequestration in situations of hysteria, agoraphobia, and anorexia cannot possibly engage in radical gender performatives of an active public sort or in other acts by which the feminist subject is robustly constituted. In contrast, healthy women who have a feminist understanding of cosmetic surgery are in a situation to deploy cosmetic surgery in the name of its feminist potential for parody and protest.

As Butler correctly observes, parody "by itself is not subversive" since it always runs the risk of becoming "domesticated and recirculated as instruments of cultural hegemony." She then goes on to ask, in relation to gender identity and sexuality, what words or performances would compel a reconsideration of the *place* and stability of the masculine and the feminine? And what kind of gender performance will enact and reveal the performativity of gender itself in a way that destabilizes the naturalized categories of identity and desire? (Butler 1990: 139).

We might, in parallel fashion, ask what sorts of performances would sufficiently destabilize the norms of femininity, what sorts of performances will sufficiently expose the truth of the slogan "Beauty is always made, not born." In response I suggest two performance-oriented forms of revolt.

The first form of revolt involves revalorizing the domain of the "ugly" and all that is associated with it. Although one might argue that the notion of the "ugly" is parasitic on that of "beauty," this is not entirely true since the ugly is also contrasted with the plain and the ordinary, so that we are not even at the outset constrained by binary oppositions. The ugly, even in a beauty-oriented culture, has always held its own fascination, its own particular kind of splendor. Feminists can use that and explore it in ways that might be integrated with a revalorization of being old, thus simultaneously attacking the ageist dimension of the reigning ideology. Rather than being the "culturally mired subjects" of Butler's analysis, women might constitute themselves as culturally liberated subjects through public participation in Ms. Ugly Canada/America/Universe/Cosmos pageants *and use the technology of cosmetic surgery* to *do so.*

Contemplating this form of revolt as a kind of imaginary model of political action is one thing; actually altering our bodies is another matter altogether. And

---

Femininity": hysteria, agoraphobia, and anorexia. What cosmetic surgery shares with these gestures is what Bordo remarks upon, namely, the fact that they may be "viewed as a surface on which conventional constructions of femininity are exposed starkly to view, through their inscription in extreme or hyperliteral form." What is different, I suggest, is that although submitting to the procedures of cosmetic surgery involves pain, risks, undesirable side effects, and living with a heightened form of patriarchal anxiety, it is also fairly clear that, most of the time, the pain and risks are relatively short-term. Furthermore, the outcome often appears to be one that generally enhances women's confidence, confers a sense of well-being, contributes to a greater comfortableness in the public domain, and affirms the individual woman as self-determining and risk-taking individual. All these outcomes are significantly different from what Bordo describes as the "languages of horrible suffering" (Bordo 1989, 20) expressed by women experiencing hysteria, agoraphobia, and anorexia.

the reader may well share the sentiments of one reviewer of this paper who asked: "Having one-self surgically mutilated in order to prove a point? Isn't this going too far?" I don't know the answer to that question. If we cringe from contemplating this alternative, this may, in fact, testify (so to speak) to the hold that the beauty imperative has on our imagination and our bodies. If we recoil from *this* lived alteration of the contours of our bodies and regard it as "mutilation," then so, too, ought we to shirk from contemplation of the cosmetic surgeons who de-skin and alter the contours of women's bodies so that we become more and more like athletic or emaciated (depending on what's in vogue) mannequins with large breasts in the shop windows of modern patriarchal culture. In what sense are these not equivalent mutilations?

What this feminist performative would require would be not only genuine celebration of but *actual* participation in the fleshly mutations needed to produce what the culture constitutes as "ugly" so as to destabilize the "beautiful" and expose its technologically and culturally constitutive origin and its political consequences. Bleaching one's hair white and applying wrinkle-inducing "wrinkle creams," having one's face and breasts surgically pulled down (rather than lifted), and having wrinkles sewn and carved into one's skin might also be seen as destabilizing actions with respect to aging. And analogous actions might be taken to undermine the "lighter is better" aspect of racist norms of feminine appearance as they affect women of color.

A second performative form of revolt could involve exploring the commodification aspect of cosmetic surgery. One might, for example, envision a set of "Beautiful Body Boutique" franchises, responsive to the particular "needs" of a given community. Here one could advertise and sell a whole range of bodily contours; a variety of metric containers of freeze-dried fat cells for fat implantation and transplant; "body configuration" software for computers; sewing kits of needles, knives, and painkillers; and "skin-Velcro" that could be matched to fit and drape the consumer's body; variously sized sets of magnetically attachable breasts complete with discrete nipple pumps; and other inflation devices carefully modulated according to bodily aroma and state of arousal. Parallel to the current marketing strategies for cosmetic breast surgeries, commercial protest booths, complete with "before and after" surgical makeover displays for penises, entitled "The Penis You Were Always Meant to Have" could be set up at various medical conventions and health fairs; demonstrations could take place outside the clinics, hotels, and spas of particularly eminent cosmetic surgeons—the possibilities here are endless. Again, if this ghoulish array offends, angers, or shocks the reader, this may well be an indication of the extent to which the ideology of compulsory beauty has anesthetized our sensibility in the reverse direction, resulting in the domesticating of the procedures and products of the cosmetic surgery industry.

In appropriating these forms of revolt, women might well accomplish the following: acquire expertise (either in fact or in symbolic form) of cosmetic surgery to challenge the coercive norms of youth and beauty, undermine the power dynamic built into the dependence on surgical experts who define themselves as aestheticians of women's bodies, demonstrate the radical malleability of the cultural commodification of women's bodies, and make publicly explicit the political role that technology can play in the construction of the feminine in women's flesh.

Conclusion

I have characterized both these feminist forms of response as utopian in nature. What I mean by "utopian" is that these responses are unlikely to occur on a large scale even though they may have a kind of ideal desirability. In any culture that defines femininity in terms of submission to men, that makes the achievement of femininity (however culturally specific) in appearance, gesture, movement, voice, bodily contours, aspirations, values, and political behavior obligatory of any woman who will be allowed to be loved or hired or promoted or elected or simply allowed to live, and in any culture that increasingly requires women to purchase femininity through submission to cosmetic surgeons and their magic knives, refusal and revolt exact a high price. I live in such a culture.

Acknowledgments

Many thanks to the members of the Canadian Society for Women in Philosophy for their critical feedback, especially my commentator, Karen Weisbaum, who pointed out how strongly visualist the cosmetic surgery culture is. I am particularly grateful to Sarah Lucia Hoagland, keynote speaker at the 1990 C-SWIP conference, who remarked at my session, "I think this is all wrong." Her comment sent me back to the text to rethink it in a serious way.

Postscript: All of me … Why Don't You Nip/Tuck/Suck/Inject/Laser ALL of me?

> As people become richer, they start to strive for more beyond the basic needs of filling their stomachs and looking for a roof over their heads. Now people will proudly admit they had done plastic surgery as it's perceived as a sign of affluence and sophistication.[8] (Zhang Wei, plastic surgeon in Shanghai)

8 At present it is estimated that China has 1 million plastic surgery clinics which employ approximately 6 million people. 30 million television viewers and 100 million Internet users watch a show called "Lovely Cinderella" in which all the contestants have undergone multiple televised cosmetic surgeries. Artificial Beauty Pageants are held to celebrate the work of cosmetic surgeons (http://www.chinadaily.com.cn and http://www.abc.net.au/news/newsitems).

Medical tourism is booming. All over the world, adolescents and adult women and men who can afford it are making travel plans for a cosmetic surgery holiday, complete with excellent medical care, reduced costs, and relaxing and rejuvenating recuperation in 5-star spas, chalets, resorts (Boasten 2005, Schult, Corey, and Schroeder 2006; http://www.internationalsurgery.com; http://medicaltourism.com; http://www.phudson.com/TOURISM/lipotourism). Costa Rica and Margarita Island off the coast of Venezuela are favored destinations in the western hemisphere; South Africa and Thailand also come highly recommended. Target countries such as the Philippines are building predicted revenue derived from medical tourism into the national budgets and estimates of Gross National Product (Nasrulla 2000, Schult et al. 2006).

What does it mean if you sign up for such a holiday?

Does it mean that you see the purchase of a new aesthetically pleasing, surgically produced body like any other commodified purchase in contemporary global economy? (Gimlin 2000, Sullivan 2001). Is such a body, indeed, a sign of sophistication? An economic necessity? An ostentatious (or discreet) display of affluence? Perhaps such a purchase signifies your participation in a form of national resistance to Anglo-centric neocolonial biopolitics (Hoefflin 1997, McCurdy and Lam 2005). Perhaps it is a rationally planned, universally applicable, biologically hard-wired strategic economic and reproductive strategy you've acted on—when affordable—to attract (and keep) the job and reproductive mate of your dreams? (Etcoff 2000). Today the alternative readings are more and more complicated. I return to them below.

My Reflective Location

I offer neither answers nor judgments. I am seeking understanding. In this search, I turn to Adele Clarke and her co-authors of the brilliant essay, "Biomedicalization: Technoscientific Transformations of Health, Illness, and U.S. Biomedicine." Clarke et al. (2007) argue that one of the basic processes of contemporary biomedicalization involves particular modes of transformations of bodies. They point out that previous modes of medicalization were directed toward regulating and disciplining a unified, relatively static body consisting of surgically targeted particular body parts such as breasts, noses, stomachs, faces, and specific sites of fat cells—in order to bring them into conformity with a single norm. They argue that normalization is no longer the sole—or even primary—focus of technoscientific biomedicine, which places greater emphasis—whether it is genetic or cosmetic—on customization, on "shifting, reshaping, reconstituting, and ultimately transforming bodies for varying purposes, including new identities" (181). Such bodies are whole bodies open to lifelong possibilities of biomedical transformation while engaged in creating new possible technoscientific "selves and identities" (192).[9] It is within this cultural/material theoretical matrix that I now, almost 20 years later, explore cosmetic surgery—and it is in this exciting, brave, and frightening transnational world that I live and continue to explore my/our ever-aging and mortal embodiment (see also Goering 2003, Sobchack 2004).

Real-izing this World

Let me make this more concrete by rejoining, in my imagination, two of the women I cited in "Women and the Knife": Miss Florida and the 49-year-old woman who wanted a face-lift, tummy tuck, and liposuction before seeing a man she hadn't seen for 28 years, hoping to find love "in later life." Let's "fast forward" 20 years into the present.

I name the first one "Marta" and the second one "Marianne." I construct Marta as a married Cuban-American and mother. When she is not busy working for her family, Marta often works long hours as the primary housekeeper for Marianne—whom I construct as the white wife of the eminently successful banker, Walter, with whom she "did find love in later life." In addition to keeping fit with her personal trainer (Brown 2002), Marianne is actively involved in progressive political and philanthropic activities in Miami. Freed from any financial worries, she is happily involved with the two grandchildren her lesbian daughter and her partner have borne and are raising.

Marianne is on her way to Thailand because she has planned a "gift for herself" in time for the winter holidays. Unlike economically privileged women in India in sequined saris and gold jewelry who request specific cosmetic surgical transformations such as a nose job or breast augmentation to celebrate Diwali, the Hindu festival of lights (Bhalla 2006), Marianne is going for a total body cosmetic makeover (Hurwitz 2005, Nash 2005). Having taken advantage of the development of body-morphing cosmetic surgery personal software based on the Visible Human Project (Waldby 2000), she has scanned into her laptop and BlackBerry recent digital photographs of her naked body from a range of perspectives and angles and has made preliminary decisions about the body she wishes to create from her current carnal resources.[10] Having spent decades as a busy vaginally oriented heterosexual,

---

9 See Hurwitz's 2005 book, *Total Body Lift: Reshaping the Breasts, Chest, Arms, Thighs, Hips, Back, Waist, Abdomen and Knees after Weight Loss, Aging, and Pregnancies*. For an emphasis on "scientific grounding" for perfect, ethnically "appropriate" cosmetically surgically created buttocks, see "The Science Behind a Beautiful Butt," in *New Beauty* (Fall/Winter, 2006). The famous plastic surgeon Tom Roberts uses scientific proportionality to create ideal normative Asian, Hispanic, Caucasian female ("athletic" or "voluptuous" ideals), and African American buttocks. For analyses of the coercive homogenizing ethnic/racial reductionism of such "culturally sensitive" practices, see Philipa Rothfield (2005). For other accounts of ethnicity and cosmetic surgery, see Gilman (1999), Kaw (1993), and Blum (2003).

10 I use this language of "resources" because, increasingly, the existing human body is seen, in dominant secular Western technoscience cultures, as a resource for harvesting

Marianne has also decided to take advantage of the elaborate restorative surgical techniques now available under the description of "vaginal rejuvenation" (http://www.tcclinic.com/toronto-preparing-vaginal-rejuvenation-pnp). As a special treat for herself (and for Walter) she has decided to have a labioplasty in order to complete her surgical "genital refinement" since the surgeons promise that "… undergoing labioplasty … can improve a woman's self esteem and general happiness" (http://www.tcclinic.com/toronto-labioplasty.php).

Now in her late 60's, Marianne has chosen the Youthful Restoration Surgical Cluster which will involve a face-lift, eyelid tightening, forehead lift, cheek and chin implants and autologous fat therapy for her wrinkles, breast tightening, general body contouring with liposuction, autologous fat transfer to her breast, lips, and buttocks, arm lifts and thigh lifts, and abdominoplasty. Since she has also lost a considerable amount of weight due to her successful gastric bypass surgery, she is also keen for the surgeon to cut off whatever excess skin can be eliminated all over her body (Hurwitz 2005).

After Marianne scanned in her personal images, she contacted plastic surgeons around the world through the Internet and used her digital images to have virtual consultations. Many women have to borrow money from the financial firm, Aestheticard, Ltd. to finance their cosmetic surgery. As a very privileged woman whose stock portfolio is doing very well Marianne easily covered the cost of this medical holiday (partially because the fees are 40–60 percent less than in North America). Knowing that the standards of medical excellence are now very high around the world in countries that compete for the coveted medical tourist dollars, Marianne consulted surgeons in Singapore, Thailand, Argentina, the Philippines, India, South Africa, Brazil, Costa Rica, and Sri Lanka. Having decided to go to Bangkok, Thailand for her surgery, she made her reservations with Cosmetic Surgery Travel LLC, the prestigious global travel and medical hospitality company (http://www.cosmeticsurgerytravel.com). The day of departure arrived. She waved goodbye to Marta knowing that her home would be in Marta's capable hands during her absence.

When she arrived, Marianne was met by her personal medical concierge at the Bangkok airport. They were then taken by limousine to the Spa-Techno-Aesthetica. Surrounded by profusely blooming gardens and musical fountains, the spa is part of a larger international Wellness complex, which also includes the similarly beautifully groomed Weight-loss Surgery and Body Contouring Centre, the Repro-Genetic Diagnostic and Enhancement Centre, and the Sex-Gender Hormonal-

---

future flesh for transplantation, grafting, or future indeterminate use. For example, autologous cellular regeneration (Isolagan) is based on myofibroblasts, which have been grown outside the body, in large quantity, from a biopsied skin sample and then injected into the scars and wrinkles of the original person. Autologous fat cell regeneration is also used for fat grafting to enlarge, for example, the size/width of penises (http://www.psurg.com; http://www.spamedica.com/service_spec/injectables_fillers.html; http://www.maxfac.com/facial/wrinkles.html).

Surgical Transformation Centre. Marianne then met the team that would provide for her every need during her stay: cosmetic surgeons, anesthetists, nutritionists, makeup artists, dermatologists, trainers, gourmet chefs, nurses, stylists, medical aestheticians, cosmetic dentists, and therapists.

While Marianne confides, privately, that she feels a certain amount of anxiety, her overriding feelings are those of excitement, determination, strength, and anticipatory personal aesthetic pleasure. At the spa, she is delighted to find congenial, sophisticated, and supportive fellow travelers in this carnal adventure (Rosen 2004). Marianne sees this surgical gift-to-herself as the rejuvenating start of the rest of her surgically enhanced and surgically maintained life. She only wishes that she had been able to lead a more comprehensive aesthetic surgical life from her youth.

Multiple Readings; Multiple Discourses

At this point, I leave my (only semi-)fictitious holiday traveler to her own adventures and return to questions which intrigue, trouble, and challenge me and many other feminist theorists as I/we try to understand real-life Mariannes. Like Leibovich (1998) and many others I wonder how I can combine my fascination, enchantment/horror, and excitement with the radical carnal metamorphosis at the heart of contemporary aesthetic technoscience with my deep feminist sense of despair based on contemporary heteronormative cultural norms and practices of cosmetic surgeons (Morgan 2005). I find, more often than not, that I live on a continually swinging hermeneutic pendulum occupying both end points and multiple intermediate positions.

When I think about Marianne, I might, with Brooks (2004), see her as a courageous and bold woman, displaying real leadership as a self-determining woman demonstrating autonomy and independence as an ideal modernist subject (Davis 2003, Jones 2008), particularly since she is not doing this under duress by her husband or coercion by her peers. Like Heyes (2006) or Jones (2008), I would stress the importance of seeing, clearly, that Marianne describes and experiences this as a reward, a gift, or a treat to herself—and this is important given the centrality of compulsory altruism in the lives of many women. On the other hand, I think it is also fair to say that in choosing the specific surgeries she is choosing, Marianne can be seen as acting out of compliance with new aesthetic total-body surgical norms (Jones 2008, Kuczynski 2006, Negrin 2002, Spitzack 1987, 1991, Wolf 1991) and choosing dangerous forms of carnal invasion and technoscientific violence leading to her body commodification in the present and in the future (Sobchack 2004).

Etcoff (2000) and Rosen (2004) might see Marianne as a sophisticated decision-theoretic strategist taking important, pro-active steps towards her continued heterosexual security and economic success status. Balsamo (1996), Brand (2000), and Davis (1997) could interpret Marianne as an exemplar of a liberated, imaginative woman, and Davis (1995, 1997, 2003), Haiken (1997), and Olesen and Olesen (2005) might celebrate the extent to which Marianne's economically privileged position makes her choices of personal empowerment through her body possible and remind us of the discourses of personal empowerment found in the empirical narrative literature. Bordo (1993) and Young (1990, 2005), on the other hand, might be inclined to see Marianne's public participation in a transnational matrix of aesthetic surgery as intensifying an already systemically oppressive "scaling of bodies" since Marianne will, clearly, take her place among a powerful aesthetic surgery elite whose embodiments establish new and powerful norms of legitimizing aesthetic self-pleasure (Kapelovitz 2002).

Sometimes I agree with the perspectives of some cyberfeminists and some corporeal feminists (Grosz 2000, Hawthorne 1999, Klein 1999) who might see Marianne as emblematic of the ideal vanguard cyber-scientific citizen of the twenty-first century, as a woman courageously and enthusiastically open to all the best that contemporary enhancement biomedicine has to offer, an ideal postmodern subject. On the other hand, like Kuczynski (2006), I have argued in the past (1996, 1998) and continue to fear that Marianne will be committed to a life of expensive, biomedical, expert dependence. I also believe that her use of autonomy-rich discourse continues to reinforce illusory neoliberal rhetoric. Such rhetoric not only directs Marianne's attention in a personal, inward direction, it also camouflages the systemic anti-liberal economic and cultural structures within which the Spa(s)-Techno-Aesthetica economically flourish and continue to market their services primarily to women as an increasingly compulsory way of constructing privileged gender in a heteronormative, racialized world. If only the "Enhanced Life" is worth living, what implications does this have for most human beings in the world who live under circumstances of oppressive poverty and global domination by the West? (Goering 2003, Little 1998).

The pendulum continues to swing. Perhaps this is as it should be as I try to think through the complex issues at the heart of the aesthetic surgery matrix (involving theories, institutions, practitioners, cultural forms, subjects and excluded "others"). As Clarke et al. remind us, with the advance of biomedicalization, "… we see new forms of agency, empowerment, confusion, resistance, responsibility, docility, subjugation, citizenship, subjectivity, and morality …" (2003: 185). What these new forms call for in terms of feminist interpretation and assessment of aesthetic surgery is an extremely complex challenge (Balsamo 1996, Jones 2002, Morgan 2004, 2005, Pitts 2003).

Meanwhile, Back at the Mansion, on the Eve of Marianne's Return …

Marta has been busy making sure that Marianne and Walter's home is in excellent shape for Marianne's return. As she polished the silver, she watched one of the shows in Marianne's DVD collection of all the seasons of *Nip/Tuck* (one of the Fox Channel's top four shows, which it broadcasts globally to South America, Europe, Africa, and the Far East [http://www.fxnetwork.com]). Now an attractive "plus size" middle-aged mother of two lovable daughters, Marta thought back to those days when she had her cosmetic surgery as Miss Florida. If she had the money, she knew what she would do now. At the top of her list would be a nose job to restore a more naturally Hispanic nose on her face—along with elastomere implants, buttock threading, and fat grafting to give her those perfect Hispanic buttocks described in Marianne's recent copy of *New Beauty* (Fall–Winter, 2006). These surgeries might make her feel more pride as a Hispanic woman (Gimlin 2006, http://www.phudson.com/ETHNIC; see also Note 9).

As Marta looked at her plump, maternal, middle-aged body in Marianne's full-length mirrors, she dreamt about how she might recapture her slim, pre-partum Miss Florida body. Having read some of Marianne's articles printed off the Internet, she knew that, today, PostPartum Comprehensive Plastic Surgery promises to make you look "… as good or better than before pregnancy" (http://www.phudson.com/postpartum.html). She would love to regain her pre-partum body—and she knew that her husband, Antonio, would love that, too. After all, it was Miss Florida that he was initially attracted to. But she also knew that that kind of total body makeover was completely unaffordable given the family's financial needs. Nevertheless, to keep her dream intact, she promised herself that she would purchase a lottery ticket on her way home. "It can't hurt to dream"—for herself and for her daughters.[11] Or can it?

References

Balsamo, Anne. 1996. *Technologies of the Gendered Body*. Durham, NC and London: Duke University Press.

Barker-Benfield, G. J. 1976. *The Horrors of the Half-Known Life*. New York: Harper and Row.

Bartky, Sandra Lee. 1988. "Foucault, Femininity, and the Modernization of Patriarchal Power," in *Femininity and Foucault: Reflections of Resistance*, edited by Irene Diamond and Lee Quinby. Boston: Northeastern University Press.

Berger, John. 1972. *Ways of Seeing*. New York: Penguin Books.

Bhalla, Nita. 2006. "Cosmetic Surgery Booms Ahead of Diwali," Reuters, 20 Oct. Available at http://www.int.iol.co.za/index.php?set_id=1&click_id=117&art_id=qw1161338941130B253 [accessed: July 25, 2008].

Blum, Virginia. 2003. *Flesh Wounds: The Culture of Cosmetic Surgery*. Berkeley: University of California Press.

Boasten, Michelle. 2005. *Lipo Tourism … The American's "Nip and Tuck" Medical Tourism Guide to Cosmetic Surgery and More Outside the US*. New York, NY: FBE Service Network.

11 See Jones (2008) for an excellent analysis of this complicated, unstable synthesis of modernist and postmodernist personal and cultural dynamics at work in what she analyzes as the powerful master narrative of "MakeOver Culture." Jones and others note that neoliberal models of agency are compatible with understanding aesthetic surgery in relational settings such as mother–daughter relationships, familial kinship identifying marks, and public displays of surgically constructed markers of ethnic affinity.

Bordo, Susan R. 1989. "The Body and the Reproduction of Femininity: A Feminist Appropriation of Foucault," in *Gender/Body/Knowledge: Feminist Reconstructions of Being and Knowing*, edited by Alison Jaggar and Susan Bordo. New Brunswick, NJ: Rutgers University Press.

Bordo, Susan R. 1993. *Unbearable Weight: Feminism, Western Culture, and the Body*. Berkeley: University of California Press.

Brand, Peg Zeglin. 2000. "Bound to Beauty: An Interview with Orlan," in *Beauty Matters*, edited by Peg Zeglin Brand. Bloomington, IN; Indiana University Press, 289–313.

Brooks, Abigail. 2004. "'Under the Knife and Proud of It': An Analysis of the Normalization of Cosmetic Surgery." *Critical Sociology*, 30(2), 207–39.

Brown, Sarah. 2002. "Artificial Intelligence. Can Features be Fashionable? ... The Evolution of Plastic Surgery and the Rise of the (Somewhat) Natural Woman." *Vogue*, 244, 247.

Butler, Judith. 1990. *Gender Trouble: Feminism and the Subversion of Identity*. New York: Routledge.

"Changing Faces." 1989. *Toronto Star*. May 25.

"China's Man-made Beauties Line Up." 2004. *ABC News Online*. 13 December. Available at http://www.abc.net.au/news/newsitems/200412/s1264103.htm. [accessed: July 25, 2008].

"Chinese Women under Knife in Race for Jobs, Husbands." 2006. *China Daily*. 13 January. Available at http://www.chinadaily.com.cn/english/doc/2006-01/13/content_51210. [accessed: March 1, 2006].

Clarke, Adele, Shim, Janet K., Mamo, Laura, Fosket, Jennifer Ruth, and Fishmann, Jennifer R. 2003. "Biomedicalization: Technoscientific Transformations of Health, Illness, and U.S. Biomedicine." *American Sociological Review*, 68(April), 161–94.

Cosmetic Facial Surgery. 2008. http://www.maxfac.com/facial/wrinkles.html. [accessed: July 25, 2008].

"Cosmetic Surgery for the Holidays." 1986. *Sheboygan Press*. New York Times News Service.

Cosmetic Surgery Travel: Exclusive Medical Vacations. http://www.cosmeticsurgerytravel.com [accessed: July 25, 2008].

Davis, Kathy. 1995. *Reshaping the Female Body: The Dilemma of Cosmetic Surgery*. New York, NY: Routledge.

Davis, Kathy. 1997. "'My Body is my Art': Cosmetic Surgery as Feminist Utopia?" in *Embodied Practices: Feminist Perspectives on the Body*, edited by Kathy Davis. London, UK: Sage Publishing.

Davis, Kathy. 2003. *Dubious Equalities and Embodied Differences: Cultural Studies on Cosmetic Surgery*. New York, NY: Rowman and Littlefield.

Dworkin, Sari. 1989. "Not in Man's Image: Lesbians and the Cultural Oppression of Body Image." *Women & Therapy* 8(1,2), 27–39.

E-sthetics: comprehensive online information about cosmetic plastic surgery. http://www.phudson.com/ [accessed: July 25, 2008].

Etcoff, Nancy. 2000. *Survival of the Prettiest: The Science of Beauty*. New York, NY: Anchor.

"Falling in Love Again." 1990. *Toronto Star*. July 23.

Foucault, Michel. 1979. *Discipline and Punish: The Birth of the Prison*, translated by Alan Sheridan. New York: Pantheon.

Gilman, Sander. 1999. *Making the Body Beautiful: A Cultural History of Aesthetic Surgery*. Princeton, NJ: Princeton University Press.

Gimlin, Debra. 2006. "The Absent Body Project: Cosmetic Surgery as a Response to Bodily Dysappearance." *Sociology*, 40(August), 699–716.

Gimlin, Debra. 2000. "Cosmetic Surgery: Beauty as Commodity." *Qualitative Sociology*, 23(1), 77–99.

"Global Broadcast Range for 'Nip/Tuck.'" *FX Network*. http://www.fxnetwork.com/. [accessed: July 25, 2008].

Goering, Sara. 2003. "The Ethics of Making the Body Beautiful: What Cosmetic Genetics Can Learn from Cosmetic Surgery," in *Genetic Prospects: Essays on Biotechnology, Ethics, and Public Policy*, edited by Verna V. Gehring. New York, NY: Rowman and Littlefield, 111–22.

Goodman, Ellen. 1989. "A Plastic Pageant." *Boston Globe*. September 19.

Griffin, Susan. 1978. "The Anatomy Lesson," in *Woman and Nature: The Roaring Inside Her*. New York: Harper & Row.

Grosz, Elizabeth. 2000. "Deleuze's Bergson: Duration, The Virtual, and Politics of the Future," in *Deleuze and Feminist Theory*, edited by Ian Buchanan and Claire Colebrook. Edinburgh, Scotland: Edinburgh University Press, 214–34.

Haiken, Elizabeth. 1997. *Venus Envy: A History of Cosmetic Surgery*. Baltimore, MD: Johns Hopkins University Press.

Haraway, Donna. 1978. "Animal Sociology and a Natural Economy of the Body Politic, Parts I, II." *Signs: Journal of Women in Culture and Society*, 4(1), 21–60.

Haraway, Donna. 1989. *Primate Visions*. New York: Routledge.

Hartsock, Nancy. 1990. "Foucault on Power: A Theory for Women?" in *Feminism/Postmodernism*, edited by Linda Nicholson. New York: Routledge.

Haug, Frigga (ed.) 1987. *Female Sexualization: A Collective Work of Memory*, translated by Erica Carter. London: Verso.

Hawthorne, Susan. 1999. "Cyborgs, Virtual Bodies and Organic Bodies: Theoretical Feminist Responses" in *Cyberfeminism: Connections, Critique, and Creativity*, edited by Susan Hawthorne and Renate Klein. North Melbourne, Victoria: Spinifex, 213–45.

Heyes, Cressida. 2006. "Psychopathology and Normalization: The Case of Cosmetic Surgery and Body Dysmorphic Disorder." Paper presented at the International Symposium: "The Body: Ethos and Ethics," Foucault Society and New School & Hunter College.

Hirshson, Paul. 1987. "New Wrinkles in Plastic Surgery: An Update on the Search for Perfection." *Boston Globe Sunday Magazine*. May 24.

Hoefflin, Steven M. 1997. *Ethnic Rhinoplasty*. New York: Springer.

Hurwitz, Dennis J. 2005. *Total Body Lift: Reshaping the Breasts, Chest, Arms, Thighs, Hips, Back, Waist, Abdomen and Knees After Weight Loss, Aging, and Pregnancies*. New York: NY: MD Publishing.

"Implants Hide Tumors in Breasts, Study Says." 1988. *Toronto Star*. July 29. Summarized from article in *Journal of the American Medical Association*, July 8.

Jones, Amelia. 2002. "Dispersed Subjects and the Demise of the 'Individual': 1990's Bodies In/As Art," in *The Visual Culture Reader*, 2nd edition, edited by Nicholas Mirzoeff. New York: Routledge, 698–710.

Jones, Meredith. 2008. *Skintight: An Anatomy of Cosmetic Surgery*. Oxford: Berg.

Kapelovitz, Dan. 2002. "Slaves to the Scalpel: Cosmetic-Surgery Junkies." *Hustler Magazine*, November. For an electronic pornographic version see: http://www.kapelovitz.com/plastic.htm [accessed: July 25, 2008].

Kaw, Eugenia. 1993. "Medicalization of Racial Features: Asian American Women and Cosmetic Surgery." *Medical Anthropology Quarterly*, 7(1), 74–89.

Klein, Renate. 1999. "The Politics of Cyberfeminism: If I'm a Cyborg Rather Than a Goddess Will Patriarchy Go Away?" in *Cyberfeminism: Connections, Critique, and Creativity*, edited by Susan Hawthorne and Renate Klein. North Melbourne, Victoria: Spinifex, 185–212.

Kuczynski, Alex. 2006. *Beauty Junkies: Inside Our $15 Billion Obsession with Cosmetic Surgery*. New York: Doubleday.

Lakoff, Robin Tolmach and Scherr, Raquel. 1984. *Face Value: The Politics of Beauty.* Boston: Routledge and Kegan Paul.

Leibovich, Lori. 1998. "From Liposuction to Labioplasty. American Women are Getting Nipped, Tucked, and Sucked in Record Numbers. What Does it Mean for Feminism?" *Salon*, January 14 . Available at http://www.salon.com/mwt/feature/1998/01/14feature.html [accessed: July 25, 2008].

Little, Margaret. 1998. "Cosmetic Surgery, Suspect Norms, and the Ethics of Complicity," in *Enhancing Human Traits: Ethical and Social Implications*, edited by Erik Parens, Mark J. Hanson, and Daniel Callahan. Georgetown, MD: Georgetown University Press.

Lowe, Marion. 1982. "The Dialectic of Biology and Culture," in *Biological Woman: The Convenient Myth*, edited by Ruth Hubbard, Mary Sue Henifin, and Barbara Fried. Cambridge, MA: Schenkman.

"Madonna Passionate about Fitness." 1990. *Toronto Star*. August 16, 1990.

Markovic, Mihailo. 1976. "Women's Liberation and Human Emancipation," in *Women and Philosophy: Toward a Theory of Liberation*, edited by Carol Gould and Marx Wartofsky. New York: Capricorn Books.

Matthews, Gwyneth Ferguson. 1985. "Mirror, Mirror: Self-image and Disabled Women." *Women and Disability: Resources for Feminist Research*, 14(1), 47–50.

McCurdy, John Jr. and Lam, Samuel M. 2005. *Cosmetic Surgery of the Asian Face*, 2nd edition. New York and Stuttgart: Thieme.

Medical Tourism. 2006. http://medicaltourism.com. [accessed: May 12, 2006].

Morgan, Kathryn Pauly. 1986. "Romantic Love, Altruism and Self-respect: An Analysis of Simone De Beauvoir." *Hypatia* 1(1), 117–48.

Morgan, Kathryn Pauly. 1989. "Of Woman Born: How Old-fashioned! New Reproductive Technologies and Women's Oppression," in *The Future of Human Reproduction*, edited by Christine Overall. Toronto: The Women's Press.

Morgan, Kathryn Pauly. 1996. "Gender Rites and Rights: The Biopolitics of Beauty and Fertility," in *Philosophical Perspectives on Bioethics*, edited by L. W. Sumner and Joseph Boyle. Toronto, ON: University of Toronto Press, 210–44.

Morgan, Kathryn Pauly. 1998. "Contested Bodies, Contested Knowledges: Women, Health, and the Politics of Medicalization," in *The Politics of Women's Health: Exploring Agency and Autonomy*, edited by Susan Sherwin and the Feminist Health Care Ethics Research Network. Philadelphia, PA: Temple University Press, 83–121.

Morgan, Kathryn Pauly. 2004. "Dysphoric/Euphoria." Critical Response to Carl Elliott's *Better than Well: American Medicine meets the American Dream.* American Philosophical Association (Pacific Division), March 27.

Morgan, Kathryn Pauly. 2005. "Gender Police" in *Foucault and the Government of Disability*, edited by Shelley Tremain. Ann Arbor, MI: University of Michigan Press, 298–328.

Murphy, Julie [Julien S.]. 1984. "Egg Farming and Women's Future," in *Test-tube Women: What Future for Motherhood?* edited by Rita Arditti, Renate Duelli-Klein, and Shelley Minden. Boston: Pandora Press.

Nash, Karen. 2005. "Many Factors Fuel Continued Cosmetic Surgery Boom: Post-Bariatric, Post-Pregnancy Patients Rise; New Materials, Less-Invasive Procedures Fuel Upswing." *Cosmetic Surgery Times*, June.

Nasrulla, Amber. 2000. "Sweet Blade of Youth: Canadian Cosmetic Surgeons are Slicing Inches Off Baby Boomers. But Doctors in Costa Rica and Poland Will Slash a Lot More Off the Price." *Financial Post* Data Group, November 18. Available at http://www.psurg.com/financialpost-2000.html [accessed: July 25, 2008].

Negrin, Llewellyn. 2002. "Cosmetic Surgery and the Eclipse of Identity." *Body and Society*, 8(4), 21–42.

New Beauty. 2006. "The Science behind a Beautiful Butt." Fall/Winter 2006, 76–85.

"New Bodies for Sale." 1985. *Newsweek.* May 27.

Olesen, R. Merrel, Oleson, Marie B. V. 2005. *Cosmetic Surgery for Dummies.* Hoboken, NJ: Wiley Publishing, Inc.

Piercy, Marge. 1980. "Right to Life," in *The Moon is Always Female*. New York: A. Knopf.

Pitts, Victoria. 2003. *In the Flesh: The Cultural Politics of Body Modification*. New York: Palgrave Macmillan.

PSURG: Cosmetic Surgicentre. 2008. http://www.psurg.com [accessed: July 25, 2008].

"The Quest to be a Perfect 10." 1990. *Toronto Star*. February 1.

"Retouching Nature's Way: Is Cosmetic Surgery Worth It?" 1990. *Toronto Star*. February 1.

Rosen, Christine. 2004. "The Democratization of Beauty." *The New Atlantis: A Journal of Technology and Society*, Spring, 19–35.

Rothfield, Philipa. 2005. "Phenomenology and Bioethics," in *Ethics of the Body: Postconventional Challenges*, edited by Margrit Shildrick and Roxanne Mykitiuk. Cambridge, MA: MIT Press, 29–48.

Schult, John, Corey, Jeff, and Schroeder, Curtis. 2006. *Beauty From Afar: A Medical Tourist's Guide to Affordable and Quality Cosmetic Care Outside the United States*. New York: Stewart, Tabori, and Chang.

Sherwin, Susan. 1984–85. "A Feminist Approach to Ethics." *Dalhousie Review*, 64(4), 704–13.

Sherwin, Susan. 1989. "Feminist and Medical Ethics: Two Different Approaches to Contextual Ethics." *Hypatia*, 4(2), 57–72.

Silver, Harold. 1989. "Liposuction isn't for Everybody." *Toronto Star*. October 20.

Sobchack, Vivian. 2004. *Carnal Thoughts: Embodiment and Moving Image Culture*. Berkeley: University of California Press.

Spamedica.com/Injectable Fillers. 2008. http://www.spamedica.com/service_spec/injectables_fillers.html [accessed: July 25, 2008].

Spitzack, Carole. 1987. "Confession and Signification: The Systematic Inscription of Body Consciousness." *Journal of Medicine and Philosophy*, 12, 357–69.

Spitzack, Carole. 1991. "The Confession Mirror: Plastic Images for Surgery," in *The Hysterical Male: New Feminist Theory*, edited by A. Kroker and M. Kroker. Montreal, PQ: New World Perspectives.

Sullivan, Deborah A. 2001. *Cosmetic Surgery: The Cutting Edge of Commercial Medicine in America*. New Brunswick, NJ: Rutgers University Press.

Toronto Cosmetic Clinic. 2008. http://www.tcclinic.com/ [accessed: July 25, 2008].

Waldby, Catherine. 2000. *The Visible Human Project: Informatic Bodies and Posthuman Medicine*. New York: Routledge.

Warren, Mary Anne. 1985. *Gendercide: The Implications of Sex Selection*. Totowa, NJ: Rowman & Allenheld.

Weldon, Fay. 1983. *The Life and Loves of a She-devil*. London: Coronet Books; New York: Pantheon Books.

Williams, John, M.D. and Williams, Jim. 1990. "Say it with Liposuction." From a press release; reported in *Harper's*, August, 1990.

Wolf, Naomi. 1991. *The Beauty Myth: How Images of Beauty are Used Against Women*. New York: William Morrow.

"Woman, 43, Dies after Cosmetic Surgery." 1989. *Toronto Star*. July 7.

Young, Iris Marion. 1990. *Justice and the Politics of Difference*. Princeton, NJ: Princeton University Press.

Young, Iris Marion. 2005. *On Female Body Experience*. New York: Oxford University Press.

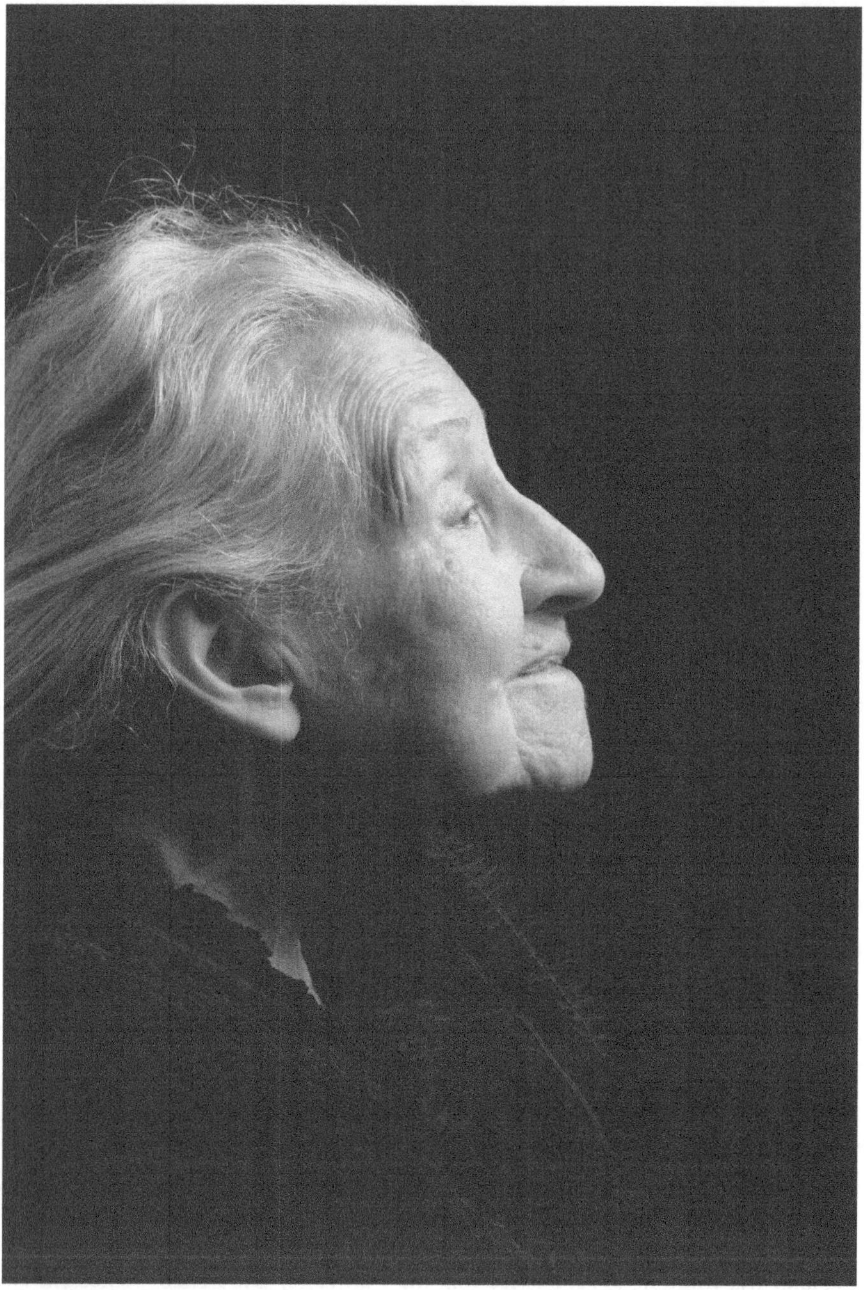

Figure 5.1 "Dorothy" 2006

Source: © Anne de Haas

Chapter 5
Scary Women: Cinema, Surgery, and Special Effects

Vivian Sobchack

> I once heard a man say to his gray-haired wife, without rancor: "I only feel old when I look at you."
>
> Ann Gerike, "On Gray Hair and Oppressed Brains"

> "I'm prepared to die, but not to look lousy for the next forty years."
>
> Anonymous woman to Elissa Melamed

Mirror, Mirror: The Terror of Not Being Young

What is it to be embodied quite literally "in the flesh," to live not only the remarkable elasticity of our skin, its colors and textures, but also its fragility, its responsive and visible marking of our accumulated experiences and our years in scars and sags and wrinkles? How does it feel and what does it look like to age and grow old in our youth-oriented and image-conscious culture—particularly if one is a woman? In an article on the cultural implications of changing age demographics as a consequence of what has been called "the graying of America," James Atlas writes: "Americans regard old age as a raw deal, not as a universal fate. It's a narcissistic injury. That's why we don't want the elderly around: they embarrass us, like cripples or the terminally ill. Banished to the margins, they perpetuate the illusion that our urgent daily lives are permanent, and not just transient things" (Atlas 1997: 59). This cultural—and personal—sense of aging as "embarrassing" and as a "narcissistic injury" cannot be separated from our objectification of our bodies as what they look like rather than as the existential basis for our capacities, as images and representations rather than as the means of our being. Thus, insofar as we subjectively live both our bodies and our images, each not only informs the other, but they also often become significantly confused.

What follows, in this context, is less an argument than a meditation on these confusions as they are phenomenologically experienced, imagined, and represented in contemporary American culture, where the dread of aging—particularly by women—is dramatized and allayed both through the wish-fulfilling fantasies of rejuvenation in certain American movies and the more general, if correlated, faith in the "magic" and "quick fixes" of "special effects," both cinematic and surgical.

This conjunction of aging women, cinema, and surgery is also the conjunction of aesthetics and ethics, foregrounding not merely cultural criteria of beauty and desirability but also their very real as well as representational consequences. As Susan Sontag writes: "Growing older is mainly an ordeal of the imagination—a moral disease, a social pathology—intrinsic to which is the fact that it afflicts women much more than men. It is particularly women who experience growing older with distaste and even shame." (Sontag 1975: 31)[1]

Thus, it is not surprising that, at 63 and as a woman with the privilege of self-reflection, I am always struggling with such distaste and shame in response to the various processes and cultural determinations of my own aging. Indeed, for a long time, despite my attempts at intellectual rationalization, cultural critique, or humor, I found myself unable to dismiss a recurrent image—one that still horrifies me as I reinvoke it. The image? It's me and her, an other—and as her subjective object of a face has aged, the blusher I've worn every morning since I was a teenager has migrated and condensed itself into two distinct and ridiculously intense red circles in the middle of her cheeks. This image—which correspondingly brings a subjective flush of shame and humiliation to my cheeks for the pity and unwilling disgust and contempt with which I objectively regard hers—is that of an aging woman who not only deceives herself into thinking she is still young enough to wear makeup, and poorly applies it, but who also inscribes on her face the caricature both of her own desire and of all that was once (at least to some) desirable. This is not only my face but also the face of clutchy and desperate Norma Desmond. It is whatever happened to Baby Jane, the child star who never grew up but did grow old: ludicrous, grotesque, overpowdered and -rouged, mascara and lipstick bleeding into and around her wrinkled eyes and mouth, maniacally proclaiming an energy that defies containment, that refuses invisibility and contempt.[2]

Although I no longer imagine the extremity of my blusher converging into shameful red circles on my cheeks or fear producing the chilling whiteface of the self-deluded Baby Jane, I still despair of ever being able to reconcile my overall sense of well-being, self-confidence, achievement, and pleasure in the richness of my present with the problematic and often distressing image I see in my mirror. Over the past several years, most of my exaggerated fantasies gone, I nonetheless have become aware not only of my mother's face frequently staring back at me from my own but also of an increasing inability to see myself with any real objectivity at all (as if I ever could). In less than a single minute I can go from utter dislocation and despair as I gaze at a face that seems too old for me, a face

---

1 Sontag's original article was published in *Saturday Review*, Sep. 1972: 29–38. Sontag's insights are echoed in the epigraphs that begin this chapter; see Gerike 1990: 38 and Melamed 1983: 30.

2 I've invoked these images before in an earlier companion piece on aging. See Sobchack 1994: 79–91. The specific film characters mentioned here—now icons for certain generations of women—occur, respectively, in *Sunset Boulevard* (Billy Wilder, 1950) and *Whatever Happened to Baby Jane?* (Robert Aldrich, 1962).

that I "have," to a certain satisfying recognition and pleasure at a face that looks "pretty good for my age," a face that I "am." Most often, however, in the middle register between despair and self-satisfaction I stand before the mirror much like "The Vain but Realistic Queen" who intones, in a wonderful *New Yorker* cartoon, "Mirror, mirror, on the wall: Who—if she lost ten pounds and had her eyes and neck done, and had the right haircut, could, in her age group—be the fairest one of all?"[3]

Whatever my stance, I live now in heightened awareness of the instability of my image of myself, and I think about cosmetic surgery a lot: getting my eyes done, removing the furrows in my forehead, smoothing out the lines around my mouth, and lifting the skin around my jaw. But I am sure I would be disappointed. I know the effects wouldn't last—and I feel, perhaps irrationally but perhaps not, that there would be awful consequences. Indeed, after reading an earlier version of this essay, a friend told me the following joke: "One night, in a vision, God visits a 75-year-old woman. 'How much time do I have left to live?' she asks him; and he replies, 'Thirty-five years.' Figuring that as long as she is going to live another 35 years, she might as well look young again, she spends the following year having a ton of cosmetic surgery: a face-lift, a tummy tuck, her nose reshaped, liposuction, a whole makeover. After all this is finally done, she is hit by a car and killed instantly. Inside the pearly gates, she angrily asks God, 'What happened? I thought you said I had another thirty-five years.' And God replies: 'Sorry, but I didn't recognize you.'" Indeed, I not only dread others not recognizing me but I also dread not recognizing myself. I have this sense that surgery would put me physically and temporally out of sync with myself, would create of me an uncanny and disturbing double who would look the way I "was" and forcibly usurp the moment in which I presently "am." There is a certain irony operative here, of course, since even without surgery I presently don't ever quite recognize myself or feel synchronous with my image when I look at it in mirrors or pictures. And so, although I don't avoid mirrors, I also don't seek them out and I'm not particularly keen on being photographed. Rather, I try very hard to locate myself less in my image than in (how else to say it?) my "comportment."

It is for this reason that I was particularly moved when I first read in *Entertainment Weekly* that Barbra Streisand (only a year younger than I am, a Brooklyn-born Jew, a persistent and passionate woman with a big mouth like me) was remaking and updating *The Mirror Has Two Faces*, a 1959 French film about a housewife who begins a new life after plastic surgery. Barbra's update was to tell the story of "an ugly duckling professor and her quest for inner and outer beauty."[4] Obviously, given that I'm an aging academic woman who has never been secure about her looks, this struck a major chord. Discussing the film's progress and performing its own surgery (a hatchet job) on the middle-aged producer, director,

3 *New Yorker*, Feb. 19 and 26, 2001: 166.

4 Jeffrey Wells, "Mirror, Mirror," *Entertainment Weekly*, Apr. 12, 1996: 8. Subsequent references will be cited in the text.

and star, *Entertainment Weekly* reported that the "biggest challenge faced by the 54-year-old" and "hyper-picky" Barbra:

> was how to present her character. In the original, the mousy housefrau undergoes her transformation via plastic surgery. But Streisand rejected that idea—perhaps because of the negative message—and went with attitude adjustment instead. Which might work for the character, but does it work for the star? "Certain wrinkles and gravitational forces seem to be causing Streisand concern," says one ex-crew member. "She doesn't want to look her age. She's fighting it." (9)

The Mirror—indeed—*Has Two Faces*. Except for the income and, of course, the ability to sing "People," Barbra and I have a lot in common.

Before actually seeing the film (eventually released in 1996), I wondered just what, as a substitute for surgery, Barbra's "attitude adjustment" might mean. And how would it translate to the superficiality of an image—in the mirror, in the movies? Might it mean really good makeup for the middle-aged star? Soft focus? Other forms of special effects that reproduce the work of cosmetic surgery? It is of particular relevance here that recent developments in television technology have produced what is called a "skin contouring" camera that makes wrinkles disappear. In a *TV Guide* article rife with puns about "vanity video" and "video collagen" we are told of this "indispensable tool for TV personalities of a certain age" that "can give a soap opera ingenue a few extra years of playing an ingenue" but was first used "as a news division innovation" to make aging news anchors look younger. According to one news director, the camera "can remove almost all of someone's wrinkles, without affecting their hair or eyes." However, for the "top talents" who "get a little lift from the latest in special effects, ... the magic only lasts as long as the stars remain in front of the camera."[5] This marvelous television camera aside, however, just how far can these special effects that substitute for cosmetic surgery take you—how long before really good makeup transforms you into a grotesque, before soft focus blurs you into invisibility, before special effects transform you into a witch, a ghoul, or a monster? Perhaps this *is* the cinematic equivalent of attitude adjustment. The alternative to cosmetic surgery in what passes for the verisimilitude of cinematic realism is a change in *genre*, a transformation of sensibility that takes us from the "real" world that demonizes middle-aged women to the world of "irreal" female demons: horror, science fiction, and fantasy.

Indeed, a number of years ago, I published an essay on several low-budget science fiction/horror films made in the late 1950s and early 1960s that focused on middle-aged female characters (Sobchack 1994). I was interested in these critically neglected films because, working through genres deemed fantastic,

---

5 J. Max Robins, "A New Wrinkle in Video Technology," *TV Guide* (Los Angeles metropolitan Edition), Sep. 28–Oct. 4, 1996: 57. The news anchors who have benefited from the camera and their ages at the time of the *TV Guide* piece were Dan Rather, 64; Peter Jennings, 58; Tom Brokaw, 56; and Barbara Walters, 65.

they were able to displace and disguise cultural anxieties about women and aging while simultaneously figuring them in your face, so to speak. For example, in *Attack of the 50-Ft. Woman* (Nathan Juran, 1958), through a brief (and laughable) transformative encounter with a giant space alien, wealthy, childless, middle-aged, and brunette Nancy achieves a literal size, power and youthful blondeness her philandering husband, Harry, can no longer ignore as she roams the countryside, wearing a bra and sarong made out of her bed linens, looking for him. In *The Wasp Woman* (Roger Corman, 1959), Janet Starlin, the fortyish and fading owner of a similarly fading cosmetics empire, can no longer serve as the model for advertising her products ("Return to Youth with Janice Starlin!") and overdoses in secret experiments with royal "wasp jelly," which not only reduces but also reverses the aging process. There are, however, side effects, which regularly turn the again youthful cosmetics queen into a murderous insect queen (with high heels, a sheath dress, and a wasp's head). And, in *The Leech Woman* (Edward Dein, 1960), blowzy, alcoholic, despised June becomes her feckless endocrinologist husband's guinea pig as they intrude on an obscure African village to find a secret "rejuvenation serum." Made from orchid pollen mixed with male pituitary fluid (the extraction of which kills its donors), the serum allows June to experience, if only for a while, the simultaneous pleasures of youth, beauty, and revenge—in the tribal ritual of her transformation, she chooses her husband as pituitary donor. *The Leech Woman* is the most blatant of these movies about ageism, not only in plot but also in dialogue. The wizened African woman who offers June her youth speaks before the ritual:

> For a man, old age has rewards. If he is wise, the gray hairs bring dignity and he is treated with honor and respect. But for the aged woman, there is nothing. At best, she's pitied. More often, her lot is of contempt and neglect. What woman lives who has passed the prime of her life who would not give her remaining years to reclaim even for a few moments of joy and happiness and now the worship of men. For the end of life should be its moment of triumph. So it is with the aged women of Nandos, a last flowering of love, beauty—before death.

In each of these low-budget SF-horror films scared middle-aged women are transformed into rejuvenated but scary women—this not through cosmetic surgery but through fantastical means, makeup, and special effects. Introduced as fading (and childless) females still informed by—but an affront to—sexual desire and the process of biological reproduction, hovering on the brink of grotesquerie and alcoholism, their flesh explicitly disgusting to the men in their lives, these women are figured as more horrible in—and more horrified by—their own middle-aged bodies than in or by the bodies of the "unnatural" monsters they become. In this regard Linda Williams's important essay, "When the Woman Looks," is illuminating. Williams argues that there is an affinity declared and a look of recognition and sympathy exchanged between the heroine and the monster in the horror film. The SF-horror films mentioned here, however, collapse the distance of this exchange into a single look of *self-recognition*. Touching on this conflation of woman and monster in its link with aging, Williams writes:

> There is not that much difference between an object of desire and an object of horror as far as the male look is concerned. (In one brand of horror film this difference may simply lie in the age of its female stars. The Bette Davises and Joan Crawfords considered too old to continue as spectacle-objects nevertheless persevere as horror objects in films like *Whatever Happened to Baby Jane?* [1962] and *Hush ... Hush, Sweet Charlotte* [1965]). (Williams 1996: 21)

Indeed, such horror and SF films dramatize what one psychotherapist describes as the culture's "almost visceral disgust for the older woman as a physical being," and they certainly underscore "ageism" as "the last bastion of sexism" (Melamed 1983: 30). These films also recall, particularly in the male—and self—disgust they generate, Simone de Beauvoir's genuine (if, by today's standards, problematic) lament:

> [W]oman is haunted by the horror of growing old. … [T]o hold her husband and to assure herself of his protection, … it is necessary for her to be attractive, to please. … What is to become of her when she no longer has any hold on him? This is what she anxiously asks herself while she helplessly looks on at the degeneration of this fleshly object which she identifies with herself. She puts up a battle. But hair-dye, skin treatments, plastic surgery, will never do more than prolong her dying youth. … But when the first hints come of that fated and irreversible process which is to destroy the whole edifice built up during puberty, she feels the fatal touch of death itself. (Beauvoir 1968: 542)

How, in the face of this cultural context, *as* a face in this cultural context, could a woman not yearn for a rejuvenation serum, not want to realize quite literally the youth and power she once seemed to have? In the cinematic—and moral—imagination of the low-budget SF-horror films I've described above, aging and abject women are thus "unnaturally" transformed. Become suddenly young, beautiful, desirable, powerful, horrendous, monstrous, and deadly, each plays out grand, if wacky, dramas of poetic justice. No plastic surgery here. Instead, through the technological magic of cinema, the irrational magic of fantasy, and a few cheesy low-budget effects, what we get is major "attitude adjustment"—and of a scope that might even satisfy Barbra. The leech woman, wasp woman, and 50-foot woman each literalize, magnify, and enact hyperbolic displays of anger and desire, their youth and beauty represented now as lethal and fatal, their unnatural ascendance to power allowing them to avenge on a grand scale the wrongs done them for merely getting older. Yet, not surprisingly, these films also maintain the cultural status quo—even as they critique it. For what they figure as most grotesque and disgusting is not the monstrousness of the transformation or the monster but rather the "unnatural" conjunction of middle-aged female flesh and still-youthful female desire. And—take heed, Barbra—the actresses who play these pathetic and horrific middle-aged women are always young and beautiful under their latex jowls and aging makeup. Thus, what these fantasies of female rejuvenation give with one hand, they take back with the other. They represent less a grand masquerade of feminist resistance than a retrograde striptease that undermines the double-edged and very temporary narrative power these transformed and empowered middle-aged protagonists supposedly enjoy—that is, "getting their own back" before they eventually "get theirs." And, as is the "natural" order of things in both patriarchal culture and SF-horror films of this sort, they do get theirs—each narrative ending with the restoration and reproduction of social (and ageist) order through the death of its eponymous heroine-monster. Attitude adjustment, indeed!

These low-budget films observe that middle-aged women—as much before as after their transformations and attitude adjustments—are pretty scary. In *Attack of the 50-Ft. Woman*, for example, as Nancy lies in her bedroom after her close encounter of the third kind but before she looms large on the horizon, her doctor explains to her husband the "real cause" of both her "wild" story of an alien encounter and her strange behavior: "When women reach the age of maturity, Mother Nature sometimes overworks their frustration to a point of irrationalism." The screenwriter must have read Freud, who, writing on obsessional neurosis in 1913, tells us: "It is well known, and has been a matter for much complaint, that women often alter strangely in character after they have abandoned their genital functions. They become quarrelsome, peevish, and argumentative, petty and miserly; in fact, they display sadistic and anal-erotic traits which were not theirs in the era of womanliness" (Freud 1950: 130).

Which brings us back again to Barbra, whom it turns out we never really left at all. In language akin to Freud's, the article on the production woes of Barbra's film in *Entertainment Weekly* performs its own form of ageist (psycho)analysis. The "steep attrition rate" among cast and crew and the protracted shooting schedule are attributed to both her "hyper-picky" "perfectionism" and to her being a "meddler" (8). We are also told: "Among the things she fretted over: the density of her panty hose, the bras she wore, and whether the trees would have falling leaves" (9). A leech woman, wasp woman, 50-foot woman—in Freud's terms, an obsessional neurotic: peevish, argumentative, petty, sadistic, and anal-erotic. Poor Barbra. She can't win for losing. Larger than life, marauding the Hollywood countryside in designer clothes and an "adjusted" attitude doesn't get her far from the fear or contempt that attaches to middle-aged women in our culture.

Perhaps Barbra—perhaps I—should reconsider cosmetic surgery. Around ten years younger than Barbra and me and anxious about losing the looks she perceived as the real source of her power, my best friend recently did—although I didn't see the results until long after her operation. Admittedly, I was afraid to: afraid she'd look bad (that is, not like herself or like she had surgery), afraid she'd look good (that is, good enough to make me want to do it). Separated by physical distance, however, I didn't have to confront—and judge—her image, so all I initially knew about her extensive face-lift was from email correspondence. (I have permission to use her words but not her name.) Here, in my face, so to speak, as well as hers were extraordinary convergences of despised flesh, monstrous acts, and malleable image (first "alienated" and later proudly "possessed"). Here, in the very prose of her postings, was the conjunction of actuality and wish, of surgery and cinema, of transformative technologies and the "magic" of "special effects"—all rendered intimately intelligible to us (whether we approve or not) in terms of mortal time and female gender. She wrote, "IT WORKED!" And then she continued:

> My eyes look larger than Audrey Hepburn's in her prime. … I am the proud owner of a fifteen-year old's neckline. Amazing—exactly the effect I'd hoped for. Still swollen … but that was all predicted. What this tendon-tightening lift did (not by any means purely "skin deep"—he actually … redraped the major neck and jaw infrastructure) was reverse the effects of gravity. Under the eyes—utterly smooth, many crow's feet eradicated. The jawline—every suspicion of jowl has been erased. Smooth and tight. Boy, do I look good. The neck—the Candice Bergen turkey neck is gone. The tendons that produce that stringy effect have been severed—forever! OK—what price (besides the $7000) did I pay? Four hours on the operating table. One night of hell due to … a compression bandage that made me feel as if I were being choked. Mercifully (and thanks to Valium) I got through it … Extremely tight from ear to ear—jaw with little range of motion—"ate" liquids, jello, soup, scrambled eggs for the first week. My sutures extend around 80% of my head: *Bride of Frankenstein* city. All (except for the exquisitely fine line under my eyes) are hidden in my hair. But baby I know they're there. Strange reverse-phantom limb sensation. I still have my ears, but I can't exactly feel them … I took Valium each evening the first week to counteract the tendency toward panic as I tried to fall asleep and realized that I could only move 1/4 inch in any direction. Very minimal bruising—I'm told that's not the rule … I still have a very faint chartreuse glow under one eye. With makeup, *voilá*! I can't jut my chin out—can barely make my upper and lower teeth meet at the front. In a few more months, that will relax. And I can live with it. My hair, which was cut, shaved and even removed (along with sections of my scalp), has lost all semblance of structured style. But that too is transitory. The work that was done by the surgeon will last a good seven years. I plan to have my upper eyes done in about three years. This message is for your eyes only. I intend, if pressed, to reveal that I have had my eyes done. Period. Nothing more.[6]

---

6 An illuminating comparison might be made between my friend's detailing of her cosmetic surgery and its aftermath with J. G. Ballard's "Princess Margaret's Face Lift," in *The Atrocity Exhibition* (1990: 111–12). Its opening paragraph reads (and note the focus again on jowls and neck): "As Princess Margaret reached middle age, the skin of both her cheeks and neck tended to sag from failure of the supporting structures. Her naso-labial folds deepened, and the soft tissues along her jaw fell forward. Her jowls tended to increase. In profile the creases of her neck lengthened and the chin-neck contour lost its youthful

But there's plenty more. And it foregrounds the confusions and conflations of surgery and cinema, technology and "magic," of effort and ease, that so pervade our current image culture. Indeed, there is a bitter irony at work here. Having willfully achieved a "seamless" face, my best friend has willingly lost her voice. She refuses to speak further of the time and labor and pain it took to transform her. The whole point is that, for the magic to work, the seams—both the lines traced by age and the scars traced by surgery—must not show. Thus, as Kathleen Woodward notes in her wonderful essay "Youthfulness as a Masquerade": "Unlike the hysterical body, whose surface is inscribed with symptoms, the objective of the surgically youthful body is to speak nothing" (1988: 133–4). But this is not the only irony at work here. At a more structural level this very lack of disclosure, this silence and secrecy, is an *essential* (if paradoxical) element of a culture increasingly driven—by both desire and technology—to extreme extroversion, to utter disclosure. It is here that cosmetic surgery and the special effects of the cinema converge and are perceived as phenomenologically reversible in what has become our current morphological imagination. Based on the belief that desire—through technology—can be materialized, made visible, and thus "realized," such morphological imagination does a perverse, and precisely superficial, turn on Woodward's distinction between the hysterical body that displays symptoms and the surgically youthful body that silences such display. That is, symptoms and silence are conflated as *the image of one's transformation* and *one's transformation of the image* become reversible phenomena. These confusions and conflations are dramatized most literally, of course, in the genre of fantasy, where "plastic surgery" is now practiced through the seemingly effortless, seamless transformations of digital morphing.

Indeed, the morphological figurations of fantasy cinema not only allegorize impossible human wish and desire but also extrude and thus fulfill them. In this regard two such live-action films come to mind, each not only making visible (and seemingly effortless) incredible alterations of an unprecedented plastic and elastic human body but also rendering human affective states with unprecedented superficiality and literalism. The films are *Death Becomes Her* (Robert Zemeckis, 1992) and *The Mask* (Chuck Russell, 1994)—both technologically dependent on digital morphing, both figuring the whole of human existence as extrusional, superficial, and plastic. *The Mask*, about the transformation and rejuvenation of the male psyche and spirit, significantly plays its drama out on—and as—the surface of the body. When wimpy Stanley Ipkiss is magically transformed by the ancient

outline and became convex" (111). For similar graphic description, see also MacFarquhar 1997: 68: "Consider the brutal beauty of the face-lift. … If you're getting a blepharoplasty (an eye job), the doctor will slice open the top of each of your eyelids, peel the skin back, and trim the fat underneath with a scalpel, or a laser. If you're also in for a brow-lift, the doctor might carve you to the bone from the top of your forehead down along your hairline; slowly tear the skin away from the bloody muck it's attached to underneath; and then stretch it back and staple it near the hairline. You may suffer blindness, paralysis, or death as a consequence, but most likely you'll be fine."

mask he finds, there is no masquerade, no silence, since every desire, every psychic metaphor, is extroverted, materialized, and made visible. His tongue "hangs out" and unrolls across the table toward the object of his desire. He literally "wears his heart on his sleeve" (or thereabouts). His destructive desires are extruded from his hands as smoking guns. Thus, despite the fact that one might describe Jim Carrey's performance as "hysterical," how can one possibly talk about the Mask's body in terms of hysterical "symptoms" when everything "hangs out" as extroverted id and nothing is repressed "inside" or "deep down"? Which makes it both amusing and apposite, then, that one reviewer says of *The Mask*: "The effects are show-stopping, but the film's hollowness makes the overall result curiously depressing."[7] Here, indeed, there is no inside, there are no symptoms, there is no silence; there is only display.

Death Becomes Her functions in a similar manner, although, here, with women as the central figures, the narrative explicitly foregrounds age and literal rejuvenation as its central thematic—youth and beauty are the correlated objects of female desire. Indeed, what's most interesting (although not necessarily funny) about *Death Becomes Her* is that plastic surgery operates in the film twice over. At the narrative level its wimpy hero, Ernest Menville, is a famous plastic surgeon—seduced away from his fiancée, Helen, by middle-aging actress Madeline Ashton, whom we first see starring in a musical flop based on Tennessee Williams's *Sweet Bird of Youth*. Thanks to Ernest's surgical skill (which we never actually *see* on the screen), Madeline finds a whole new career as a movie star. Here, J. G. Ballard, in a chapter of his *The Atrocity Exhibition* called "Princess Margaret's Face Lift," might well be glossing Madeline's motivations in relation to Ernest in *Death Becomes Her*. Ballard writes: "In a TV interview … the wife of a famous Beverly Hills plastic surgeon revealed that throughout their marriage her husband had continually re-styled her face and body, pointing a breast here, tucking in a nostril there. She seemed supremely confident of her attractions … as she said: 'He will never leave me, because he can always change me'" (Ballard 1990: 111). *Death Becomes Her* plays out this initial fantasy but goes on to exhaust the merely human powers of Madeline's surgeon husband to avail itself of "magic"—both through narrative and "special" morphological effects. Seven quick years of screen time into the marriage, henpecked, alcoholic Ernest is no longer much use to Madeline. Told by her beautician that he—and cosmetic surgery—can no longer help her, the desperate woman seeks out a mysterious and incredibly beautiful "Beverly Hills cult priestess" (significantly played by onetime Lancôme pitchwoman, Isabella Rossellini), who gives her a youth serum that grants eternal life, whatever the condition of the user's body.

At this point the operation of plastic surgery extends from the narrative to the representational level. Indeed, *Death Becomes Her* presents us with the first digitally produced skin—and the "magic" transformations of special computer

7 CineBooks' Motion Picture Guide, review of *The Mask*, dir. Chuck Russell, *Cinemania 96* CD-ROM (Microsoft, 1992–95).

graphic and cosmetic effects instantaneously nip and tuck Madeline's buttocks, smooth and lift her face and breasts with nary a twinge of discomfort, a trace of blood, or a trice of effort, and reproduce her as "young." Indeed, what Rossellini's priestess says of the youth serum might also be said of the cinematic effects: "A touch of magic in this world obsessed by science." Thus, in the service of instant wish fulfillment, this phrase in the narrative disavows not only the extensive calculations of labor and time involved in its own digital effects but also the labor and time entailed by the science and practice of cosmetic surgery.

The film's literalization of anxiety and desire in relation to aging is carried further still. That is, inevitably, the repressed signs of age return and are also reproduced and literalized along with the signs of youth and beauty. When rejuvenated Madeline breaks her neck after being pushed down a flight of stairs by Ernest, she lives on (although medically dead) with visible and hyperbolic variations of my friend's despised "Candace Bergen turkey neck." (Her celebration of the fact that "the tendons that produce that stringy effect have been severed—forever!" certainly resonates here in the terrible, but funny, computer graphic corkscrewing of Madeline's neck after her fatal fall.) And, after Madeline shoots the returned and vengeful Helen (who has also taken the serum), Helen walks around with a hole in her stomach—a "blasted" and "hollow" woman, however youthful. ("I can see right through you," Madeline says to her.) Ultimately, the film unites the two women—"Mad" and "Hel"—in their increasingly unsuccessful attempts to maintain their literally dead and peeling skin, to keep from "letting themselves go," from "falling apart"—which, at the film's end, they quite literally do.

In both *The Mask* and *Death Becomes Her* cinematic effects and plastic surgery become reversible representational operations—literalizing desire and promising instant and effortless transformation. Human bodily existence is foregrounded as a material surface amenable to endless manipulation and total visibility. However, there is yet a great silence, a great *invisibility*, grounding these narratives of surface and extroversion. The labor, effort, and time entailed by the real operations of plastic surgery (both cinematic and cosmetic) are ultimately disavowed. Instead, we are given a screen image (both psychoanalytic and literal) that attributes the laborious, costly, and technologically based reality that underlies bodily transformation to the non-technological properties of, in the one instance, the mask, a primitive and magical fetish, and in the other, a glowing potion with "a touch of magic." Of course, like all cases of disavowal, these fantasies turn in and around on themselves like a Möbius strip to ultimately break the silence and reveal the repressed on the same side as the visible screen image.

That is, on the screen side, the technological effects of these transformation fantasies are what we came for, what we want "in our face." But we want these effects without wanting to see the technology, without wanting to acknowledge the cost, labor, time, and effort of its operations—all of which might curb our desire, despoil our wonder, and generate fear of pain and death. As Larissa MacFarquhar notes: "Surely, the eroticizing of cosmetic surgery is a sign that the surgery is no longer a gory means to a culturally dictated end but, rather, an end in itself" (1997:

68). Indeed, like my friend who wants the effects of her face-lift to be seen but wants the facts of her costly, laborious, lengthy, and painful operation to remain hidden, our pleasure comes precisely from this "appearance" of seamless, effortless, "magical" transformation. Yet on the other repressed side, we are fascinated by the operation—its very cost, difficulty, effortfulness. We cannot help but bring them to visibility. There are now magazines, videos, and websites devoted to making visible not only the specific operations of cinematic effects but also surgical effects. (Perhaps the most "in your face" of these can be found on a website called—no joke—"Dermatology in the Cinema," where dermatologist Dr. Vail Reese does a film survey of movie stars' skin conditions, both real and cinematic.)[8] These tell-all revelations are made auratic by their previous repression and through a minute accounting of the technology involved, hours spent, effort spent, dollars spent. My friend, too, despite her desire for secrecy, is fascinated by her operation and the visibility of her investment. Her numeracy extends from money to stitches but is most poignant in its temporal lived dimensions: four hours on the operating table, one night of hell, a week of limited jaw motion, time for her hair to grow back, a few months for her upper and lower jaws to "relax," three years before she will do her eyelids, seven years before the surgeon's work is undone again by time and gravity. The "magic" of plastic surgery (both cinematic and cosmetic) costs always an irrecoverable—and irrepressible—portion of a mortal life.

And a mortal life must *live through* its operations, not magically, instantaneously, but *in time*. It is thus apposite and poignant that, off screen, Isabella Rossellini, who plays and is fixed forever as the eternal high priestess of youth and beauty in both *Death Becomes Her* and old Lancôme cosmetic ads, has joined the ranks of the onscreen "wasp woman," Janet Starlin. After 14 years as the "face" of Lancôme cosmetics, she was fired at age 42 for getting "too old."[9] Unlike the wasp woman, however, Rossellini can neither completely reverse the aging process nor murder those who find her middle-aged flesh disgusting. Thus, it is also apposite and poignant that attempts to reproduce the fantasies of the morphological imagination in the real world are doomed to failure: medical cosmetic surgery never quite matches up to the seemingly effortless and perfect plastic surgeries of cinema and computer. This disappointment with the real thing becomes ironically explicit when representational fantasies incorporate the real to take a documentary turn. Discussing the real face-lift and its aftermath of a soap opera actress incorporated into the soap's televised narrative, Woodward cites one critic's observation that "the viewer inspects the results and concludes that they are woefully disappointing." (Woodward 1988: 135)[10]

---

8 See: http//:www.skinema.com [accessed: October 24, 2003].

9 For more on the Lancôme episode and Rossellini's bitterness about it see Rossellini 1997.

10 Woodward is citing film and cultural critic Patricia Mellencamp.

This disappointment with the "real thing" also becomes explicit in my friend's continuing emails. Along with specific descriptions of her further healing, she wrote:

> Vivian, I'm going through an unsettling part of this surgical journey. When I first got home, the effect was quite dramatic—I literally looked twenty years younger. Now what's happened: the swelling continues to go down, the outlines of the "new face" are still dramatically lifted. BUT, the lines I've acquired through a lifetime of smiling, talking, being a highly expressive individual, are returning. Not all of them—but enough that the effect of the procedure is now quite natural and I no longer look twenty years younger. Maybe ten max. … I'm experiencing a queasy depression. Imagining that the procedure didn't work. That in a few weeks I'll look like I did before the money and the lengthy discomfort. Now I scrutinize, I imagine, I am learning to hate the whole thing. Most of all, the heady sense of exhilaration and confidence is gone. In short, I have no idea any longer how the hell I look.

Which brings me back to myself before the mirror—and again to Barbra, both behind and in front of the camera. There is no way here for any of us to feel superior in sensibility to my friend. Whether we like it or not, as part of our culture, we have all had "our eyes done." As Jean Baudrillard writes: "We are under the sway of a surgical compulsion that seeks to excise negative characteristics and remodel things synthetically into ideal forms. Cosmetic surgery: a face's chance configuration, its beauty or ugliness, its distinctive traits, its negative traits—all these have to be corrected, so as to produce something more beautiful than beautiful: an ideal face." (Baudrillard 1993: 45)[11] With or without medical surgery we have been technologically altered, both seeing differently and seeming different than we did in a time before either cinema or cosmetic surgery presented us with their reversible technological promises of immortality and idealized figurations of magical self-transformation—that is, transformation without time, without effort, without cost.

To a great extent, then, the bodily transformations of cinema and surgery inform each other. Cinema *is* cosmetic surgery—its fantasies, its makeup, and its digital effects able to "fix" (in the doubled sense of repair and stasis) and to fetishize and to reproduce faces and time as both "unreel" before us. And, reversibly, cosmetic surgery *is* cinema, creating us as an image we not only learn to enact in a repetition compulsion but also must—and never can—live up to. Through

11 Of special interest in surgically constructing the ideal face is the French performance artist, Orlan, who has publicly undergone any number of surgeries in an ironic attempt to achieve the forehead of Mona Lisa, the eyes of Psyche (from Gérôme), the chin of Botticelli's Venus, the mouth of Boucher's Europa and the nose from an anonymous sixteenth-century painting of Diana. On Orlan and the connection between special effects and cosmetic surgery see Duckett 2000: 209–23.

their technological "operations"—the work and cost effectively hidden by the surface "magic" of their transitory effects, the cultural values of youth and beauty effectively reproduced and fixed—we have become subjectively "derealized" and out of sequence with ourselves as, paradoxically, these same operations have allowed us to objectively reproduce and "realize" our flesh "in our own image." These days, as MacFarquhar puts it, "sometimes pain, mutilation, and even death are acceptable risks in the pursuit of perfection"—and this because the plasticity of the image (and our imagination) has overwhelmed the reality of the flesh and its limits. Indeed, as of 1996, "three million three hundred and fifty thousand cosmetic surgical procedures were performed, and more than one and a half million pounds of fat were liposuctioned out of nearly three hundred thousand men and women." (MacFarquhar 1997: 68)[12]

Over email, increments of my friend's ambiguous "recovery" from realizing her fantasies of transformation and rejuvenation seemed to be in direct proportion to the diminishing number of years young she felt she looked: "Vivian, I've calmed down, assessed the pluses and minuses and decided to just fucking go on with it. Life, that is. They call it a 'lift' for a reason. … The face doesn't look younger (oh, I guess I've shaved five to eight years off), but it looks better. OK. Fine. Now it's time to move on." But later the fantasy of realization reemerges—for the time being, at least, with real and sanguine consequences: "Vivian, the response has been terrific—everybody is dazzled, but they can't quite tell why. It must be the color I'm wearing, they say, or my hair, or that I am rested. At any rate, I feel empowered again."

In sum, I don't know how to end this—nor could I imagine at the time of my friend's rejuvenation how, without cosmetic surgery, Barbra would end her version of *The Mirror Has Two Faces*. Thus, not only for herself, but also for the wasp woman, for my friend, for Isabella Rossellini, and for me, I hoped that Barbra—both on screen and off—would survive her own cinematic reproduction. Unfortunately, she did not. "Attitude adjustment" was overwhelmed by image adjustment in her finished film: to wit, a diet, furious exercise, good makeup, a new hairdo, and a Donna Karan little black dress. Despite all her dialogue, Barbra had nothing to say; instead, like my friend, she silenced and repressed her own middle-aging—first, reducing it to a generalized discourse on inner and outer beauty and then displacing and replacing it on the face and in the voice of her bitter, jealous, "once beautiful," and "much older" mother (played by the still spectacular Lauren Bacall). Barbra's attitude, then, hadn't adjusted at all.[13]

---

12 In regard to the meaning of these statistics (and I don't fully agree with her), MacFarquhar writes: "It doesn't make sense to think about cosmetic surgery as a feminist issue these days, since more and more men—a fifth of all patients in 1996—are electing to undergo it" (68).

13 For a particularly devastating but accurate (and funny) send-up of *The Mirror Has Two Faces*, see the pseudonymous Libby Gelman-Waxner's "Pretty Is as Pretty Does," *Premiere* 10, no. 6 (Feb. 1997). Reading the film's central thematic as asking and

Susan Bordo ponders "the glossy world " of media imagery that "feeds our eyes and focuses our desires on creamy skin, perfect hair, bodies that refuse awkwardness and age. It delights us like visual candy, but it also makes us sick with who we are and offers remedies that promise to close the gap—at a price" (Bordo 1997: B8). I finally did get to see my rejuvenated friend in the flesh. She looked pretty much the same to me. And, at the 1996 Academy Awards (for which the song in *The Mirror Has Two Faces* received the film's only nomination), Barbra was still being characterized by the press as "peevish" and "petty." And that wasn't all, poor woman (money and voice aside). Two years after linking Barbra with her SF-horror film counterparts and ironically figuring her as marauding the countryside as a middle-aged monster in designer clothes, I found my imagination elaborately realized in a 1998 episode of the animated television series, *South Park.* Here was featured a huge "MechaStreisand" trashing the town like Godzilla. Tellingly, one of the South Park kids asks: "Who is Barbra Streisand?" and is answered thus: "She's a really old lady who wants everybody to think she's forty-five." This coincidence may seem uncanny but, indeed, suggests just how pervasively middle-aged women, particularly those with power like Streisand, are demonized and made monstrous in our present culture.

I, in the meantime, have become more comfortable in my ever-aging skin. I'm old enough now to feel distant from the omnipresent appeals around me to "look younger" and to "do" something about it. Indeed, after my friend's surgery I vowed to be kinder to my mirror image. In the glass (or on the screen), that image is, after all, thin and chimerical, whereas I, on my side of it, am grounded in the fleshy thickness and productivity of a life, in the substance—not the reproduced surface—of endless transformation. Thus, now each time I start to fixate on a new line or wrinkle or graying hair in the mirror, now each time I envy a youthful face on the screen, I am quick to remember that on my side of the image I am not so much ever aging as always becoming.

Postscript: (Not Quite) Post-Mortem

More than a decade after publishing the essay above, I've been asked to revisit it. No longer "middle-aged" (I'm 65 as I write this), I observe that I'm less angst-ridden about aging than I was ten years ago. Indeed, I'm now quite comfortable in my own skin—which I have not had stretched and tanned (through surgical or

responding to Streisand's increasingly desperate question "Is Barbra pretty?," Gelman-Waxner also recognizes the displaced age issue—and, dealing with the confrontation scene between daughter and mother in which the latter reveals her jealousy and finally admits her daughter's beauty, she writes: "Watching a 54-year-old movie star haranguing her mother onscreen is a very special moment; it's like seeing the perfect therapy payoff, where your mom writes a formal note of apology for your childhood and has it printed as a full-page ad in the *Times*" (38).

other means) into the horror film "leather face" one sees on many older women who live, as I do, in Los Angeles. Nor have I lost sight (or use) of my blusher or become so over-powdered as to resemble Baby Jane—whom I valorized above for her anger, spite, and manic glee. I also haven't become invisible; indeed, I smile at the thought that such a fate ever occurred to me. Comfortable in my own skin (a condition more of good health than of looks), I know who I am: I recognize myself in the mirror.

I'm aware, of course, that I'm one of the lucky women who have "realized" themselves fully, had relationships and a child, and achieved financial independence, a certain degree of fame, and a great deal of "presence." I'm seen now as "dignified," "serene," "centered" and, yes, "powerful." Note that "hot" and "sexy" are not on this list (although, on occasion, they do crop up, albeit not together). I don't really mind, however. Perhaps because I'm surrounded by a whole host of people (young and old) who are preoccupied with being "hot" and "sexy," and who wander around reeking desire, I feel I'm well out of it. Theirs seems to me such a *reduction* of desire to neediness and emptiness and I, quite frankly, feel *full*.

Certainly, when it comes to women, ours is still an ageist culture. (You don't have to live in Los Angeles to recognize this.) But things are looking up to some degree. Here, I am not only thinking of aging women stars who keep buff, unlined, and gorgeous as 30-year-olds but with character—although more power to them! At least nowadays, they don't have to appear in horror films—stories and roles relegated to a younger set (now often twenty-somethings and single mothers). They're neither scary nor scared and that's a good thing. However, I am also banking on the "graying" of America, the power of healthy, aging, *women* "baby-boomers" to make a fuss, to use their money and smarts to insist on equality, attention, and admiration. Thus, it is not the cop-out of a "senior" woman to suggest that, as I age, my desire and desirability have different—and broader—contours than they did when I was younger; gentled, they radiate from an expansiveness of my "being" rather than from the relaxation of my flesh. Indeed, today, I am kinder to both myself and others and accept those sags, wrinkles, and imperfect bodies as—and because of—what they are; signs of life and not the stuff of horror films.

References

Atlas, James. 1997. "The Sandwich Generation." *New Yorker*, Oct. 13.

Ballard, J. G. 1990. "Princess Margaret's Face Lift," in *The Atrocity Exhibition*, new rev. ed. San Francisco: Re/Search, 111–12.

Baudrillard, Jean. 1993. "Operational Whitewash," in *The Transparency of Evil: Essays on Extreme Phenomena*, trans. James Benedict. New York: Verso.

de Beauvoir, Simone. 1968. *The Second Sex*, trans. H. M. Parshley. New York: Bantam.

Bordo, Susan. 1997. "In an Empire of Images, the End of a Fairy Tale." *The Chronicle of Higher Education*, Sep. 19.

Duckett, Victoria. 2000. "Beyond the Body: Orlan and the Material Morph," in *Meta-Morphing: Visual Transformation and the Culture of Quick Change*, edited by Vivian Sobchack. Minneapolis: University of Minnesota Press, 209–23.

Freud, Sigmund. 1950. "The Predisposition to Obsessional Neurosis," in *Collected Papers*, vol. 1, edited by Ernest Jones, trans. Joan Riviere. London: Hogarth and the Institute of Psycho-Analysis.

Gerike, Ann. 1990. "On Gray Hair and Oppressed Brains" In *Women, Aging and Ageism*, edited by Evelyn R. Rosenthal. New York: Haworth.

MacFarquhar, Larissa. 1997. "The Face Age." *New Yorker*, July 21.

Melamed, Elissa. 1983. *Mirror, Mirror; The Terror of Not Being Young*. New York: Linden Press/Simon and Schuster.

Rossellini, Isabella. 1997. *Some of Me*. New York: Random House.

Sobchack, Vivian. 1994. "Revenge of *The Leech Woman*: On the Dread of Aging in a Low-Budget Horror Film," in *Uncontrollable Bodies: Testimonies of Identity and Culture*, edited by Rodney Sappington and Tyler Stallings. Seattle: Bay Press, 79–91.

Sontag, Susan. 1975. "The Double Standard of Aging." Reprinted in *No Longer Young: The Older Woman in America*. Ann Arbor: The Institute of Gerontology, University of Michigan/Wayne State University Press.

Williams, Linda. 1996. "When the Woman Looks," in *The Dread of Difference: Gender and the Horror Film*, edited by Barry Keith Grant. Austin: University of Texas Press.

Woodward, Kathleen. 1988. "Youthfulness as Masquerade." *Discourse*, 11(1), 119–42.

PART 2
Representing Cosmetic Surgery

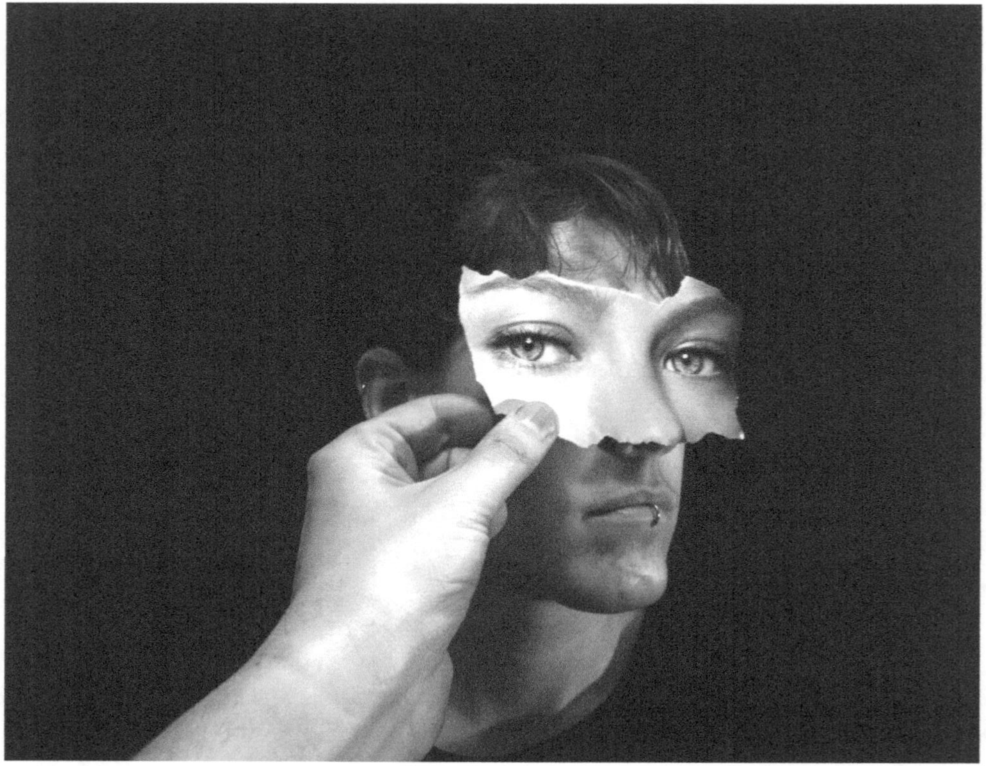

Figure 6.1 "Modular Face" 2007

Source: © Carrie Cizauskas

Chapter 6
Agency Made Over? Cosmetic Surgery and Femininity in Women's Magazines and Makeover Television

Suzanne Fraser

A successful television comedy actress features under a banner that reads "Tortured lives." Her "shock confession" includes repeat cosmetic surgery and extreme dieting, but her circumstances hardly invite pity:

> "I've always dreamt of looking beautiful. And now, with a pocketful of money and an opportunity to wear the most gorgeous designer clothing, I'm not going to blow my chance," says Patricia, who earns $11 million a year for her role [in *Everybody Loves Raymond*]. (*New Idea*, 2002)

Is Patricia a victim or a hero? Is she vain, and if so, is that OK? Posed broadly, these questions formed part of the basis for the analysis of cosmetic surgery discourse I conducted in my 2003 book, *Cosmetic Surgery, Gender and Culture*. In that book I explored three themes central to cosmetic surgery discourse, nature, agency, and vanity, and analyzed the ways each theme informed the others, and more generally, how gender norms came to be both reproduced and disrupted in the playing out of these themes. I traced the themes through four areas of cosmetic surgery discourse—medical literature, feminist analyses, regulatory discourse, and women's magazine coverage. Since this work was published, a new, highly visible area of cosmetic surgery discourse has emerged—that of makeover television. This new media phenomenon invites fresh analysis from feminists interested in women's engagement with the body and beauty in contemporary culture. It also invites us to draw links with existing discourses of gender and beauty, especially those relating to cosmetic surgical practices.

This chapter aims to address both these invitations, and to this end is divided into two parts. The first and longer presents part of the argument on agency in magazine coverage of cosmetic surgery made in my original work.[1] Following this, I look briefly at the rise of makeover television, and consider the relevance of these arguments to this new phenomenon. Do the insights provided in my original analysis shed any light on makeover television, or has this new form seen a shift in popular culture representations of cosmetic surgery such that these observations no longer apply? I conclude by arguing that while makeover television does not merely reproduce the approaches to cosmetic surgery and women's agency evident in the magazines I examined, some of the observations made about magazines do illuminate the preoccupations of these programs and of contemporary notions of beauty, agency, and vanity. In the process, the comparison I make reveals the limits of "progress" models of gender politics in the West, and highlights the extent to which gender discourse is constituted via class discourse, as well as via the demands of contemporary media forms.

Femininity, Agency and Women's Magazines

The notion of agency plays a central role in cosmetic surgery discourse, particularly in relation to questions of women's power, subjectivity, and choice in undergoing surgery. Here I trace the circulation of ideas of agency in magazine material on cosmetic surgery and reflect on how they shape contemporary concepts of femininity. How should these notions of agency be theorized and investigated? One useful method for analysis is that offered in Potter and Wetherell's (1987) poststructuralist work on textual repertoires. According to Potter and Wetherell, identifiable patterns can be reconstructed from discourse; patterns individuals "tap into" to present themselves in socially viable or coherent ways. These patterns are termed discursive or linguistic repertoires. In drawing on poststructuralist theories of discourse and the subject, Potter and Wetherell's approach offers important advantages for my analysis. According to the authors, discursive or linguistic repertoires should not be mistaken for tools which intentional subjects take up to "reveal" themselves. Rather, they are resources through which subjects are produced. This perspective suits my needs in that I do not wish to treat the many statements of agency and motive found in the magazine material naively as offering "real" insights into the subjectivities of cosmetic surgery participants. Instead, I see these comments and the articles they are drawn from as indicators of magazine culture; of magazine constructions of cosmetic surgery and its consumers, not of "extra-textual" subjects. My interest is in how women's magazines represent and constitute subjects, so I am not positioning magazines as a reliable means of accessing how people "really" feel, even in general terms. In short, I interpret the repertoires in the texts as offering culturally coherent positions, rather than revealing underlying truths or realities about individual subjects.

1 Due to space constraints, aspects of this argument have been edited heavily. Please turn to the 2003 book for a full elaboration of the material presented here.

The question of agency is central to this methodological issue. Some feminist research into cosmetic surgery has treated the utterances of recipients as offering access to the "real" reasons why women undergo surgery. From this starting point debates about the comparative agency or victimhood of recipients—as revealed by their descriptions of their motives and feelings—almost inevitably arise. In taking a different approach and treating discussions about motives as reliant on available linguistic repertoires, however, comparisons such as this are no longer appropriate. Equally, judgments about the "authenticity" or "truthfulness" of certain statements about motives and experiences are irrelevant. Where language is seen as a means of *producing a viable subject* rather than expressing an originary one, attempting to excavate a priori motives for language use does not make sense. Most relevant are questions about the type and range of repertoires available to individuals, the options or models for producing the self they offer, and what these indicate about gender and culture.

In conducting my analysis, it is important to emphasize that the magazines I look at cannot be said to offer any homogeneous approach to cosmetic surgery. These publications are varied in terms of readership, sponsorship, and tone. Most of the more lengthy articles about cosmetic surgery I analyze are primarily aimed at informing the reader about the possibilities of cosmetic surgery, emphasize best-case results, and engender a generally positive attitude towards cosmetic surgery for women.[2] A different group of pieces look at cosmetic surgery in relation to celebrities, offering a variety of perspectives.[3] The primary tone in which these articles are written is one of mild titillation where the reader is invited to wonder at the strange, sometimes sad and often extravagant cosmetic surgery experiences of famous people. Other kinds of articles also appear regularly. These include entirely negative pieces about breast implant tragedies or (rare) critical feminist pieces which argue for self-acceptance.[4] Most recently, articles began to offer cosmetic

---

2 See for instance, "Lunchtime Lifts," *Marie Claire Australia*, February 1998, pp. 154–164; *She* Cosmetic Surgery Supplement, December 1994; "Future Perfect," *Elle*, February 1997, pp. 48–52; "Cosmetic Surgery Changed My Life!" *For Me*, June 9, 1997, pp. 12–17; "Borrowing Time," *Vogue Australia*, January 1996, pp. 37–39; "Look at me now!" *Cosmopolitan*, March 1994, pp. 60–63. Cosmetic surgery has even been offered as prizes, for example, "Win cosmetic treatments worth $20,000," *She Australia*, June 1999, p. 120, although the 1999 Health Care Complaints Commission Inquiry into Cosmetic Surgery Report recommended that the NSW government refuse permits to competitions that offer such prizes. See *The Cosmetic Surgery Report: Report to the NSW Minister for Health—October 1999*, HCCC, 1999, p. iv.

3 For example, "Fantastic Plastic," *Who Weekly*, November 4, 1996, p. 87; "Melanie Griffith looks stunning thanks to plastic surgery," *Women's Weekly*, August 1997, pp. 10–13; "Breasts: fake vs flesh," *New Weekly*, June 9, 1997, pp. 48–51.

4 See "Mirror Mirror on the Wall," *New Woman*, March 1996, pp. 107–109; "Scarred For Life," *Who Weekly*, May 10, 1993, pp. 24–27; "What Price Perfection?" *Mode*, October/November 1993, pp. 128–132; "Breast Implants: Beauty or Barbarity?" *Ita*, February 1992, pp. 18–23.

surgery as a prize in competitions, and a regular column on cosmetic surgery was launched in another magazine.[5] Across this variety, however, it is possible to identify distinct patterns in meaning making, although these patterns are at times disrupted. For instance, while most articles on cosmetic surgery procedures assume that pursuit of beauty is a natural and inevitable priority for women, occasional pieces assert that personality, not appearance, is what matters, and that the pursuit of beauty should be of secondary importance. Here, the existence of broad assumptions upon which debate about cosmetic surgery is conducted can be identified, although these assumptions are not universal. Thus, for example, while it is not uncommon to encounter two separate pieces on cosmetic surgery within one magazine, and find them completely at odds on questions of cosmetic surgery's legitimacy or desirability, they may share other more far-reaching perspectives on the meaning and character of women's agency. Indeed, as my analysis of the repertoires of agency will show, significant common ground can be identified in terms of fundamental agency concepts that help shape notions of gender.

Within feminist discussions of cosmetic surgery, the question of agency tends to be conceptualized via a continuum that places passive victimhood at one end and autonomous individualism on the other. Some feminist work, such as Germaine Greer's book *The Whole Woman* (1999), offers an account of cosmetic surgery that leans heavily toward the former end, while other studies, like Kathy Davis's important *Reshaping the Female Body* (1995), focus on an individual agency more in keeping with the latter. What all of these works share is a view of agency as inhering in the individual.[6] Using Nikolas Rose's *Inventing Our Selves* (1996), this section will look more closely at this idea, relating our current understandings of the self and agency to modern forms of liberal democratic governance. In order to open up space for a critical perspective on the use of agency repertoires in women's magazines, I explore agency using the alternative model found in Rose's study of the emergence and development of the "psy" disciplines in the West.

The modern Western version of the self has been described by Clifford Geertz in the following terms:

> [t]he Western conception of the person as a bounded, unique, more or less integrated motivational and cognitive universe, a dynamic center of awareness, emotion, judgement and action, organised into a distinctive whole and set contrastively against other wholes and against a social and natural background is, however incorrigible it may seem to us, a rather peculiar idea within the context of the world's cultures. (Cited in Rose, 1996: 5)

The view Geertz describes here is no less incorrigible in the work of feminist writers than in any other context. This is partly because the attribution of agency and selfhood

5 See *The Australian Women's Weekly*.

6 This argument is elaborated fully in chapter 4 of *Cosmetic Surgery, Gender and Culture*.

to women has been central to their acquisition of legal and political rights. Indeed, among some feminist scholars, poststructuralist deconstructions of the unified, bounded subject have been greeted with suspicion. Why deconstruct the very subject women have only recently laid claim to? There is no doubt that the taking up of what might be seen as a classically masculine model of the subject/citizen by feminists has many uses and should not be eschewed as a matter of principle. It is important, however, to remember that this account of the subject is only one of many; that along with its advantages, it also has limitations. According to Rose, the sovereign subject of liberal individualism benefits democratic forms of government in that it represents subjectification as essentially voluntary and self-defined:

> [t]he forms of freedom we inhabit today are intrinsically bound to a regime of subjectification in which subjects are not merely "free to choose" but *obliged to be free*, to understand and enact their lives in terms of choice under conditions that systematically limit the capacities of so many to shape their own destinies. (Rose 1996: 17)

In other words, contemporary society relies on a model of the subject that does more than privilege individual decision-making, action, and reward; it demands it. In this model individuals are able to claim all personal successes as their achievements alone, but they must also take responsibility for all failures, even those in which broader factors clearly play a part, such as unemployment, illness and so on. This formulation of responsibilities is by no means seamlessly expressed within culture, but there is no doubt it constitutes a major trend. Part of this trend, Rose argues (1996: 160), is the constitution of the proper subject as an "enterprising" self able to manage risk and opportunity individually, with suitable recourse to the wisdom of experts: "we are condemned to make a project out of our own identity and we have become bound to the powers of expertise." For Rose, this is not a process of suppression but of production. He argues that current forms of regulation are shaped around this notion of the self as "enterprising"; as the improvable, transformable object of psy practices of "self-help" (1996: 154). As we will see, this enterprising self finds countless echoes in the cosmetic surgery coverage examined here.

As I have noted, liberal forms of agency are not without value. At the same time, it is important to recognize other possibilities for conceptualizing agency, both to denaturalize our assumptions and to analyze and potentially dismantle some of their negative effects. In relation to processes of subjectification, Rose states that they should be understood as operating within "a complex of apparatuses, practices, machinations and assemblages within which human being has been fabricated, and which presuppose and enjoin particular relations with ourselves" (1996: 10). Where the subject is defined as a cultural product, attributes of the subject such as agency are properly understood as cultural as well. This statement is an initial step away from conventional notions of agency as internal, or ontologically intrinsic to the subject, and toward notions that see it as fundamentally external to the subject.

It also suggests another, equally important, point—that the subject is, in any case, a fragmentary, non-unified one. Thus, Rose argues that individual subjects "live their lives in a constant movement across different practices that subjectify them in different ways. Within these different practices, persons are addressed as different sorts of human being, acted upon as if they were different sorts of human being" (1996: 35). This subject does not "exercise" an agency implanted by culture and which she or he then possesses, rather the subject is *produced through* the various forms of agency available at any given moment. This observation gives rise to a key question for analyzing the constitution of cosmetic surgery and agency in magazines. How varied *are* the forms of agency, or agency repertoires, available in this material?[7] As I will argue, they tend to adhere to a familiar binary framework that polarizes the victim and the agent.

Perhaps the most frequently encountered approach to agency found in magazine articles constitutes the use of cosmetic surgery to negotiate personal and professional relationships as a form of agency in itself. Here cosmetic surgery is presented as the very kind of "practice of the self" (Foucault 1988) Rose identifies, through which the individual establishes an ethical relationship with her- or himself in the process of self-governance. In contrast, cosmetic surgery is also often represented within women's magazines as suspect, illegitimate, and dangerous. In some cases a woman's willingness to undergo surgery is presented as evidence that she may be psychologically disordered, or, more simply, that she has been fooled into believing that her body is inadequate or unsightly and that her life will be significantly improved by surgery. Here, the woman is constructed as lacking precisely that ethical relationship to herself that would allow for a conscious reflection upon her desires and conduct. This argument is often made in articles that adopt a feminist tone, and it sometimes underpins the terms in which recipients themselves construct their own motives in both feminist and "non-feminist" pieces. Broadly, then, undergoing cosmetic surgery is seen by some as evidence of agency and by others as evidence of its absence or its opposite—victimhood. To take a closer look at these articulations of agency and victimhood I will now explore four agency repertoires found in the magazine articles.

A Very Good Investment

A key agency repertoire operating in magazine discourse treats cosmetic surgery as part of every career woman's collection of tools for achieving success. As such, the use of cosmetic surgery is cast as a sign of empowerment, ambition, and freedom. Face-lifts, collagen injections, and skin treatments such as dermabrasion

7 The term "agency" is a specifically academic one. As such, it is rarely if ever used explicitly in women's magazines, although it is often invoked implicitly in this context. (Jane Ussher suggests that feminism has helped reshape magazine discourse around the issue of agency. See Ussher 1997: 64.) In order to trace the occurrence of agency repertoires, I examine the use of concepts around women's power, rather than look only for specific terms.

are framed as useful rejuvenating procedures, and liposuction, rhinoplasty, and breast augmentation are seen as improving a woman's general appeal, and so her career prospects and even her job performance. This approach to cosmetic surgery assumes that a woman can (and even should) control her professional destiny by controlling or manipulating her appearance. Here, the obligation to make an enterprise of the self is clearly constructed. So for example, we read:

> For most actresses whose faces are their fortune, remodelling is not just vanity, it is a career move. ("Stay Young Hollywood Style," *New Idea*, 8 June 1996, p. 32)

> In a world where good looks often equal success, some executives are heading for the cosmetic surgeon in a bid to score the top jobs … all [recipients] essentially want to improve self-esteem and this enables them to function effectively in their careers. In this sense, cosmetic surgery is a very good investment. ("Could Cosmetic Surgery Save Your Career?" *She*, March 1996, p. 48)

> This time it's for my career … as I am expected to look a certain way. ("I Had Cosmetic Surgery to Look Like a Barbie Doll," *Cleo*, December 1993, p. 80)

These statements echo a long-standing stereotype in which women compete, and are judged, on the basis of their appearance. Perhaps one innovation these statements effect, however, is the location of competitiveness in the realm of careers, in addition to its location in the traditional realm of romantic relationships. In doing this, they also directly challenge the idea that for women, attention paid to the appearance equals vanity. Nevertheless, by promoting this method of competition in the workplace, magazines construct another familiar form of femininity, one open to the imputation that career success has been achieved through illegitimate means.[8]

Other articles take a rather different approach to this issue, positioning the recipient as a negotiator of circumstances beyond her control. Women are presented as conscious of the unjust demands placed upon them in the workplace, and as choosing reluctantly to meet these demands in order to accrue the benefits they deserve. One woman states:

> It irked me that men are so caught up with what you look like but I had a financial interest in fixing my appearance … On one level, I abhor the fact that I'm batting my eyelashes to get the sales when it's my brain I should be using. On the other hand, it worked. I've never been better off. ("Could Cosmetic Surgery Save Your Career?" *She*, March 1996, p. 50)

8 Rosemary Pringle (1998) notes that in the workplace "women are perceived as using sex to their advantage," though in reality, "[t]hey are much less likely to initiate sexual encounters and more likely to be hurt by sex at work" (94).

Elsewhere, another woman argues that:

> I didn't make the rules—they were already in place when I was growing up ... I just want to play the game to the best of my ability and come out a winner. ("I had plastic surgery to look like a Barbie Doll," *She* Cosmetic Surgery Supplement, December 1994, p. 80)

In this case, agency inheres in the process of negotiating values taken to be immutable and beyond the individual's power to change or reject. The possibility of collective change is ignored here, in favor of resignation to individual forms of negotiation and compromise. Working on the self, rendering oneself an enterprise, is again emphasized.

Interestingly, financial gain is often posed in the magazines as more legitimate an explanation for undergoing surgery than beauty or "vanity" alone, and it may be that this indicates a change in the way femininity is understood in culture, in that beauty has traditionally been presented as valuable for women primarily as a means of acquiring attention from men and a loving relationship, rather than as a tool for direct material gain. This legitimizing of women's interest in money and success demonstrates that certain feminist values such as financial independence are now readily deployed in popular culture discussions of cosmetic surgery, and suggests that conventional femininity as represented within these pages may in some ways be expanding.

Doing It for Me

Many of the articles I examined discuss cosmetic surgery in terms of the individual's right to make changes that improve her own well-being. As such, these pieces directly challenge assumptions that women undertake surgery as a result of pressure from partners. This challenge constitutes another common agency repertoire: the assertion that women become recipients not for the sake of others, but for their own self-respect and happiness. An extreme example of this approach is found in an article detailing the breast implant surgery of British television celebrity and former wife of rock musician Bob Geldof, Paula Yates. The introductory text states that:

> [i]t was a symbolic act for 36-year-old Paula. During her nineteen years with Bob Geldof, she was tortured by deep-rooted insecurity about her less-than-spectacular bust. She felt unfeminine and longed for a womanly cleavage. But Bob—whom Paula has described as a "control freak"—sneered at cosmetic surgery and put a ban on any such plans. ("New Breasts are the Best!" *New Weekly*, April 29, 1996, p. 18)

Here, the power of the husband to ban certain activities is contrasted with the image of Yates as "tortured" and "longing" (1996: 18). Yates is definitely the victim until her marriage dissolves. At this point, cosmetic surgery becomes a means of asserting a new independence and strength of character: "[n]o sooner had Paula broken free of the marital shackles than she was on the phone to a plastic surgeon" (1996: 18). Indeed, Yates is reported as saying, "Bob wouldn't let me have the operation, but after I left I felt free to do as I pleased" (1996: 18).

A number of magazine interviews with women cosmetic surgery recipients emphasize this same sense of empowerment in undergoing surgical procedures in spite of resistance from those around them. In some cases, the value of undergoing cosmetic surgery is explicitly linked to the sense that such surgery must be for oneself alone, and not to please others. Thus one woman states:

> It's been great for my self esteem and confidence and I couldn't recommend it enough for anyone wanting it. It's got to be done for yourself. Don't do it for a partner. ("Get Real! Silicone Sucks," *New Weekly*, June 9, 1997, p. 49)

Yet, in an indication of how contradictory many articles can be, the piece in which this statement appears is structured around a football commentator and his evaluations of the breasts of film stars. Of course, trying to unpick the degree to which women (or men) make "autonomous" decisions about such a public aspect of the self as appearance is in some ways nonsensical. The undeniable status of appearance as social belies the possibility of autonomous decisions about it. Yet the notion of "doing it for oneself" recurs over and over in magazine material on cosmetic surgery, reflecting the contemporary preoccupation with the self as entirely independent and self-defining, as internally located, rather than as a product of culture.

Importantly, however, this notion tends to reconfigure femininity along more independent lines than traditional formations. As in the presentation of ambition and career progress as a legitimate concern for women, this refiguring of the feminine subject as self-defining, autonomous, and independent departs from traditional notions of femininity as essentially dependent and relational. Again, gender is constituted in relatively innovative ways here.

Weighing the Risks Against the Rewards

Also central to the discourse of agency that saturates much cosmetic surgery coverage in women's magazines is the notion that the individual is able to evaluate the relative risks and rewards of undergoing surgery and, it is implied, has adequate access to information in order to make an informed decision. Thus one woman, familiar with stories of cosmetic surgery failure through her work in the media, states that she:

> "weighed up the validity of the stories and decided to accept the risks" in the decision to undergo breast augmentation. ("You can change your looks," *For Me*, June 9, 1997, p. 12)

Another woman acknowledges the dangers of breast augmentation, observing that,

> apparently, they are still unsure of the long-term effects of the saline implants, but that's the risk you take. ("I've Had Eleven Operations," *Cosmopolitan* Cosmetic Surgery Special, nd, p. 84)

It is not made clear on what grounds this participant decided to take the "risk" of breast augmentation. The discourse of justified risk appears to be regarded as adequate explanation in itself.

This emphasis on "risk" reflects the ascendancy of risk analysis as an industry in the latter three decades of the twentieth century. Originally used to refer to potential outcomes both good and bad,[9] risk has since become synonymous with the negative. Mary Douglas (1992: 15) argues that the term "risk analysis" relies on a spurious claim to the possibility of "a scientifically objective decision about exposure to danger" and allows doctors to "let the patient choose for herself." In her view, this approach is of most benefit to surgeons who face high rates of malpractice litigation. Similarly, Deborah Lupton (1995: 79) notes that risk discourse is directly related to contemporary individualism. Paralleling Rose's identification of the "enterprising self," she sees it as "an extension of one's life as an enterprise and the belief that individuals should plan for the future and take judicious steps to ensure protection against misfortune, retaining responsibility for their affairs." Here it is interesting to consider how the discourse of risk contributes to the image of women not only as rational decision-makers weighing up risks and benefits (along the lines of the claim to scientific choices noted above), but also as somewhat heroic in their willingness to take risks. Certainly, while critical analysis of the notion of risk tends to concentrate on the contemporary injunction to manage one's life effectively through *minimizing* risk, cosmetic surgery departs from this model in promoting the calculated and purportedly intrinsically edifying practice of *risk-taking*.[10]

Manipulation and Victimhood

In contrast to the magazine accounts of women as determined, fearless, and rational consumers of cosmetic surgery, however, a portrayal of cosmetic surgery recipients as hapless victims of social pressure and advertising also emerges.

The latter view of women as pawns characterizes some of the anti-cosmetic surgery material found in women's magazines—and is not entirely unexpected given the nature of some pro-surgery material. In one article entitled "I Did it All

9 According to Mary Douglas the term first came into use during the seventeenth century. See Douglas (1992: 23).

10 John Adams notes the connections between risk taking and heroism in his *Risk* (1995: 2).

for Antonio," film star Melanie Griffiths is interviewed about her marriage, her work, and her appearance. Having recently undergone cosmetic surgery, Griffiths states,

> [b]eing married to Antonio Banderas was enough of a motivation for me to get it together … I've got to look pretty damn good, you know. ("I Did It All For Antonio," *Australian Women's Weekly*, August 1997, p. 11)

It may be that this remark is meant humorously: it is in some respects ambiguous. The remainder of the article strikes a serious tone, however, suggesting that this comment should be read seriously too. This approach is distinctly at odds with the tendency to construct cosmetic surgery as entirely about career opportunities, material gain, or other self-focused motives. Pleasing her husband is presented as Griffiths's primary and unabashed motive.

As I noted earlier, this construction of the relationship between women and cosmetic surgery renders conclusions about women as victims less surprising than they might otherwise appear. As one article explains,

> Many are able to look beyond the shifting trends in body shape, the risks of the operation and fears about the safety of silicone, to the world of opportunity it seemingly offers. It's easy to convince yourself that a nip, a tuck and a suck will make you more taut, more sexy, more beautiful. ("Plastic Surgery: what if you could try before you buy?" *Cleo*, July 1992, p. 76)

Taking a different tack, but equally invested in the notion of the victim, another article asks,

> Could there be hundreds of women out there who have been suffering in silence and on their own for years and years over their breast implants? ("Breast Implants: Beauty or Barbarity?" *Ita*, February 1992, p. 23)

The gendered nature of these agency/victimhood repertoires becomes especially clear when articles about cosmetic surgery for men are examined. Several articles argue that while women have been succumbing to the pressure to pursue beauty through surgery for years, men are beginning to follow suit. One piece on penis extension surgery, entitled "Men Who Have Cosmetic Surgery: would you respect him in the morning?" treats men who undergo the procedure as the victims of media pressure in a manner reminiscent of discussions of women and cosmetic surgery. A surgeon is reported as saying,

> I suspect a lot of insecure people are being brought out of the woodwork by these ads [for penis extensions]. ("Men Who Have Cosmetic Surgery," *Cleo*, December 1993, p. 20)

The article positions susceptibility to pressure and feelings of insecurity as feminine and, as its title suggests, implies that cosmetic surgery and the associated vulnerability is for women only. In this way, a series of associations is built which tends to feminize male recipients of surgery. Here, the representation of cosmetic surgery as feminine not only constructs femininity, but also masculinity (and the gender binary itself) by problematizing in specific ways those men who do participate in surgical alteration.

In that passivity and victim status are both key attributes of traditional femininity and of accounts of cosmetic surgery participation, there is a sense in which framing women as potential victims serves to reinforce their place in cosmetic surgery practice. Given this, our next question might be whether *any* reference to victimhood in the conventional sense serves to reinscribe women as open to (physical and psychological) manipulation, and cosmetic surgery as an inevitable extension of this. If so, this presents a series of problems for feminists working to have the problems women have faced as a result of cosmetic surgery recognized. Without recourse to repertoires for presenting some women as poorly or unsafely treated, the need to address real problems such as side effects or unsuccessful outcomes becomes difficult to articulate.

Transcending Agency Versus Victimhood

Clearly the victim repertoires circulating through magazine coverage of cosmetic surgery offer a range of advantages and disadvantages in terms of gender representation and self-representation. The available agency repertoires are equally risky. As I have shown, assertions of agency are common in women's magazines, reconfiguring femininity along some unfamiliar lines, but frequently invoking established ideas based on feminine action through appearance. Thus, while the pitfalls of invoking the victim are many, an exclusive emphasis on agency has its disadvantages as well. It tends, for example, to undermine the need for legislative and other safeguards around the cosmetic surgery industry. Given these dilemmas, how should feminists proceed in analyzing cosmetic surgery? Crucially, this debate is fixed in a binary mode which conceptualizes agency as inhering within the individual and which offers only two options—victim *or* agent. As I have already noted, in many magazine discussions of cosmetic surgery, agency is posed directly against victimhood. Either the recipient is an entirely free individual with completely self-generated desires and values, or else she is a mindless pawn, easily swayed by what she encounters in popular culture and by the wishes of sexist partners. Here, victim and agent become ontological categories, so that again the degree or type of agency the participant exhibits is seen to emanate from within. Located in the individual, agency or the lack of it becomes an individual quality or failing. In thinking through cosmetic surgery, it is necessary to build new approaches to agency that do not contrast it with victimhood and do not take for granted the ontological assumptions of internal origins and coherence questioned by Rose and others. In this way, more sophisticated conceptions of agency, offering greater analytical purchase, will be developed.

Cosmetic Surgery Made Over?

How do the forms of feminine agency operating in the women's magazines I examined square with the representations of femininity and agency at work in the relatively new arena for cosmetic surgery, makeover television? There is no doubt that many similarities can be identified across the two forms (for example, the "natural look" repertoire identified by Weiss and Kukla in Chapter 7 is almost identical to that found in the magazine material I originally examined (Fraser 2003: 64–76)). To think systematically through the relationship between magazines and makeover television on the issue of agency, I will draw on three key repertoires found in the material presented above. These are:

- Cosmetic surgery as a means of enhancing competitiveness in both career and romance contexts
- "Doing it for oneself" as the central value, with risk-taking framed as an intrinsically edifying form of agency
- The repudiation of vanity as a legitimate motive for cosmetic surgery.

An exploration of the growing literature on makeover television suggests some correspondence and some divergence between the magazine material of the late 1990s and early 2000s and the newer medium of makeover television. This range is perhaps not surprising in that women's magazines can be seen as offering some early expression of makeover culture and values, even as it differs from makeover television in important ways. To clarify this overlap it is important first to spell out what might be meant by the term "makeover culture." Meredith Jones (2008: 12) defines it as centrally organized around the value of continual improvement. Jones distinguishes the "makeover" from the more familiar "transformation" by arguing that transformation entails a shift from one static condition to a new static condition, whereas makeover entails a constant state of becoming. Thus she notes that "Good citizens of makeover culture improve and transform themselves ceaselessly."

How pronounced is this shift in focus from transformation to makeover? As noted at the outset of this chapter (that is, in my original discussion of agency repertoires in cosmetic surgery discourse), Rose argues that current forms of regulation are shaped around a notion of the self as "enterprising"; as the improvable, transformable object of psy practices of "self-help" (1996: 154). Here the word "enterprising" indicates a self committed to constantly generating value, and to seeking change as intrinsically yielding value. Women's magazines have long framed cosmetic surgery as a tool for this enterprising self, that is, for the self as always in motion, always seeking betterment. Indeed, cosmetic surgery is only one area in which women's magazines promote ceaseless change and improvement. Their continual provision of advice on more traditional beauty-related activities such as makeup application and clothing choice, and on other key feminine responsibilities such as mothering technique and housekeeping, has always constituted the feminine self as intrinsically in need of constant revision and upgrading. Clearly this is required by the format. Magazines are a form of serial—unless we are always in need of updating and change, one issue (presumably the first) would be all we would need to buy.

Jones, of course, does not suggest that makeover culture is an entirely new phenomenon. She sees it as adding "another layer to cosmetic surgery discourse. Fantasies of transformation remain dominant, now accompanied by a new and potent ally" (2008: 57). Together, she argues, two powerful languages—those of magic and labor—create makeover culture. Interestingly, it is in relation to this last idea, that of labor, where differences emerge between the discourse of cosmetic surgery in magazines and that in makeover television. Before examining this difference, however, it is worth drawing out the elements of continuity between the repertoires identified above and those evident in makeover television.

First, as Cressida Heyes has pointed out in her analysis of *Extreme Makeover* (2007: 24), makeover television poses autonomy and self-satisfaction (though not as an expression of selfishness) as the central motivations for participants. As Heyes puts it, "choosing cosmetic surgery 'for oneself' rather than for others is represented as an authentic and pure motivation that can be ontologically distinguished from social pressures." Clearly this emphasis on self-motivation echoes the women's magazines analyzed above, although the differing media formats generate an important variation in this framing, specifically in relation to the idea of work. Indeed, and this is my second point, also evident in both contexts is the balancing or modulating of self-satisfaction with the values of hard work and the willingness to take a risk. In the television program *The Swan*, for instance, cosmetic surgery recipients compete with each other for the accolade of being "the ultimate swan." This accolade is based, as Heyes notes, on "work ethic, growth and achievements" (2007: 26). Likewise, she notes, *Extreme Makeover* emphasizes "corporeal hard labor" (2007: 26; see also Jones, 2008: 12). Suffering, in this framework, is also constituted as work—as a means of earning the right to a makeover. Weber (2005: 7), for example, notes that "it is the suffering that makes these subjects worthy."

Thirdly, and I make this point partly in response to the emphasis in the programs on hard work, both forms (magazines and television programs) continually turn away from imputations of vanity. This is explicitly expressed in the magazine material presented above, but tends to be more indirectly managed in makeover television. In the book (2003) from which my discussion of magazines is taken, I argue that accusations of vanity "haunt" cosmetic surgery discourse. I would extend this observation here to interpret the stories of struggle and hard work that characterize the narrative trajectories of makeover television as motivated by a perceived need to pre-empt audience condemnation of the participants as vain, and to present them instead as deserving, so as to maximize the audience's identification with them. Indeed, as Jones (2008: 52) argues in relation to *Extreme*

Makeover, "the program's subjects are not vain but instead worthy because of having suffered hardship."

Yet this point of overlap (the focus on work to circumvent accusations of vanity) also constitutes a point of divergence. The magazines I analyzed consistently treated career aspirations and the desire for success and financial benefit as legitimate motivations for surgery, and as proof that vanity was not motivating women's actions. In this sense, notions of work and the "earning" of transformation were often quite explicitly linked with paid work. Makeover programs, however, negotiate the terrain of work and deservingness rather differently. As Heyes (2007: 26) observes, women participants rarely if ever cited career aspirations as a reason for undergoing a makeover. What is behind this reticence, or difference in emphasis? I would argue that the answer lies in the encounter between the genre's strategic reliance on formats in which surgery is "won" and on key aspects of working class culture, especially as they bear on women. By constituting themselves as competitions in which surgery is won, the programs tend to attract economically disadvantaged participants, and a large following among viewers whose own access to surgical makeovers is limited by financial constraints. As Heyes (2007: 21) points out in relation to *Extreme Makeover*:

> The show predominantly features the working-class and lower middle-class white women aged between 25 and 45 who are increasingly the target market for cosmetic surgery as well as, presumably, a significant part of the viewing audience; or, as the producers' vernacular puts it, "We are looking for people who America will love and root for."

These participants and viewers are less likely to relate to accounts of motivation based on notions of career progress and success in that their own access to opportunities for taking up high-paying, high-status, high-satisfaction work are minimal. In an important sense, that is, the "career" is a middle-class construct and preoccupation (see McDowell 2006 for a discussion of the polarization of contemporary employment opportunities and conditions). Given this, the programs understandably tend to draw on the idea that transformation is earned through suffering, sacrifice, and hard emotional work rather than through dedication to professional demands and hard work in the paid employment context.

What are the implications of this difference in emphasis and values for the constitution of femininity via cosmetic surgery discourse? As I noted at the outset, cosmetic surgery discourse generates particular, historically and culturally specific iterations of femininity and masculinity. In concluding my original discussion of women's magazines and their constructions of femininity, I noted that their reliance on career repertoires helped constitute femininity along relatively new lines, authorizing women's interest in the public sphere and in ambition and professional success. Makeover television departs noticeably from this by focusing solely on personal growth and intimate relationships as motivations for surgery. In doing so, it reproduces femininity in relatively traditional terms.

These developments are salutary for those inclined to see gender politics in the West as inevitably following a progressive trajectory. I have noted elsewhere, as have many feminists, that gender is co-constituted in relation to other axes of identity such as race and class (2003: 39). Makeover television is a good example of this. Arguably, then, we can characterize the effects of makeover television in the following broad terms: in enacting an encounter between the gendered technologies of cosmetic surgery, particular elements of working class experience, economics and politics, and the unique demands of the "TV competition" genre, femininity is iterated in rather less diverse terms than in earlier magazine iterations.[11] To return to the insights offered by Rose's work on subjectification, we can formulate this process in the following way: magazines and makeover television constitute "different practices that subjectify [cosmetic surgery participants and audiences] in different ways" (1996: 35), in the process generating different modes of agency through which aspects of this subjectification are achieved. Here, agency emerges not from within individuals, but in the encounter between material phenomena, subjects-in-the-making, and cultural constructs such as gender and class. Given the range of influences on the ways in which gender is constituted in the media, and given the distributed nature of agency, we cannot assume this contraction in diversity will necessarily continue. New considerations and influences will surely emerge, taking the media and its femininities, in new directions.

Acknowledgments

The first part of this chapter is adapted from my book, *Cosmetic Surgery, Gender and Culture* (Palgrave, 2003). I thank Mark Davis for providing valuable feedback on an earlier draft of this chapter.

References

Adams, J. 1995. *Risk*. London: UCL Press.

Davis, K. 1995. *Reshaping the Female Body: The Dilemma of Cosmetic Surgery*. New York and London: Routledge.

Douglas, M. 1992. *Risk and Blame: Essays in Cultural Theory*. London and New York: Routledge.

11 Admittedly this formulation does not capture other relevant considerations such as the broader implications of makeover programs as "reality television," and the US origins of these programs as opposed to the origins of the magazine material in Australian publications. Space constraints prevent me form exploring these issues further, but in relation to the latter point I should note that many articles published in Australian magazines are originally sourced overseas, including the US, so the degree to which the Australian context differs from the US is probably relatively small.

Foucault, M. 1988. *Technologies of the Self.* Amherst: University of Massachusetts Press.
Fraser, S. 2003. *Cosmetic Surgery, Gender and Culture*. Basingstoke: Palgrave.
Greer, G. 1999. *The Whole Woman*. London: Doubleday.
Heyes, C. 2007. "Cosmetic Surgery and the Televisual Makeover: A Foucauldian Feminist Reading." *Feminist Media Studies*, 7(1), 17–32.
Jones, M. 2008. *Skintight: An Anatomy of Cosmetic Surgery*. Oxford and New York: Berg.
Lupton, D. 1995. *The Imperative of Health: Public Health and the Regulated Body*. London: Sage.
McDowell, L. 2006. "Reconfigurations of Gender and Class Relations: Class Differences, Class Condescension and the Changing Place of Class Relations." *Antipode*, 38(4), 825–50.
Potter, J. and Wetherell, M. 1987. *Discourse and Social Psychology: Beyond Attitudes and Behaviour*. London: Sage.
Pringle, R. 1998. *Secretaries Talk: Sexuality, Power and Work*. Sydney: Allen & Unwin.
Rose, N. 1996. *Inventing Our Selves: Psychology, Power and Personhood*. Cambridge: Cambridge University Press.
Ussher, J. 1997. *Fantasies of Femininity: Reframing the Boundaries of Sex*. Harmondsworth: Penguin.
Weber, B. 2005. "Beauty, Desire and Anxiety: the Economy of Sameness in ABC's Extreme Makeover." *Genders*, No. 41. Available at: http://www.genders.org/g41/g41_weber.html.

Women's Magazine Articles

Australian Women's Weekly 1997. "I Did It All For Antonio." August.
Cleo 1992. "Plastic Surgery: What if you could try before you buy?" July.
Cleo 1993. "I Had Cosmetic Surgery to Look Like a Barbie Doll." December.
Cleo 1993. "Men Who Have Cosmetic Surgery: Would you respect him in the morning?" December.
Cosmopolitan n.d. "I've Had Eleven Operations." Cosmetic Surgery Special.
Elle 1997. "The Future Perfect: The Age of the Superbody." February.
For Me 1997. "You can change your looks." June 9.
Ita 1992. "Breast Implants: Beauty or Barbarity?" February.
Mode 1993. "What Price Perfection?" October/November.
New Idea 1996. "Stay Young Hollywood Style." June 8.
New Idea 2002. "'I starve myself' (And I've had cosmetic surgery too)." October 19.
New Weekly 1996. "New Breasts are the Best!" 29 April.
New Weekly 1997. "Get Real! Silicone Sucks." June 9.
She 1994. "I had plastic surgery to look like a Barbie Doll," in Cosmetic Surgery supplement, December.
She 1996. "Could Cosmetic Surgery Save Your Career?" March.

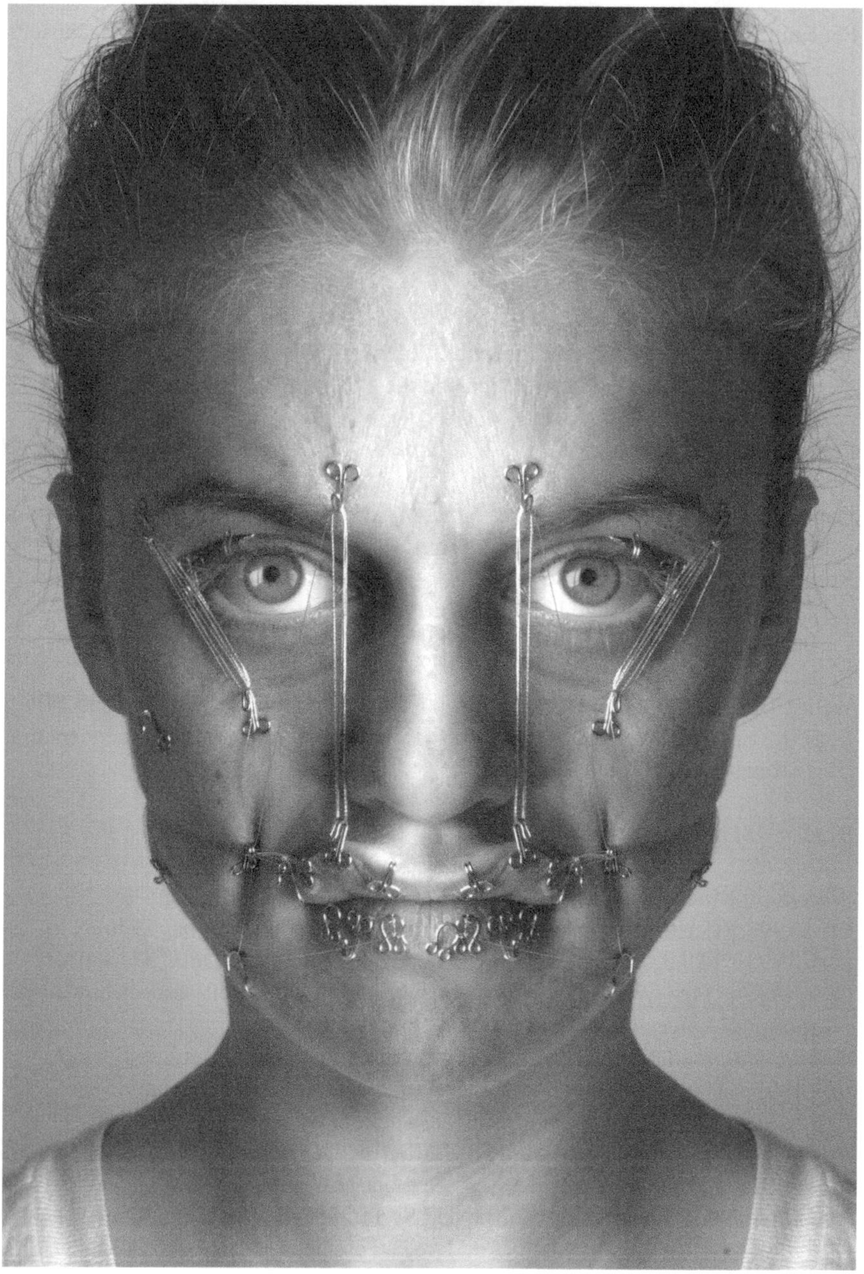

Figure 7.1 "Hook and Eyes" 2007

Source: © lucyandbart

Chapter 7
The "Natural Look": Extreme Makeovers and the Limits of Self-Fashioning

Dennis Weiss and Rebecca Kukla

In this chapter we treat *Extreme Makeover* as an exemplary text for the purpose of critically examining the conceptual ground of the debate over the ethics of "radical" bodily transformation. Situating *Extreme Makeover* as part of a constellation of discourses revolving around biotechnology, human enhancement, and the limits of self-fashioning, we argue that in interesting and contradictory ways the show challenges familiar frameworks in this debate. Highlighting the constructed nature of beauty and femininity while it simultaneously reinforces the production of a "natural look," *Extreme Makeover* visually displays tensions that also exist in two popular philosophical positions on human enhancement: a libertarian position that naturalizes our capacity for transformation and an essentialist position that imposes ethical limits on those transformations in the name of nature. We argue that an examination of these positions through a close reading of *Extreme Makeover* points to conceptual difficulties in their normative deployment of nature. These conceptual tensions can also be found in some feminist theorizing about cosmetic surgery. We argue that addressing these tensions requires greater attention to the nature of norms, the natural, and how the natural functions in this performative context, and use *Extreme Makeover* as a springboard for concretizing a feminist understanding of the notion of "naturalness."

Reading *Extreme Makeover*

Extreme Makeover is a show whose very title seems to promise radical transformations, celebrating a vision of an age of voluntaristic control over our bodies, and through them, our identities. The show premiered in 2002 and over three seasons featured close to 100 individuals undergoing makeovers. The typical structure of the show featured two, sometimes three individuals selected for makeovers. The narratives of the makeover candidates were presented through a video montage introducing the candidates, their family and friends, and highlighting how the candidates' looks led to a lack of self-esteem or to insecurity, and how particular elements of their body have gotten in the way of their happiness. Many of the individuals chosen to participate in extreme makeovers suggested that the makeover would change their lives far beyond simply making them better looking. The candidates were flown to Los Angeles and taken by limousine to meet their Beverly Hills "Extreme Team" of cosmetic surgeons, dentists, and stylists. Candidates were separated from family for six to eight weeks, during which they underwent a litany of procedures including liposuction, breast augmentation, tummy tucks, chin implants, rhinoplasty, upper and lower eyelid surgery, and face-lifts. Participants also commonly underwent LASIK eye surgery, dental procedures including veneers and teeth whitening, Botox injections, makeup, hair, and wardrobe restyling, and fitness training. While the surgical element was often emphasized as the most important part of the makeover process, each episode spent at most 60 seconds on the surgery itself. Substantially more time was spent on the recovery period. At the end of the show, candidates were flown home for a final "reveal," in which family and friends were assembled to witness the coming out and register excitement and surprise at the transformation. Without exception, these loved ones were shown as delighted by the changes. Notably, while the episodes stressed the language and logic of transformation, and while family members always showed amazement at the extent of the change, most episodes closed with loved ones commenting that the procedures allowed the subject's "true self" to be revealed. In the tradition of makeover stories since Cinderella, it always turned out that the transformed self is somehow *more* authentic than the self it replaced, a point often remarked upon in analyses of the makeover genre (Tait 2007, Heyes 2007, Banet-Weiser and Portwood-Stacer 2006). *Extreme Makeover* was just one of a series of similar shows appearing at roughly the same time that seemingly celebrated human malleability and voluntaristic self-production. Shows such as *The Swan*, *Plastic Surgery Before and After*, and *I Want a Famous Face*, concretize and make available for mass consumption what Susan Bordo has characterized a culture of plastic bodies, in which the body is indefinitely malleable and transformable. As Bordo pointed out in "Material Girl," in a culture of organ transplants, life-extension machinery, microsurgery, and artificial organs, we have now arrived at a "new, postmodern imagination of human freedom from bodily determination" (Bordo 1993: 245). It is precisely this cultural imagination hinted at in Oprah Winfrey's take on the *Extreme Makeover* phenomenon, as she suggested while introducing one of two shows devoted to this genre of makeover narratives: "There is a new television show that takes makeovers to a whole new level. It's called 'Extreme Makeover,' and when they say extreme, they really mean it. These are makeovers like you have never seen before." These are, Oprah promises, "radical transformations … Nothing is off limits" (Hudson 2003). A similar response is evident in Sander Gilman's defense of *Extreme Makeover* in a *New York Times* op-ed piece that appeared during the show's run. Defending our right to shape ourselves, Gilman asserts that *Extreme Makeover* "is just another name for life in the 21st century" (Gilman 2002).

On the surface, *Extreme Makeover* seems to signal just such a paradigm shift as Bordo references in "Material Girl." The show, with its emphasis on the *extreme* nature of the makeover, signals that this is about more than a few beauty secrets meant to freshen up one's looks. It can be read as partaking in a constellation of discourses all of which underscore the power of new medical and bio-technologies to transform the self, even the species—a power regularly celebrated by proponents of human enhancement such as the extropians and the transhumanists (Bostrom 2005); by magazine covers, including *Newsweek* ("Building a New Human"), *Popular Science* ("Body of the Future"), *Scientific American* ("Your Bionic Future"), and *Wired* ("Beyond the Body: The Science of Human Enhancement"); and a host of books debating the coming era of the posthuman.[1] The human potential for self-transformation becomes the normative lynchpin for such libertarian proponents of biotechnology as John Harris, Gregory Stock, and Nicholas Agar, each of whom has argued that human beings have always embraced technology to overcome the limits of the body or biology, changing our nature and transcending biological limits. According to these authors, our capacity to change is itself part of human nature; science and technology provide us with the means for controlling and improving upon nature and biology. On this reading of *Extreme Makeover*, the implicit message of the show is that, as Gregory Stock puts it, "remaking ourselves is the ultimate expression and realization of our humanity" (Stock 2002: 197). *Extreme Makeover* exemplifies a libertarian endorsement of human malleability and voluntaristic self-production. Participants on the show take their destiny into their own hands, undergoing projects of transformation that will lead to fulfillment and happiness.

This reading of *Extreme Makeover* seemingly aligns the show with at least some dominant strains of feminist theory in highlighting the body as an artifact constructed by culture. No longer are we beholden to a given nature once we recognize that nature itself is a cultural construction, now to be remade through the powers of science and technology. As Bordo pointed out in a 1985 essay on anorexia nervosa,

> the body, far from being some fundamentally stable, acultural constant to which we must *contrast* all culturally relative and institutional forms, is constantly "in the grip," as Foucault puts it, of cultural practices. … there is no "natural" body. … Our bodies, no less than anything else that is human, are constituted by culture. (Bordo 1993: 142)

1 These include Francis Fukuyama's *Our Posthuman Future: Consequences of the Biotechnology Revolution*, Joel Garreau's *Radical Evolution: The promise and peril of enhancing our minds, our bodies—and what it means to be human*, Nicholas Agar's *Liberal Eugenics: In Defense of Human Enhancement*, Gregory Stock's *Redesigning Humans: Our Inevitable Genetic Future*, John Harris's *Enhancing Evolution: The Ethical Case for Making Better People*, Bill McKibben's *Enough: Staying Human in an Engineered Age*, Jurgen Habermas's *The Future of Human Nature*, and the President's Council on Bioethics report *Beyond Therapy: Biotechnology and the Pursuit of Happiness*.

The body as socially constructed, Bordo argues, owes much to the activist feminism of the late 1960s and early 1970s that challenged biological determinism and essentialism (Bordo 1997: 196). Already in 1970, Shulamith Firestone in *The Dialectic of Sex* was encouraging women to embrace technology in order to transcend and re-make nature. Her views resonate with more contemporary feminist figures who seek to appropriate cosmetic surgery as a tool of political critique. As Llewellyn Negrin notes in "Cosmetic Surgery and the Eclipse of Identity," for several feminist writers,

> the revolutionary potential of cosmetic surgery lies in its capacity to highlight the fact that the body is a cultural construct rather than a natural entity, which is fixed and immutable. They see it as a tool that can be used to deconstruct the notion of a unified and unchanging self, replacing it with a performative conception of the self as being in a constant state of transmutation. (Negrin 2002: 29)

Ruth Holliday and Jacqueline Sanchez Taylor argue that from a "post-feminist" standpoint, which foregrounds agency and identifies sexual assertiveness with power and autonomy, "aesthetic surgery," rather than producing normalized bodies is more about differentiation and distinction (Holliday and Sanchez Taylor 2006: 188). They argue that for many consumers of aesthetic surgery enhancements are more about standing out rather than blending in and may produce a proliferation of difference.

> This idea is supported by recent "ideal bodies" represented in popular magazines that foreground racial "mixing" … we can also consider the number of "non-normative" surgeries that are increasingly taking place—transsexual surgery, operations to make the patient more like a tiger, amputations, as well as breast implants in men or shaped collarbone implants adding interest to any body. (Holliday and Sanchez Taylor 2006: 189)

In taking us into the surgical hall and bearing the open body to the latest medical and technical interventions, *Extreme Makeover* underscores that the body is far from fixed and immutable and can be reconstructed. And yet even a cursory glance at any episode of *Extreme Makeover* suggests that any apparent promise of a celebration of voluntarism lies unfulfilled, for the show reinforces a deeply conventional picture of what bodies should look like. For all that philosophers like Agar and Stock celebrate our immanent transformation into posthuman chimeras, it is remarkable just how ordinary the makeovers on *Extreme Makeover* actually are. As Alex Kuczynski reports for the *New York Times*, "As the patients make their appearances, week after week, viewers have … begun to notice an eerie Stepford-spouse similarity. 'They all get a chin implant, all get a brow lift, all get their lips done,' said Dr. Z. Paul Lorenc, a New York plastic surgeon" (Kuczynski 2004: 4). Friends, family, and participants on *Extreme Makeover* routinely describe the participants as having achieved a particular look. Throughout the three seasons of the show, one regularly heard comments such as: "She looks like she belongs in Hollywood." "She looks like a movie star." "I felt like a woman. I feel feminine. It's nice." "I feel sexy." "I feel like a little princess." And, in the case of one male participant, "I'm movie star handsome. I've got an action hero face now." If we really are free to design our own natures, it is remarkable the extent to which we choose to fashion ourselves in pretty familiar ways. We do not pursue makeovers in order to make ourselves into unique works of art, expressions of our will and power over nature. We most often pursue them in order to achieve an unremarkable look exemplifying a conventional standard of glamour and beauty.[2] Indeed, a number of feminist critics of cosmetic surgery, including Bordo (1997), Heyes (2007), and Tait (2007) have pointed out that while such shows appropriate the language of self-transformation and authenticity, they do so by enforcing a homogenized look in which race, class, and disability are all effaced and subjects seek a culturally dominant feminine or masculine look.

The show severs any naive link between the "constructed" and the "voluntaristically produced," while offering the complex message that normative, "natural" bodies can be the product of artifice and technology. Despite the glorification of medical and technological alterations of the body on *Extreme Makeover*, the show's utilization of the rhetoric of nature is surprisingly pervasive. The surgeons and other professionals on the show regularly brag about how "natural" their finished products are and the "naturalness" of a result is a recurrent measure of its success. Participants almost invariably aim for a "natural look." In a startling television moment, one participant on *I Want a Famous Face* claimed that her surgical goal was to have "Kate Winslet's natural beauty" for herself. As one of the surgeons appearing regularly on *Extreme Makeover* explained it, "You want it to look really natural, refreshed, and not have the surgical element where people say something's happened" (*The Oprah Winfrey Show* 2003). One family member commented upon witnessing a final reveal, "She just looked naturally beautiful. She came out looking like a movie star" (*Extreme Makeover*). The extreme team isn't embracing our artificiality in order to redesign our humanity, but in order to put in place another natural norm.

Reading *Extreme Makeover* as a libertarian argument for the de-naturalization of the body, a celebration of technical intervention and the culturally plastic body, thus seems too simplistic in light of the actual choices participants on the show make and their desire to achieve a "natural look." Perhaps then the show calls for a more cautionary reading one that highlights the growing dangers of our enchantment with human enhancement and biotechnology. Such a reading is favored by Leon Kass, the Chair of the United States President's Council on Bioethics from 2002 to 2005. Agreeing with feminist concerns over the normalizing and homogenizing power of cosmetic surgery in a consumer culture, Kass extends these concerns to

2 Kathy Davis has argued in detail that cosmetic surgery patients in general seek normalcy rather than beauty. See Davis 1995 and 2003.

enhancement technologies more generally: "As with cosmetic surgery, Botox, and breast implants, the enhancement technologies of the future will likely be used in slavish adherence to certain socially defined and merely fashionable notions of 'excellence' or improvement, very likely shallow, almost certainly conformist" (Kass 2003). Kass and other critics of human enhancement technologies, such as Francis Fukuyama and George Annas, draw on substantive notions of nature or human nature to justify limits on human self-fashioning and argue that human nature alone provides a ground on which to judge the acceptable limits of human transformation. Kass remarks, "If we can no longer look to our previously unalterable human nature for a standard or norm of what is good or better, how will anyone know what constitutes an improvement?" (Kass 2002: 132) Fukuyama's *Our Posthuman Future* offers a similar response to biotechnology, suggesting that human beings have deeply rooted instincts and a human nature that ought to have a special role in defining for us what is right and wrong (Fukuyama 2003: 7). Nature, Fukuyama suggests, imposes limits (2003: 38) and can serve as a ground for morality (2003: 115). Our sentimental, "gut-level" repugnance to technological projects of self-transformation is, Kass claims, "the emotional expression of deep wisdom, beyond reason's power to fully articulate it" (Kass 2002: 150). Human life elicits feelings of awe and respect that serve to demarcate the natural from the unnatural. Human dignity embraces the worthiness of embodied human life and "therewith of our natural desires and passions, our natural origins and attachments, our sentiments and aversions, our loves and longings" (Kass 2002: 18–19).

Reading *Extreme Makeover* from what we can call this "essentialist" perspective, we might think that as our participants are ushered from the American heartland to glitzy west-coast Beverly Hills, to be remade according to the latest fads and artificial standards of the Hollywood beauty and movie industries, what we witness is not the incipient birth of the posthuman, but rather the inhuman—the undignified descent into a realm where we are, as Kass puts it, so enchanted and enslaved by technology that we "have lost our awe and wonder before the deep mysteries of nature and life" (Kass 2002: 144). Rather than revealing the coming of a liberated age of autonomous self-creation, perhaps *Extreme Makeover* is more indicative of the lengths we twenty-first-century humans are willing to go to deny the natural aging process, our finitude and mortality, and the limits imposed on us by nature. In its display of human viscera, *Extreme Makeover* discloses our misguided attempts to control our future and transcend our biology.

Here too we have a position that has some resonance with a variety of approaches in feminist theory. Consider Kathryn Morgan's influential article "Women and the Knife." Like Kass, Morgan situates cosmetic surgery in a broader "era of biotechnology" and, again like Kass, worries that we are witnessing the "metaphysical neutralizing of man." "We have arrived at the stage of regarding ourselves as both technological subject and object, transformable and literally creatable through biological engineering. The era of biotechnology is clearly upon us and is invading even the most private and formerly sequestered domains of human life, including women's wombs" (Morgan 1991: 30). The increasing normalization of cosmetic surgery together with a host of other technical interventions in the body transforms the body into "an increasingly artificial and ever more perfect object" and transforms "the natural" from a barrier into a frontier (1991: 31). Patients and their surgeons opt for the apparent over the real and youthful appearance triumphs over "aged reality" (1991: 28). Morgan too, like Kass, seemingly draws on "gut-level" responses to the pathologies of cosmetic surgery. The opening of her essay contrasts passages about cosmetic surgery with images of surgical knives. She asks the reader: "Now look at the needles and at the knives. Look at them carefully. Look at them for a long time. *Imagine them cutting into your skin*" (1991: 26). A mere examination of these surgical knives is perhaps meant to provoke a counter-response to those passages celebrating cosmetic surgery.

Bordo situates cosmetic surgery more broadly in the "emergence of a culture of infinitely malleable 'plastic' bodies" (Bordo 1997: 9) and warns that "some of the paths our culture is following today are at the edges of a Brave New World that we ought to think twice about entering—as individuals and as contributors to the shaping of our culture" (Bordo 1997: 15). While Bordo insists that "all human bodies are culturally worked on, adorned, shaped, evaluated ..." (Bordo 1997: 17) and that "our knowledge of biology is always mediated by the conceptual frameworks—cultural as well as scientific paradigms—that we bring into the laboratory" (Bordo 1997: 179), in responding to questions (Hekman 1998) about her theory of the body she points to an evolution in her thinking toward a position "more agnostic and humble ... about the role of biology and evolution" (Bordo 1997: 179), motivated in part perhaps by her aging. "For myself, today I am less inclined than I used to be to dismiss the claims of geneticists. As I grow older and fall prey to the same disorders as everyone else in my family, I feel my own genetic inheritance more acutely than I did when I was younger and naively convinced of my power to 'resist' becoming anything like my father and mother" (Bordo 1997: 180). In "Braveheart, Babe, and the Contemporary Body," Bordo recommends that we learn to "accept and accommodate the small changes that happen gradually over the years," hold on perhaps to the ideal of aging beautifully and gracefully (Bordo 1997: 45), and see lines and wrinkles as the "markers of the accumulated experience and accomplishment of our lives," (Bordo 1997: 47). Bordo prefers to "get used to aging gradually" so that she can be "prepared and respond consciously and with dignity ... I'd rather be a vibrant old woman than embalm myself in a mask of perpetual youth" (Bordo 1997: 49). While Bordo describes this as individual preference, it is hard not to read it as the "natural" choice rather than simply one more norm that might be available were this the less normalizing, more heterogeneous and diverse culture for which Bordo is advocating.

While it is clear that neither Bordo nor Morgan would embrace the rather stark essentialism of Kass or Fukuyama, *Extreme Makeover* raises intriguing questions for some of the common elements in their critiques of cosmetic surgery and human enhancement technologies. Why prefer aged reality to youthful appearance? Why prefer the ideal of aging beautifully and gracefully to fighting it, kicking and screaming? Why not resist one's genetic inheritance or embrace synthetic beauty ideals (Tait 2007)? Here too standards of the "natural" are seemingly functioning to establish normative limits of the acceptable, though they wouldn't seem to be functioning very well, from the evidence provided by the show itself. Repugnance, whether engendered by projects of self-transformation or needles and knives, is certainly not much in evidence on the show. *Extreme Makeover* is one of many shows in which individuals are represented as voluntarily and gladly participating in their makeovers. They are represented as liking their makeovers and feeling transformed by them, both externally and internally. They look forward with eager anticipation to "beginning their new lives," a refrain heard regularly on the show. As one participant commented in an update several months after her final reveal, "I am becoming the person I always wanted to be. I'm so happy. I'm so glad." Claims to the effect that embracing these technological makeovers robs human beings of their dignity and inspires "our" repugnance do not entirely convince in light of such enthusiasm. On the shows themselves and in the many talk shows and newspaper and magazine articles examining them, there is very little of the gut-level repugnance Kass suggests "naturally" exists. One wonders whose gut-level reactions are trustworthy sources of "wisdom," according to Kass—certainly not those of the participants on these shows, apparently. Kass neither explains why we should trust *any* gut-level reactions as moral compasses, nor how we should decide, non-circularly, whose to trust.

The repeated reversion to the language of the "natural" on *Extreme Makeover*—the seeming need for participants, surgeons, family, and friends to accept the new bodies just insofar as they can somehow be counted as "natural" bodies that disclose the *authentic* looks of the participants—suggests that the show bears a complex relationship to essentialism. After all, Kass and his compatriots are not opposed to *all* technological interventions into the body. As an MD, Kass is in favor of the capacity of medicine to "cure" the body, but rules as "unnatural" any sort of "enhancements" of the body. Hence he too apparently appeals to a conception of the natural that is somehow consistent with artifice and intervention. While Kass and the makers of *Extreme Makeover* would clearly draw the line between "treatments" and "enhancements" in very different places, perhaps they share a broad-strokes ontology. *Extreme Makeover* can be read as offering cosmetic surgery as a "treatment" that allows the restoration/creation of a "natural look" revealing a "true self," but as excluding any modifications of the self that do not uphold such a narrative. The human nature essentialists want to preserve *natural norms* for human bodies. Yet they certainly recognize that it is never the case that all *Homo sapiens* will incarnate these norms; medicine can and should step in when it comes to "curing" abnormality, but it should never try to change what counts as normal. Meanwhile, *Extreme Makeover* apparently shares this conservative stance. It offers makeovers designed to make participants who suffer from aesthetic "ailments" (portrayed as direct causes of psychological and social ailments, such as low self-esteem, unemployability, and inability to catch the eye of a man) become "normal"—just "naturally beautiful." It offers "cures," but never challenges to established norms.

Clearly *Extreme Makeover* functions to problematize facile accounts of the natural as they appear in a variety of discourses about cosmetic surgery and human enhancement. The show exists as part of a constellation of practices and discourses that revolve around our sense of the natural while obscuring precisely what is meant by "the natural." Gaining greater conceptual clarity of this realm requires a more focused attention on this concept, to which we now turn.

Nature, Order, Monstrosity

Feminists and disability theorists generally have used Foucauldian accounts of normalization and discipline in order to challenge the fiction of a given natural body.[3] Yet there is a different conception of naturalness at work in the ontology and ideology of *Extreme Makeover*, since we have seen that here the normative call for the discipline and modification of the body is combined somehow with appeals to the natural body and the natural look as normative standards. Feminist theory has primarily shown us what the natural is *not*, namely a pure space independent from or prior to culture. It has done much less to help us understand what the natural *is*, insofar as this notion has life within institutions of body normalization. Clearly, a more nuanced analysis of this conceptual terrain is necessary.

When we leave philosophical accounts aside and attend carefully to how the notion of naturalness is invoked in everyday discourse, we notice that our conception of the "natural" is multivalent and multiply ambiguous. In ordinary language, we delineate the "natural" in at least three different ways, which can be quickly brought out by pointing out their different contrast classes:

First, something can be "natural" in the sense that it has not been changed or intervened upon by human hands, so that the "unnatural" is the "artificial" or the "manipulated." In this sense, your "natural" hair color is different from the "unnatural" color that you went to the salon to achieve.

Second, the concept of nature proper to Enlightenment science is appropriately contrasted with the *supernatural*, the "spooky," or the divine: that which stands outside the system of causal law. In this sense, we can debate whether the likeness of the Virgin Mary that recently appeared on a grilled cheese sandwich that was auctioned off on eBay for US$28,000 was a natural or a supernatural occurrence (while no one debates that the grilled cheese sandwich was produced by human hands). According to the standard scientific world picture, there is *nothing* that is actually unnatural in this sense. The natural/artificial distinction is orthogonal to the natural/supernatural distinction.

Third, we often deem "natural" that which displays or embodies proper orderliness, where the "unnatural" is the disfigured, deformed, or monstrous

3 For example, see Butler 1997, 2005, and Sawicki 1991.

Naturalness, on this third conception, is measured by aesthetic criteria such as harmony, symmetry, and fit. In this sense, hermaphrodism or homosexuality might be judged "unnatural," even if they are neither supernatural nor the product of artificial interventions. On this third picture of the natural, naturalness is actually quite compatible with artificial interference: gay adolescents are sometimes shipped off to correction camps so as to *make* their desires more "natural," and children with ambiguous genitalia or facial deformities are surgically altered so as to excise their "unnatural," aberrant features. This sense of the natural is the hardest to make precise, and unlike the other two it directly and definitionally carries normative weight (although the other two are of course given various normative valences as well). The natural, in this version, sets norms that govern appropriate transformations, but not by demanding that we refrain from intervening upon or modifying that which is given. Rather, it makes acceptable those modifications that enhance and embody natural order and it makes unacceptable those that disfigure and deform. We deem steroid use in athletes "unnatural" because it doesn't make for a proper, balanced, and orderly game that accords with our aesthetic sensibility, but we are happy to pump men full of drugs so that they don't experience "unnatural" impotence and women full of hormones so that they don't experience "unnatural" infertility or body hair or mood swings.

Despite its fuzziness, this last notion of the natural is at least as live in our cultural discourse and intuitions as the first two. Indeed, notwithstanding their nominal appeals to a supposed "biological" basis for their judgments, essentialists such as Kass actually seem to be appealing to something closer to this third conception of nature—nature as order and freedom from monstrosity, rather than nature as defined within science or nature as that which has not been artificially altered. As Chair of the President's Bioethics Council, Kass made it explicit that it is not *artifice* that makes a body "unnatural," since after all medical treatment always involves the intentional manipulation of the body. "Nevertheless," he writes, "the 'naturalness' of means matters. [The problem] lies not in the fact that … assisting drugs and devices are artifacts, but in the danger of violating or deforming the nature of human agency and the dignity of the naturally human way of activity" (Kass 2003: 292–3). The "naturally human way of activity" is that which promotes "human flourishing," and Kass defines such flourishing in terms of the proper, orderly fit between the inner and outer self. Although he offers no theory of how to tell when the inner and outer self match, he does worry repeatedly that through enhancement, someone might end up with a deceptive body that is not properly *hers*; through enhancement, we risk losing our "full humanity," becoming "'better' by no longer fully being ourselves" (Kass 2003: 129). Hence the "unnatural" is here associated with the hybrid, the chimerical, and the disorderly as opposed to the artificial or the supernatural.

Kass's "feelings of repugnance" can be read as markers of the boundaries of this aesthetic notion of the natural order—that is, as reactions that track our aesthetic sense of the perverse and the monstrous in contrast to the orderly and appropriate. But where Kass recommends taking these feelings as transparent measures of a naturally given moral order, in fact it seems that our aesthetic sense of natural order—which is certainly not grounded in anything like a coherent or comprehensive definition of the "properly ordered"—is often a sedimentation of strongly entrenched social norms that vary dramatically by region, era, ethnicity, and more. Our gut-level feeling that incest or cannibalism is repugnant may have some biological basis and be relatively fixed—although it is unclear why that would mean we should accord it any objective moral weight. But examples of culturally specific variations in these "gut reactions" run rampant. Generations of Americans raised within a culture of racial segregation felt that miscegenation was repugnant and "unnatural" in just this aesthetic sense; now such a reaction is unimaginable to most of us. The majority of citizens in some parts of the United States still have this repugnancy reaction to seeing members of the same sex kiss, while many of us in the rest of North America have just as intense a repugnancy reaction to the cultural trappings of those very parts of the country. In India, a sizeable and respectable minority value human urine as a tasty and healthful beverage.[4] In areas and subcultures where male circumcision is the norm, many people find foreskins disgusting, while in other places, the idea of chopping off a piece of the beloved penis is greeted with horror. Since such reactions appear heavily molded by our cultural training and implicit social expectations, they stand in need of constant political critique, rather than as mute and immediate measures of normative propriety.[5] There is nothing inherently wrong with understanding the "natural" in terms of aesthetic standards of orderliness as opposed to monstrosity, but it seems dangerous indeed to allow any slippage between aesthetic and moral norms in this case.

At this point we can restate the surprising ideological similarity between the human nature essentialists and the imagery of *Extreme Makeover* in more precise terms. For it seems that we ought to read the show, not as opening room for creation of *unnatural* bodies at all, but rather as promoting modifications of the *given* body that will allow it to achieve a heightened, perfect naturalness—a proper fit with our (culturally inculcated) sense of appropriate order. Participants come to the show in order to receive bodies that look as they naturally should, with disorderly monstrosities and perversions such as bulges of fat, hooked noses, and drooping jaw lines excised. In particular, they come in order to receive bodies that are gendered in the way that bodies "naturally" ought to be, free of any boundary-crossing traits such as a weak chest or inappropriate body hair. And they come, finally, in order to achieve that elusive "natural" fit between their inner and outer selves. In the rhetoric of the show, as in the rhetoric of cosmetic surgery more

4 Thanks to Kaila Kukla for providing this example.

5 Of course, our point here is the narrowly epistemological one concerning the status of our gut feelings of repugnance as transparent moral measures based on their supposed ability to measure "the natural"; we are making no argument whatsoever for moral relativism.

generally,[6] the interventions allow the "true" self to show itself non-deceptively on the surface of the body—this "true self" is presented as one that has been hidden, whether by hard living, low self-esteem, an accident, or some other cause, and is waiting to emerge by way of a technological "cure" that reunifies self and body.[7] By marshalling the rhetoric of the "true self" and its eventual unveiling through surgery, we ground the validity of the intervention in an appeal to natural order and the excision of hybrids, misfits, and misleading surfaces that are severed from the insides they cloak.

Our notions of the proper natural order and its monstrous counterpart often code various pervasive eugenic intuitions with broader social implications, whether or not we are willing to name them. It is common for these shows to portray procedures that "de-Africanize" or "de-Semiticize" participants, such as straightening hair and paring down noses. However we suspect that there would be little tolerance, either within the show or by its audience, for a participant who wanted to "Africanize" or "Semiticize" her appearance. The show is rife with examples of women taking steps to further feminize their bodies, but it would be an unlikely location to witness gender reassignment surgery—although this might make for an interesting test case, because one can imagine the show using the rhetoric of the "true self" to portray this performance as an exercise in upholding rather than dismantling a "natural" gender identity.

When we ask about the normative "limits" of human self-fashioning, it is tempting to look for a *quantitative* answer. We may think that some changes are "too extreme" or going "too far," whereas others are small enough to be acceptable. If we assume the size of a transformation is some measure of its acceptability, then even the title of the show—*Extreme Makeover*—suggests that it comes down firmly on the side of a radically permissive attitude towards these limits. However, what we have seen is that it is the *content* and not the *size* of the transformation that determines its social palatability. After all, liposuction counts as an acceptable modification, whereas the injection of abdominal fat does not, even though both modifications are exactly the same "size." The show offers transformations that are extreme in size, but conservative in kind. Just as the doctors who balk at human "enhancement" are generally not opposed to radical medical interventions that they read as *corrections* of the body, so, at the aesthetic level, the current culture of cosmetic surgery tolerates corrections of "unnatural" disorderly bodies, but not challenges to our conceptions of bodily order. The purpose of the surgical and technological interventions on *Extreme Makeover* is to produce "that natural look." The show makes vivid the extent to which the production of the "natural," orderly, normalized body depends upon intentional interventions and modifications. In this, it diverges from the rhetoric of the President's Council. But despite what we might interpret as the show's greater honesty on this front, it relies on a deeply

6 As one cosmetic surgery patient put it, "I'm basically a small-breasted type. That's just who I am" (Davis 2003: 77).

7 For a similar point, see Gilman 1998.

similar conception of the natural, the "normal," and the normative significance of each. Like the human nature essentialists, the show idealizes a world in which the tools of medicine produce normalized bodies with unchallenging identities that look and function just as bodies "naturally should."

Toward a Feminist Account of the Limits of Self-Fashioning

A feminist perspective can make us wary of claims that our nature is fixed, and equally of claims that our natures can be engineered and remade without constraint, in acts of pure individual freedom. Instead, feminist theorizing demands that we remain sensitive to the ways in which we are constructed in and by culture, and cognizant of the concrete social and political context of our schemes for self-fashioning. It calls upon us to recognize that our nature is not innocent, but rather saturated with social baggage. An understanding of the relationship between our judgments of "naturalness" and our enculturated, aesthetic standards of orderliness can serve as the ground for a feminist critique of both the essentialists' picture of a universal set of standards for human nature, and the libertarian denial of any substantive concept of the natural. We can insist that our notions of the natural are potent and rich, and pose significant constraints upon what we as a culture can normatively tolerate, while denying that this means that these notions need to be transhistorical and socially unencumbered in order to be real.

But highlighting these warnings does not yet guide us in making normative judgments about *which* acts of bodily self-transformation are actually problematic, liberating, etc. The fashioning and transformation of the body—even when performed on national television—is not yet a tool of liberation or of oppression, of the perversion of human nature or its enhancement. We need to proceed by turning a critical eye to the origin and social meaning of the particular desires that are encouraged and gratified by particular procedures and in particular settings. The hard work will lie in unpacking the subtle differences between our possible relationships to various projects of self-transformation—the differences between complicity, creative co-option, resistance, inauthenticity, colonialism, and so forth. Teasing out these different relationships to social possibilities and their different political and ethical implications is philosophically challenging, and it cannot be done except by beginning with detailed attention to the particular social norms being negotiated. This is just the kind of applied ethical work being done not only by feminists, but also by many writers in queer studies, fat studies, disability studies, race studies, and so forth.

Our location in social space constrains both our transformative imagination and the standards of bodily acceptability that we navigate. It also gives ethical meaning to the kinds of control we exercise over our bodies. We become human only in and among other humans. Our choices, our plans for self-transformation and self-fulfillment only make sense in a particular social and dialogical context. The producers of *Extreme Makeover* have built a narrative recognition of this dialectic; each episode concludes with the final coming out, the reintroduction of the makeover participant to her family and friends. Makeovers, as the show implicitly acknowledges, are never pursued as ends in themselves, but rather only make sense in the context of our socially situated relations to other people.

References

Agar, Nicholas. 2004. *Liberal Eugenics: In Defence of Human Enhancement*. Malden: Blackwell Publishing.

Annas, G. 2005. *American Bioethics: Crossing Human Rights and Health Law Boundaries*. New York: Oxford University Press.

Banet-Weiser, Sarah and Portwood-Stacer, Laura. 2006. "'I Just Want To Be Me Again!' Beauty Pageants, Reality Television and Post-feminism." *Feminist Theory*, 7(2), 255–72.

"Beyond the Body." 2007. *Wired*. 15(1).

"Body of the Future." 1999. *Popular Science* Special Issue: The Bioengineered Human. October 1999.

Bordo, Susan. 1993. *Unbearable Weight*. Berkeley: University of California Press.

Bordo, Susan. 1997. *Twilight Zones*. Berkeley: University of California Press.

Bostrom, Nick. 2005. "A History of Transhumanist Thought." *Journal of Evolution and Technology*, 14(1), 1–25.

"Building a New Human." 2000–01. *Newsweek* Special Edition. December 2000–February 2001.

Butler, Judith. 1997. *Bodies that Matter*. New York: Routledge.

Butler, Judith. 2005. *Foucault and the Government of Disability*. Ann Arbor: University of Michigan Press.

Davis, Kathy. 1995. *Reshaping the Female Body: The Dilemma of Cosmetic Surgery*. New York: Routledge.

Davis, Kathy. 2003. *Dubious Equalities and Embodied Differences: Cultural Studies on Cosmetic Surgery*. Lanham, MD: Rowman and Littlefield.

Firestone, Shulamith. 1970. *The Dialectic of Sex*. New York: William Morrow & Co.

Fisher, Garth. 2003. Appearing on *The Oprah Winfrey Show*, August 11.

Fukuyama, Francis. 2003. *Our Posthuman Future: Consequences of the Biotechnology Revolution*. New York: Farrar, Straus and Giroux.

Garreau, Joel. 2005. *Radical Evolution: The Promise and Peril of Enhancing our Minds, our Bodies—and What it Means to be Human*. New York: Doubleday.

Gilman, Sander. 1998. *Creating Beauty to Cure the Soul: Race and Psychology in the Shaping of Aesthetic Surgery*. Durham, NC: Duke University Press.

Gilman, Sander. 2002. "Plastic Surgery Goes Prime Time." *New York Times*, December 21.

Habermas, J. 2004. *The Future of Human Nature*. Cambridge: Polity Press.

Harris, John. 2007. *Enhancing Evolution.* Princeton: Princeton UP.
Hekman, Susan. 1998. "Material Bodies," in *Body and Flesh,* edited by Donn Welton. Malden, MA: Wiley-Blackwell, 61–70.
Heyes, Cressida J. 2007. "Cosmetic Surgery and the Televisual Makeover." *Feminist Media Studies*, 7(1), 17–32.
Holliday, Ruth and Taylor, Jacqueline Sanchez. "Aesthetic Surgery As False Beauty." *Feminist Theory*, 7(2), 179–95.
Hudson, Diane A. 2003. *The Oprah Winfrey Show.* Chicago: Harpo, Inc., August 11.
Kass, Leon. 2002. *Life, Liberty, and the Defense of Dignity.* San Francisco: Encounter Books.
Kass, Leon. 2003. "Ageless Bodies, Happy Souls." *The New Atlantis.* Spring 2003. Available at: http://www.thenewatlantis.com/docLib/TNA01-Kass.pdf
Kuczynski, Alex. 2004. "The World—On Order: Brad Pitt's Nose." *The New York Times*, May 2.
Mastrangelo, Karen-Leigh (Producer). *Extreme Makeovers*, Season 1, Episode 4.
McKibben, Bill. 2004. *Enough: Staying Human in an Engineered Age.* New York: Owl Books.
Morgan, Kathryn Pauly. 1991. "Women and the Knife: Cosmetic Surgery and the Colonization of Women's Bodies." *Hypatia*, 6(3), 25–53.
Negrin, Llewellyn. 2002. "Cosmetic Surgery and the Eclipse of Identity." *Body & Society*, 8(4), 21–42.
President's Council on Bioethics. 2003. *Beyond Therapy: Biotechnology and the Pursuit of Happiness.* Washington: Reagan Books.
Sawicki, Jana. 1991. *Disciplining Foucault.* New York: Routledge.
Stock, Gregory. 2002. *Redesigning Humans: Our Inevitable Genetic Future.* Boston: Houghton Mifflin.
Tait, Sue. 2007. "Television and the Domestication of Cosmetic Surgery." *Feminist Media Studies*, 7(2), 119–35.
"Your Bionic Future." 1999. *Scientific American* Quarterly. 10(3).

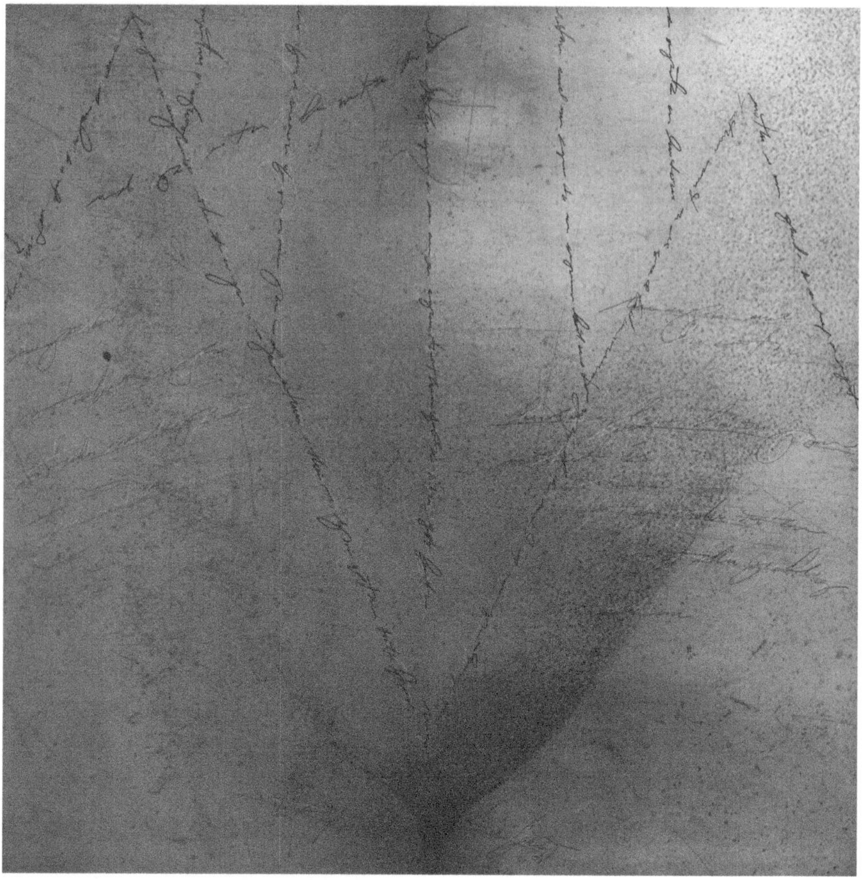

Figure 8.1 "Anatomy Lesson" 2007

Source: © Katherine Sanderson

Chapter 8
Selling the "Perfect" Vulva

Virginia Braun

In the 1970s, armed with mirrors, specula and torches, Western women learned to love their genitalia. The feminist personal/political project of genital looking aimed to demystify their genitals, and to empower women in their sexual and other lives (Ruzek 1978). It intended to reverse the iconography of women's genitalia, from something unknown, shameful, and disgusting, into something representing power, identity, and pleasure (Ardener 1987). The project has been more publicly enacted through explicit female genital displays in feminist art (Ardener 1987, Frueh 2003), and books containing vulval images (Blank 1993, Corinne 1989, Dodson 1996), compellingly demonstrating the diversity of vulval appearance. Following those heady days of second-wave feminism, which appeared to make women's genital appearance "all alright," the vulva largely disappeared from public discourse, until a play, *The Vagina Monologues* (Ensler 1998), wrenched it back into public consciousness. And, distressingly, *The Vagina Monologues* revealed that all was not well "down below." It appears "pudendal disgust is [still] a social reality" (Tiefer 2008: 475) and "ugliness … looms large in both cultural and women's consciousness of vaginas" (Frueh 2003: 145). *The Vagina Monologues* became a significant movement, globally, and in the USA, but at the same time as Ensler (1998) and thousands of women were proclaiming a message of vaginal pride, solidarity, and empowerment, thousands of other women appear to have been seeking "empowerment" in a very different way—through cosmetic surgery to alter the appearance (and function) of their genitalia.[1]

This chapter focuses on such so-called "designer vagina" surgery, defining the field and analyzing public discourse in the form of websites from surgeons who offer these procedures. Located within a framework that sees material and experiential bodies as shaped by the discursive and representational, I argue that these sites work in multiple ways to sell both vulval distress and transformation. Certain morphologies are pathologized, implicitly and explicitly; others are valorized. Women are invited into a medicalized regime of self-assessment and intervention to achieve the perfect vulva.

---

1 I am talking about a specific group of surgeries here, "chosen" to "enhance" the female genital appearance of women. I am *not* talking about gender reassignment surgeries, or surgeries on intersex individuals—although these are mostly "entirely cosmetic in function" (Chase 2005: 131)—or "traditional" genital cuttings.

The Emergence of the "Designer Vagina"

The media term "designer vagina" refers to a range of procedures designed to *enhance* the appearance and/or function of parts of a woman's vulva and vagina. This female genital cosmetic surgery (FGCS) has diversified in both site of alteration and technique of surgery, with all parts of women's genitalia subject to potential aesthetic (and "functional") enhancement. Labia minora are reduced in size and thickness, and made "symmetrical." Labia majora are filled out, the mons pubis reduced, the vagina "tightened," and the perineum "smoothed." The clitoral hood is reduced, the hymen reconstructed, and the "G-spot" "amplified." There is a seemingly endless array of genital "improvements" the could-be consumer can "choose" to purchase. These procedures are on the increase (Braun 2005, Liao and Creighton 2007), with a greater number of surgeons offering FGCS, and a greater number of women having surgery. The surgery has been identified as "basically where breast augmentation was 30 years ago" (Gurley 2003: 2).

Although some of these procedures have been performed—for aesthetic purposes—for at least 30 years, the idea of *aesthetic* surgical genital alteration was only born into *public* discourse in the late 1990s, with the emergence of surgeon websites, surgeon advertisements in various media, and extensive media coverage such as women's magazine articles, television, and Internet-based commentary. Since that emergence, public discourse has increased phenomenally. Today, Google produces nearly 85,000 hits for the exact phrase "designer vagina," and "designer vagina" has its own entry in the online encyclopedia, *Wikipedia* (http://en.wikipedia.org/wiki/Designer_vagina). In contrast to public discourse, there is limited medical literature, with no scientifically thorough, systematic studies of outcome, functional or aesthetic. Most medical literature reports one or two cases to show technique for labial reductions (e.g., Alter 1998, Giraldo Gonzalez and de Haro 2004); a few report outcome over a series of cases (de Alencar Felicio 2007, Pardo, Solà, Ricci, and Guilloff 2006, Rouzier, Louis-Sylvestre, Paniel, and Haddad 2000); one has reported patient motivations (Miklos and Moore 2008). There has been some debate regarding ethics of FGCS (Goodman et al. 2007, Liao and Creighton 2007, Tiefer 2008, Tracy 2007) and critique from professional bodies (The American College of Obstetrics and Gynecology 2007, The Royal Australian and New Zealand College of Obstetricians and Gynaecologists 2008). There has also been increasing critical academic feminist engagement (e.g., Adams 1997, Allotey, Manderson, and Grover 2001, Braun 2005, S. W. Davis 2002, Frueh 2003, Green 2005, Jeffreys 2005, Jordan 2004, Manderson 2004, McNamara 2006, Sullivan 2007, Tiefer 2008).

On one level, FGCS seems incredible; on another, perfectly understandable. In addition to the general diversification and normalization of cosmetic surgery that has recently occurred in many Western countries (Blum 2003, Brooks 2004),[2]

2 For instance, in the USA there was a 17% increase in the number of cosmetic surgeries performed in 2004 from 2003, with an increase of 44% for *all* cosmetic procedures

current and past (Western) genital practices shed light on the emergence of the "designer vagina." For instance, the apparently common practice of the "husband stitch" (Kitzinger 1994) involved an "extra" stitch to tighten the vagina post-birth. Jahoda's (1995) account of a woman whose doctor said "by the way, I put in an extra stitch for you" (258) *to her husband* is not unusual; nor are jokes about the vagina being "made new" or "tailor made" (Pizzini 1991). A noted benefit of cesarean sections, promoted in Brazil to keep the vagina "honeymoon fresh" (MacNair 1992; Orr 1998), is that they "prevent vaginal sagging" (Adams 1997: 67; also Manderson 2004; Robinson 1998). American sex therapist Jennifer Berman reportedly commented at a professional sex therapists' meeting in 2004 that she had elected for cesarean delivery, as "why ruin a perfectly good set of genitals in childbirth" (Karen Hicks, Personal Communication, September 2005). The rhetoric of childbirth as "ruining" the genitals is one that features frequently. These practices demonstrate that women's genitals have been constructed as potentially inadequate or damageable, and improvable (through medical intervention). (For more discussion on vaginal tightness, see Braun and Kitzinger 2001.)

More contentiously, continuities can be seen between FGCS and "traditional" female genital cuttings (Braun in press; Sullivan 2007). Despite some important differences, and rhetoric that constructs them as entirely different (see Braun in press), there *are* continuities between Western women's "chosen" FGCS, and non-Western women's genital "mutilation" (e.g., see Adams 1997, Green 2005, Sullivan 2007). Both are aimed at producing a culturally "appropriate," and desirable, genital appearance, and one which is "properly" gendered. Even at the material level, there are *degrees* of similarity in some procedures: where the vagina is targeted, both involve tightening; where labia minora are affected, both involve reduction. Finally, both reflect cultural pressures and expectations of appropriate, and sexually/relationally desirable, femininity and womanhood (Green 2005, McNamara 2006). It seems "the motivations that impel African-rooted FGOs and American labiaplasties should not be envisaged as radically distinct" (S. W. Davis 2002: 24). (For more discussion around this, see Allotey et al. 2001, Braun in press, S. W. Davis 2002, Essén and Johnsdotter 2004, Manderson 2004, Sullivan 2007; see also Jeffreys 2005, Sheldon and Wilkinson 1998.)

Sites of Discourse

Surgeon websites are part of the proliferation of discourse on female genital cosmetic surgery. These sites cannot be seen in isolation from other discourse on the topic, or about women's bodies, sexualities, and identities. However, they are distinct: they have a particular function—to promote the surgeon(s), clinic(s),

("Cosmetic procedures in 2004" 2005).

and surgeries to could-be clients, and are important to analyze for this reason.[3] In this chapter, I critically examine the content of 20 surgeon websites (which amounted to over 400 printed pages), which were accessed in 2005. They are a convenience sample of the first hits from Google searches and sites of high profile surgeons, combined with specific sampling for geographic dispersion. Ten are from US locations; the rest from other English-speaking countries (see Appendix 1). Although a significant proportion of this surgery *is* occurring in the US, the "global village" produced by both easy information access and transfer (e.g., the Internet), and increasingly affordable air travel, mean that this must be analyzed as a global, or at least Western-global, phenomenon. One site claims to have "patients come to South Florida from all over the world, Europe, Asia, South America, Canada, as well as from all over the United States" (US1).[4] Another tells of patients from "over 35 US states and 20 countries" and a "franchise" of associated (and technique-trained) surgeons all through the Americas, Asia, and Europe (US9). Others (e.g., US4, US6) offer televised live surgery on the *E* program *Dr 90210* (http://www.eonline.com/On/Dr90210/), to an audience that could, theoretically, be anywhere.

My analysis is situated in relation to others who have theorized the influence of society and social expectation on the experiences and practices of bodies (e.g., Bordo 1993), and who have argued that women's bodies are deeply implicated in practices of oppression and liberation (K. Davis 1997). It is located within feminist social constructionism (Burr 1995, Tiefer 1995), and recognizes bodies as material as well as discursive. I theorize practices as enabled (and constrained) by language and, specifically, discursive formulations around an area. Experience—emotional, physical, perceptual—is socially constructed, rather than essential or inherent, as are "knowledge and practices of the body" (Manderson 2004: 299), and, indeed, the meanings and "truth" of anatomy itself (e.g., Laqueur 1990). Surgeon website discourse, then, contributes to the ongoing construction of experiential as well as material bodies, to the production of desires, and practices around these desires.

My analysis focuses on the ways "right" and "wrong" genitalia are demarcated and flesh pathologized on these sites. I discuss the use of psychological discourse and (psychological) truth claims, and consider the implications of all these for women's embodied subjectivity and desires. It is important to note that there is no single narrative across all sites, or even within sites: they are not as uniform as this analysis could be taken to suggest.

3 Cosmetic surgeons are being advised in how best to market themselves through this medium (Rohrich 2001), pointing to its potential significance.

4 Websites have a country of origin reference code (US: United States; UK: United Kingdom; CA: Canada; AU: Australia; NZ: New Zealand), and an identification number. Details of each website, including location and URL, are in Appendix 1.

Surgical Stories: Ambiguity, Pathologization, and the Promise of Perfection

The sites reinforce and create a range of sociocultural norms around women's sexuality and their genitalia, and work to pathologize genital diversity. The sites target an assumed heterosexual woman whose sexual life revolves around intercourse. In some instances, there is even a conflation of the "sensual side of sexual gratification" (US7) with a *not*-"loose" vagina, reducing sex and sexual/sensual pleasures to intercourse, friction, and an oh-so-tight fit. Pleasure, here, is located *within* the vagina, for women.[5] When discussed sexually physiologically (rather than sexually psychologically), the labia minora are typically framed as causing an "interference" (US2) in sex; in one site, however, they have *no* sexual potential (and thus there is no sexual risk from surgery[6]): "the labia have no means of providing pleasurable stimulation. The labia minora are not involved in the process of sexual excitement" (US8). This demarcating of sexual problems, sensations, and pleasures is a feature of these sites. They provide women with a vocabulary of (potential) problems and their bodily locations.

Surgeon websites are involved in the demarcation of "wrong" and "right" female genital morphology. While psychology is a key dimension, the *materiality* of the body is problematic. The problems are specified: an "oversized and overstretched" (UK4) vagina with "weak, loose, vaginal muscles" (UK2) signals the "Loss of the Optimum Structural Architecture of the Vagina" (US9), clearly requiring "rejuvenation"; "thinned" (AUS2), "sagging" (NZ1), or "flat or small" (US9) labia majora are to be repaired; "large or asymmetric" (AUS1), "elongated or unequal" (NZ1), or "slightly bulky" (UK1) labia minora with "hyperpigmented ends" (US9) are to be "corrected." The concept of "large" or "enlarged" seems to act as shorthand for labia minora that extend beyond the labia majora, although "protrusion" (US4) is also clearly identified as a problematic state. Though a linking with "abnormality" in some sites—as in a "protuberant and abnormal appearance" (US10)—protrusion is framed as inherently (aesthetically) abnormal (when it is "normal," see Lloyd, Crouch, Minto, Liao and Creighton 2005).

Demarcations of "problem" states *suggest* desirable states, but (desired and actual) outcomes of such "beautification" (US5) surgery are also frequently specified. "Small, beautiful, comfortable" (US8) labia minora, with a "sleeker,

---

5 Hall (2001) makes the point that FGCS procedures like this both reinforce the centrality of vaginal penetration in women's sexual pleasure, and also make female bodies conform to cultural expectations—make bodies fit sex, rather than sex fitting bodies (Braun 2005).

6 Sexual or other risk was not a pervasive discourse. Some sites did discuss a range of risks, although often "risk" was framed as something to talk to the surgeon about, in person—and thus as something to consider at a later stage (when possibly more committed to surgery?). Typically, the surgery was framed as "relatively minor" (US2), and thus inherently not particularly risky. The underplaying of risk has been noted elsewhere in relation to cosmetic procedures (Rothman and Rothman 2003).

thinner, more comfortable and more appealing size and shape" (US10) are desired. A "tight" (US9) vagina that produces "friction" (US2) is required. A key discourse is that of "youthfulness" (AUS2): the "nice" vulva is a young-looking vulva, a "tight" vagina one that feels "young." This valorization of youth, associated with both cosmetic surgery discourse (Fraser 2003) and consumer culture (Featherstone 1991), "locks" anatomy and aesthetics into a certain point in development, constructing any subsequent change as bad. With aging inevitable, it works to construct a potentially infinite client base for surgeons.

Language offers a rich and subtle level at which "truth" and "reality" are constructed. For all the demarcation of problems, "ambiguous" language invites uncertainty. Although a "loose" (UK2) vagina, "saggy" (NZ1) labia majora, or "large" (US6) "thick" (US7) labia minora are typically presented as self-evident truths, these adjectives are anything but: is *any* level of "protrusion" a problem? How much "asymmetry" *is* acceptable? What counts as "loose"? They require a comparison state to be meaningful; they rely on the invocation of an opposite (implicitly right) state to make sense. "Small," "symmetrical," or "contained" labia minora become the standard of *normal* that "large" labia transgress. The sites rarely contain any measures of what actually counts as "large" or "thick"[7] or "loose." Even where "abnormality" is explicated—as in "oversized" (US3), "abnormally enlarged" (UK5), or "hypertrophic" (US10) labia minora there are, again, no indications as to what constitutes these particular "conditions." In this way, a wide range of appearance is potentially medicalized, inviting or inducing anxiety in women.

An effect of such ambiguous characterizations is that, for example, any labial protuberance potentially becomes constructed as anatomically abnormal. These ambiguous descriptions work in concert with descriptions of what is desirable,[8] existing genital shame and anxiety (S. W. Davis 2002, Green 2005), and broader sociocultural accounts (Braun and Wilkinson 2001), to *allow* (invite) "abnormality" and psychological discomfort to be experienced along a range of labia minora sizes and shapes. Variation becomes pathologized. In this context, with websites framing "contained" labia minora as "normal" and desirable, and genital concerns as something "many women" (US4) experience, linguistic ambiguity means many women may assume their genitals are "abnormal," and then desire and seek surgical "correction." With such ambiguity, surgeons invite anxiety (S. W. Davis 2002), and widen their potential client base.

Medicalization and pathologization of particular states occurs in other ways. The language is of "excess" vaginal (US2) or labial (US6) tissue, of "unwanted skin" (UK2) and "redundant vaginal mucosa" (US9). The discourse is one of damaged

---

7 US4 offers up 5–6 cm as an outer limit ("in some cases …"), which generally fits with Lloyd et al's (2005) data from 50 women, while CA1 shows one image with stretched labia beside a (fuzzy) ruler, which looks to measure just over 3 cm long.

8 There is a long cultural history of associating "large" labia minora with pathology and deviance (Gilman 1985, Terry 1995).

bodies and repair: "correction" (US2) or "treatment" (US9) of an identifiable "condition" (US4) or "problem" (US2), which stems from an identifiable *cause*. FGCS is thus constructed as *legitimate* surgery with a "restorative or healing function" (Jordan 2004: 338). The main causes of "damage" (US9) are aging and childbirth, although injury, weight loss, and genetics also feature. The language of decay—"shrunken or atrophied labia majora or minora" (US8)—leaves no doubt that aging is bad. Surgery is about "restoration" (US7) and "rejuvenation" (US5), the return of youth, which constructs the pre-surgical genitalia as existing in a damaged and/or not-right, not-normal, state. Surgery restores them to a (better than before) state of rightness. What the surgeon discourse produces is an account where a certain anatomical state and aesthetic is right, and the one a woman should want, and where her body is a battleground between this state and common, everyday forces designed to destroy it. As part of an established representation of women's genitalia as a site of vulnerability (Braun and Wilkinson 2001, 2003), this constitutes their very nature as always *potentially* (if not already) problematic, with the loss of "optimal architectural integrity" (US7) a constant possibility—albeit one with a solution. The websites tend to engage in a process of medicalizing genital appearance and change, taking the "natural" process of aging (and birth) and creating pathology in need of surgeon intervention. The message is that women cannot be complacent about their genitalia. Women are situated within a (culturally pervasive) discourse of risk; here the risk is to themselves, from their bodies.

Another way genital "deviance" is constructed is through the use of before-and-after photos found on ten (mostly US) sites, which, while demonstrating the "skill" of the surgeon, also display "desirable" and "undesirable" vulvas. In the context of a wider "self-surveillance world of images" (Featherstone 1991: 179), any woman can look at these "before" photographs and, if perceiving *any* vulval resemblance, potentially (re)define and (re)experience her vulva as undesirable and wrong. She can identify "desirable" vulval morphology: the "neat," "tidy," contained, almost pre-pubescent (Manderson 2004), vulva, "the clean slit" (S. W. Davis 2002: 12). This "clean aesthetic designates looseness and bulges as unsightly generosities of flesh—a mess" (Frueh 2003: 145). In its containment, the surgical vulva (and tightened vagina) is the antithesis of the leaky, uncontained abject body (Kristeva 1982), which the "messy" vulva (and the "loose" vagina) embodies, and which appears to haunt the imaginary of many women. In this sense, these images do not exist in isolation from broader cultural discourse on desirable and undesirable vulval/vaginal states.[9] They must also be considered in conjunction with the vulvas of mainstream pornography, which has been normalized in recent

9 Further, Featherstone (1991) points out that the images that surround us in consumer culture are not only about stimulating "false needs" (193), they also "harness and channel genuine bodily needs and desires" (193). FGCS images may stimulate dissatisfaction and desire for surgery, but this dissatisfaction, or hints of it, often pre-dates the images of surgery.

times (e.g., Häggström-Nordin, Sandberg, Hanson, and Tydén 2006), and is where women apparently identify the desirable vulva (Braun 2005, S. W. Davis 2002, Green 2005, Jeffreys 2005, Liao and Creighton 2007). One website stated: "Many people have asked us for an example of an aesthetically pleasing vulva. We went to our patients for the answer and they said the playmates of Playboy" (US9).

I have discussed the way certain genital morphologies are constructed as pathological or "wrong," and certain genital morphologies are constructed as desirable. Though such discursive constructions, surgery is rendered a reasonable and rational desire; it becomes more so through invocations of psychology.

Psychology and the Truth of Our Bodies, Our Selves

While these surgeries are about bodily states, they are also framed as about psychology, and *emotional* states. A recourse to psychology is not surprising, as there are intimate links between psychology, marketing, and consumption (Bowlby 1993), and psychology, appearance, and cosmetic surgery (marketing) (Jordan 2004). Readers are informed that a woman's perceptions of her genitals can have "devastating effects on her life. It can threaten her self-esteem, reduce her sexual desire and excitement, ruin her love life, or cause vaginal discomfort" (US5). Dislike of her genital appearance "may cause severe embarrassment with a sexual partner or loss of self-esteem" (US8), and "may impact on their relationships" (AUS1). Furthermore, the surgery itself is framed as a *psychological* intervention: "after labiaplasty, your self-esteem and anatomic form will be corrected" (US6); the woman will have "greater self-esteem … and improved confidence" (US8). Vaginal tightening "can enhance intimacy" (US2). The idea is that "cosmetic surgery is more than enhancing the way you look; it is about transforming the way you feel" (UK4). A discourse of psychological and sexual transformation was evident throughout: one site claimed that "many women are now seeking cosmetic vaginal surgery to recreate sexual excitement, restore self-esteem and rejuvenate their love lives" (US5). A patient testimonial on another described her surgery as "a wonderful success that I cannot describe in words … the visual appearance of before and after is amazing and has brought solace and acceptance to my life as well as my mind, body, and spirit" (US9). This discourse of (psychological) transformation is a feature of FGCS (see Braun 2005) and cosmetic surgery (e.g., Blum 2003, Haiken 1997, Jordan 2004, Sullivan 2001) discourse, where cosmetic surgery becomes *psycho*therapy (Fraser 2003, Gilman 1998, 1999).

In articulating the changes the patient will/may experience, these sites employ a range of medical, psychological, and sexual truth-claims about bodies and surgical and psychological outcomes;[10] only one (US9) cites *any* research to back

10 These truth claims are not always consistent between and even within sites (e.g., US8).

up these claims.[11] While my analytic focus is primarily on the "truths" constructed through these sites, the "validity" of such truth-claims should also be mentioned, as some are questionable, and others blatantly wrong.[12] One often-repeated claim is that vaginal tightening "typically tones vaginal muscle" (UK2). It does not; it brings the muscles closer together, and removes "excess" vaginal tissue, but the *tone* of the muscles remains unchanged. This supposed toning, and resultant "greater strength and control" (US8), apparently increases "sexual gratification" (US9) for the woman, and her (male) partner: vaginal tightening "is a direct means of enhancing one's sexual life again" (US8). Such (apparently unfounded, Green 2005, Walsh 2005) claims for increased sexual pleasure are concerning in the context of studies of other gynecological surgeries that report deterioration of sexual function in some women, along with no benefits, sexually, in others (Helström and Nilsson 2005, Lemack and Zimmern 2000). Similarly, the claim on one site that "the clitoris can be surgically reduced in size while maintaining sensitivity" (US6) needs to be assessed in light of evaluations of clitoral surgeries on intersex infants, where people often report sexual difficulties (Minto, Liao, Woodhouse, Ransley, and Creighton 2003). Finally, in relation to psychologically transformative truth-claims, although some research indicates that cosmetic surgery (in general) can be beneficial in relation to body image and self-esteem (Honigman, Phillips, and Castle 2004), results are far from conclusive and "overall, there are more questions than answers regarding the psychological effects of cosmetic surgery" (Dittman 2005: 30; see also Sarwer 2005).

Selling the Perfect Vulva

Any analysis of the "designer vagina," and surgeon websites, needs to be situated within the greater targeting of women as sexual consumers that has recently occurred (Attwood 2005) and, indeed, a broader analysis of bodies, consumption and (women's place within) consumer culture (Featherstone 1991, Jagger 2000). With "designer vagina" surgery, the female body (again) becomes the site of/for sexual consumption, with the (heterosexual) woman herself as both agent and object in this process. The websites invite women into a process where their genitalia and sexual practices are redefined, as surgically improvable. They situate

11 US9 describes Masters and Johnson's (1966) research on female and male sexual response to claim that women are "multiorgasmic" and sexually superior to men, and invokes them in its claim that friction is necessary for "female sexual gratification." Masters and Johnson's scientific demonstration of the centrality of the clitoris to female sexual pleasure is absent; pleasure is located in the almighty vagina.

12 This is not entirely surprising. Reports of examinations of information about various medical conditions available on the web range from "mostly correct" (Sandvik 1999) to "poor" (Soot, Moneta, and Edwards 1999), although one would expect surgeon sites to be accurate.

women within what Adams (1997) has referred to as the surgical aesthetic: "the theory and practice that deals with the surgical transformation of women's bodies from a 'natural' state of inadequacy and ugliness into a potentially 'ideal' state of beauty and perfect functioning" (60). These sites rely on a simultaneous tension between (future) sexual empowerment and liberation for women, and the presence or production of genital anxiety. They are typically about selling transformation: a better future through a "tidier" vulva, a tighter vagina, or a smoother perineum. This better future is one where her self-confidence and self-esteem have improved, and her sex life is fantastic (Braun 2005). They invoke a self-improving subject, who desires *and deserves* bodily perfection. Cosmetic surgery is a legitimate way to get this: it is "an honest investment in self-improvement" (CA1). Whether women should be "improving" their bodies (selves), through surgery, is not raised as a question. The story is one of transformation, but also of transcendence: the woman can transcend age, childbirth(s), or genetics, and create her perfect body—with the surgeon's help. Her body is both "scourge and salvation" (Jordan 2004: 339) of her present and future well-being.

While these websites clearly advertise a product they want people to purchase (Green 2005), they do not *just* market surgery. They also "educate" women. Some explicitly locate themselves as educational (e.g., CA1, US7), and as different from those engaged in "aggressive marketing" (CA1), but the line is blurry. In "marketing" procedures, women are "educated" of surgical solutions to potentially unknown defects in their bodies. In "educating" women about (potential) problems, causes, and treatments, and likely outcomes, women are invited into an ongoing regime of self-examination and concern (e.g., see Bartky 1988) about this part of their bodies, and invited to "correct" any "problems." Surgery becomes an appropriate way to address bodily "anomalies" (Manderson 2004) *and* psychological concerns (Braun 2005). Through educating women "what to look for" (e.g., AUS1) in surgery and a surgeon, these sites also invite the would-be consumer to purchase from them, as only a *good* doctor would consider putting such information on their website.[13] So advertising *is* education, and "education" *is* advertising.

From a feminist constructionist perspective, these sites are deeply problematic, as they contribute to the construction of women's genitals as a (potential) site of distress, and of *legitimate* distress. The information they contain does not occur in a cultural vacuum; they produce and reproduce various discourses that already exist about women's sexuality and women's bodies/genitalia (Braun and Kitzinger 2001, Braun and Wilkinson 2001, 2003), agency and choice, and cosmetic surgery. An "ideal patient" haunts these sites—a woman who is informed, thoughtful, critical,

13 Surgeon marketing is a key aspect of plastic surgery (Jordan 2004), and sites market their surgeons quite diversely, through claims of surgeon expertise, innovation, and experience, through reference to their "pioneering" (US9) and "lead[ing]" (US6) roles in FGCS, and through claims of "state of the art" (US3) equipment and facilities. Although the marketing is not blatant—they do not say "you must have surgery"—the message is that *should* a woman choose surgery, this is a surgery.

a decision-maker, certainly not a cultural dupe. They invoke feminist rhetoric (see also S. W. Davis 2002) around choice, and empowerment, to offer a positive identity for the woman who chooses surgery—a rational, informed agent, making an active decision about her (future) sexual and psychological well-being (see also Braun in press). Agency (and choice), a common discourse around cosmetic surgery (K. Davis 1995, 2003, Fraser 2003), is clearly evident here. They also invoke a dominant neoliberal Western discourse of individualism.[14] The woman is encouraged to let her own desires be known, to (actively) work with the surgeon, who designs the surgery to achieve "the results you desire" (UK5). However, ultimately, as with much cosmetic surgery discourse and practice (Morgan 1991), they promote conformity to a specific genital aesthetic, and work to normalize it. Although not a single story, these sites sell the perfect vulva and perfect vagina as a route to a better you, and better sex; at the same time, they (re)produce the potentially imperfect vulva and vagina.

14 Although I have focused on wealthy Western countries, FGCS is not just a Western phenomenon—it occurs in many other locations (e.g., Argentina, Indonesia, South Africa). Further research is needed to examine the different, and shared, meanings and practices of genitalia and FGCS in different global locations.

Appendix 1: List of surgeon websites analyzed, and surgeon location

Code	Surgeon/Surgery name	Location	URL
AUS1	Dr Mark Kohout	Sydney & Orange, NSW, Australia	http://www.drmarkkohout.com.au
AUS2	Image Cosmetic Surgery Centre	Melbourne, Australia	http://www.imagecentre.com.au http://www.aesthetica.com.au
CA1	Cosmetic Surgicentre	Toronto, Canada	http://www.psurg.com
NZ1	Appearance Gynaecology	Auckland, New Zealand	http://www.appearancegynae.co.nz
UK1	Surgicare Group	UK (Manchester & Nationwide)	http://www.surgicare.co.uk
UK2	Cosmetic Surgery Consultants	Various, UK	http://www.cosmeticsurgeryconsultants.co.uk
UK3	Cosmetic Surgery Advisory Services	Guildford & Brighton, UK	http://www.cosmeticsurgeryservices.com
UK4	Transform Medical Group	Nationwide, UK	http://www.transforminglives.co.uk
UK5	Chris J. Inglefield	London, UK	http://www.plasticsurgery-cji.co.uk
UK6	Dr Erik Scholten	London, UK	http://www.plasticsurgery4u.co.uk
US1	Dr Pamela Loftus	Boca Raton, Florida, USA	http://www.labiaplasty.org
US2	Pacific Centre for Plastic Surgery	Los Angeles, CA, USA	http://www.horowitzmd.com
US3	The Body Sculpting Center	Scottsdale, AZ, USA	http://www.bodynew.com
US4	Dr Robert Rey	Los Angeles, CA, USA	http://www.drrobertrey.com
US5	Cosmetic Surgery, PA	Ft Lauderdale, FL, USA	http://www.cosmeticsurgery2.com
US6	Gary J Alter	Los Angeles, CA, & New York, NY, USA	http://www.altermd.com http://www.labiaplastycenters.com
US7	Various	USA	http://www.lasertreatments.com
US8	Labiaplasty Surgeon (3 clinics, 2 surgeons)	Los Angeles, CA; Ft Lauderdale, FL, USA	http://www.labiaplastysurgeon.com
US9	Laser Vaginal Rejuvenation Institute of Los Angeles	Los Angeles, CA, USA	http://www.drmatlock.com
US10	Liberty Women's Health Care	New York, NY, USA	http://www.libertywomenshealth.com

References

Adams, A. 1997. "Moulding Women's Bodies: The Surgeon As Sculptor," in *Bodily Discursions: Gender, Representations, Technologies* edited by D. S. Wilson and C. M. Laennec. New York: State University of New York Press, 59–80.

de Alencar Felicio, Y. 2007. "Labial Surgery." *Aesthetic Surgery Journal*, 27(3), 322–8.

Allotey, P., Manderson, L., and Grover, S. 2001. "The Politics of Female Genital Surgery in Displaced Communities." *Critical Public Health*, 11(3), 189–201.

Alter, G. J. 1998. "A New Technique for Aesthetic Labia Minora Reduction." *Annals of Plastic Surgery*, 40(3), 287–90.

The American College of Obstetricians and Gynecologists. 2007. "Vaginal 'Rejuvenation' and Cosmetic Vaginal Procedures" (Committee Opinion Piece No. 378). *Obstetrics & Gynecology*, 110, 737–8.

Ardener, S. 1987. "A Note on Gender Iconography: The Vagina," in *The Cultural Construction of Sexuality* edited by P. Caplan. London: Routledge, 113–42.

Attwood, F. 2005. "Fashion and Passion: Marketing Sex to Women." *Sexualities*, 8(4), 392–406.

Bartky, S. L. 1988. "Foucault, Femininity, and the Modernization of Patriarchal Power," in *Feminism & Foucault: Reflections on resistance* edited by I. Diamond and L. Quinby. Boston: Northeastern University Press, 61–86.

Blank, J. 1993. *Femalia*. San Francisco: Down There Press.

Blum, V. L. 2003. *Flesh Wounds: The Culture of Cosmetic Surgery*. Berkeley: University of California Press.

Bordo, S. 1993. *Unbearable Weight: Feminism, Western Culture, and the Body*. Berkeley: University of California Press.

Bowlby, R. 1993. *Shopping with Freud*. London: Routledge.

Braun, V. 2005. "In Search of (Better) Female Sexual Pleasure: Female Genital 'Cosmetic' Surgery." *Sexualities*, 8(4), 407–24.

Braun, V. In press. "'*The women are doing it for themselves*': The Rhetoric of Choice and Agency Around Female Genital 'Cosmetic Surgery'." *Australian Feminist Studies*.

Braun, V. and Kitzinger, C. 2001. "The Perfectible Vagina: Size Matters." *Culture Health & Sexuality*, 3, 263–77.

Braun, V. and Wilkinson, S. 2001. "Socio-Cultural Representations of the Vagina." *Journal of Reproductive and Infant Psychology*, 19, 17–32.

Braun, V. and Wilkinson, S. 2003. "Liability or Asset? Women Talk About the Vagina." *Psychology of Women Section Review*, 5(2), 28–42.

Brooks, A. 2004. "'Under the Knife and Proud of It:' "An Analysis of the Normalization of Cosmetic Surgery." *Critical Sociology* 30(2): 207–39.

Burr, V. 1995. *An Introduction to Social Constructionism*. London: Routledge.

Chase, C. 2005. "'Cultural Practice' or 'Reconstructive Surgery'? U.S. Genital Cutting, the Intersex Movement, and Medical Double Standards," in *Genital*

Cutting and Transnational Sisterhood: Disputing U.S. Polemics edited by S. James, M. and C. C. Robertson. Urbana, IL: University of Illinois Press, 126–51.

Corinne, T. 1989. *Cunt Coloring Book*. San Francisco: Last Gasp.

"Cosmetic Procedures in 2004." 2005. *APA Monitor*, 36(8), 31.

Davis, K. 1995. *Reshaping the Female Body: The Dilemma of Cosmetic Surgery*. New York: Routledge.

Davis, K. 1997. "Embody-ing Theory: Beyond Modernist and Postmodernist Readings of the Body," in *Embodied Practices: Feminist Perspectives on the Body* edited by K. Davis. London: Sage, 1–23.

Davis, K. 2003. *Dubious Equalities and Embodied Differences: Cultural Studies on Cosmetic Surgery*. Lanham, MD: Rowman & Littlefield.

Davis, S. W. 2002. "Loose Lips Sink Ships." *Feminist Studies*, 28(1), 7–35.

Dittman, M. 2005. "Plastic Surgery: Beauty or Beast?" *APA Monitor*, 36(8), 30.

Dodson, B. 1996. *Sex for One: The Joy of Selfloving*. New York: Random House.

Ensler, E. 1998. *The Vagina Monologues*. New York: Villard.

Essén, B. and Johnsdotter, S. 2004. "Female Genital Mutilation in the West: Traditional Circumcision Versus Genital Cosmetic Surgery." *Acta Obstetricia et Gynecologica Scandinavica*, 83(7), 611–13.

Featherstone, M. 1991. "The Body in Consumer Culture," in *The Body: Social Processes and Cultural Theory* edited by M. Featherstone, M. Hepworth, and B. S. Turner. London: Sage, 170–96.

Fraser, S. 2003. *Cosmetic Surgery, Gender and Culture*. Basingstoke, UK: Palgrave Macmillan.

Frueh, J. 2003. "Vagina Aesthetics." *Hypatia*, 18(4), 137–58.

Gilman, S. L. 1985. *Difference and Pathology: Stereotypes of Sexuality, Race and Madness*. Ithaca, NY: Cornell University Press.

Gilman, S. L. 1998. *Creating Beauty to Cure the Soul*. Durham, NC: Duke University Press.

Gilman, S. L. 1999. *Making the Body Beautiful: A Cultural History of Aesthetic Surgery*. Princeton, NJ: Princeton University Press.

Giraldo, F., Gonzalez, C., and de Haro, F. 2004. "Central Wedge Nymphectomy with a 90-degree Z-plasty for Aesthetic Reduction of the Labia Minora." *Plastic and Reconstructive Surgery*, 113(6), 1820–1825.

Goodman, M. P., Bachmann, G., Crista, J., Fourcroy, J. L., Goldstein, A., Goldstein, G., and Sklar, S. 2007. "Is Elective Vulvar Plastic Surgery Ever Warranted, and What Screening Should Be Conducted Preoperatively?" *The Journal of Sexual Medicine*, 4, 269–76.

Green, F. J. 2005. "From Clitoridectomies to 'Designer Vaginas': The Medical Construction of Heteronormative Female Bodies and Sexuality through Female Genital Cutting." *Sexualities, Evolution & Gender*, 7(2), 153–87.

Gurley, G. 2003. "My Vagina Monologue." *New York Observer*, October 26, 2.

Häggström-Nordin, E., Sandberg, J., Hanson, U., and Tydén, T. 2006. "'It's Everywhere!' Young Swedish People's Thoughts and Reflections About Pornography." *Scandinavian Journal of Caring Sciences*, 20, 386–93.
Haiken, E. 1997. *Venus Envy: A History of Cosmetic Surgery*. Baltimore, MD: The Johns Hopkins University Press.
Hall, L. A. 2001. "The Clitoris," in *The Oxford Companion to the Body* edited by C. Blakemore and S. Jennett. Oxford: Oxford University Press, 160–162.
Helström, L. and Nilsson, B. 2005. "Impact of Vaginal Surgery on Sexuality and Quality of Life in Women with Urinary Incontinence or Genital Descensus." *Acta Obstetricia et Gynecologica Scandinavica*, 84(1), 79–84.
Honigman, R. J., Phillips, K. A., and Castle, D. J. 2004. "A Review of Psychosocial Outcomes for Patients Seeking Cosmetic Surgery." *Plastic and Reconstructive Surgery*, 113, 1229–37.
Jagger, E. 2000. "Consumer Bodies," in *The Body, Culture and Society* edited by P. Hancock, B. Hughes, E. Jagger, K. Paterson, R. Russell, E. Tulle-Winton, and M. Tyler. Buckingham, UK: Open University Press, 45–63.
Jahoda, S. 1995. "Theatres of Madness," in *Deviant Bodies: Critical Perspectives on Difference in Science and Popular Culture* edited by J. Terry and J. Urla. Bloomington, IN: Indiana University Press, 251–76.
Jeffreys, S. 2005. *Beauty and Misogyny: Harmful Cultural Practices in the West*. London: Routledge.
Jordan, J. W. 2004. "The Rhetorical Limits of the 'Plastic Body'." *Quarterly Journal of Speech*, 90(3), 327–58.
Kitzinger, S. 1994. *The Year After Childbirth: Surviving and Enjoying the First Year of Motherhood*. Toronto: HarperCollins.
Kristeva, J. 1982. *Powers of Horror: An Essay in Abjection* (trans. L. S. Roudiez). New York: Colombia University Press.
Laqueur, T. 1990. *Making Sex: Body and Gender from the Greeks to Freud*. Cambridge, MA: Harvard University Press.
Lemack, G. E. and Zimmern, P. E. 2000. "Sexual Function after Vaginal Surgery for Stress Incontinence. Results of a Mailed Questionnaire." *Urology*, 56(2), 223–7.
Liao, L.-M. and Creighton, S. 2007. "Requests for Cosmetic Genitoplasty: How Should Healthcare Providers Respond?" *BMJ*, 334, 1090–1092.
Lloyd, J., Crouch, N. S., Minto, C. L., Liao, L.-M., and Creighton, S. 2005. "Female Genital Appearance: 'Normality' Unfolds." *British Journal of Obstetrics and Gynaecology*, 112, 643–6.
MacNair, P. 1992. "Cutting Both Ways," *The Guardian*, February 4, 18.
Manderson, L. 2004. "Local Rites and Body Politics: Tensions Between Cultural Diversity and Human Rights." *International Feminist Journal of Politics*, 6(2), 285–307.
Masters, W. H. and Johnson, V. E. 1966. *Human Sexual Response*. Boston: Little, Brown and Company.

McNamara, K. R. 2006. "Pretty Woman: Genital Plastic Surgery and the Production of the Sexed Female Subject." *Gnovis*. Available at http://www.gnovisjournal.org/journal/pretty-woman-genital-plastic-surgery-and-production-sexed-female-subject.

Miklos, J. R. and Moore, R. D. 2008. "Labiaplasty of the Labia Minora: Patients' Indications for Pursuing Surgery." *The Journal of Sexual Medicine*, 5(6), 1492–5.

Minto, C. L., Liao, L.-M., Woodhouse, C. R. J., Ransley, P. G., and Creighton, S. M. 2003. "The Effect of Clitoral Surgery on Sexual Outcome in Individuals Who Have Intersex Conditions with Ambiguous Genitalia: A Cross-Sectional Study." *The Lancet*, 361, 1252–7.

Morgan, K. P. 1991. "Woman and the Knife: Cosmetic Surgery and the Colonization of Women's Bodies." *Hypatia*, 6(3), 25–53.

Orr, D. 1998. "Hands Out!" *The Guardian*, November 19, 7.

Pardo, J., V. Solà, P. A. Ricci, and Guilloff, E. 2006. "Laser Labioplasty of Labia Minora." *International Journal of Gynaecology and Obstetrics*, 93, 38–43.

Pizzini, F. 1991. "Communication Hierarchies in Humour: Gender Difference in the Obstetrical/Gynaecological Setting." *Discourse & Society*, 2, 477–88.

Robinson, A. 1998. "Hard Labour: Tough Choices." *The Guardian*, August 18, 14–15.

Rohrich, R. J. 2001. "The Web and Your Cosmetic Surgery Practice." *Plastic & Reconstructive Surgery*, 107(5), 1253–4.

Rothman, S. M. and Rothman, D. J. 2003. *The Pursuit of Perfection: The Promise and Perils of Medical Enhancement*. New York: Vintage.

Rouzier, R., Louis-Sylvestre, C., Paniel, B. J., and Haddad, B. 2000. "Hypertrophy of the Labia Minora: Experience with 163 Reductions." *American Journal of Obstetrics and Gynecology*, 182(1, part 1), 35–40.

The Royal Australian and New Zealand College of Obstetricians and Gynaecologists. 2008. "Vaginal 'Rejuvenation' and Cosmetic Vaginal Procedures," *New College Statement C-Gyn 24*. Melbourne: The Royal Australian and New Zealand College of Obstetricians and Gynaecologists.

Ruzek, S. B. 1978. *The Woman's Health Movement: Feminist Alternatives to Medical Control*. New York: Praeger.

Sandvik, H. 1999."Health Information and Interaction on the Internet: A Survey of Female Urinary Incontinence." *BMJ*, 319, 29–32.

Sarwer, D. B. 2005. "Invited Discussion: Quality of Life and Self-esteem Outcomes after Rhytidoplasty." *Annals of Plastic Surgery*, 54(4), 515–16.

Sheldon, S. and Wilkinson, S. 1998. "Female Genital Mutilation and Cosmetic Surgery: Regulating Non-Therapeutic Body Modification." *Bioethics*, 12(4), 263–85.

Soot, L. C., Moneta, G. L., and Edwards, J. M. 1999. "Vascular Surgery and the Internet: A Poor Source of Patient-Oriented Information." *Journal of Vascular Surgery*, 30(1), 84–91.

Sullivan, D. A. 2001. *Cosmetic Surgery: The Cutting Edge of Commercial Medicine in America*. New Brunswick, NJ: Rutgers University Press.

Sullivan, N. 2007. "'The Price to Pay for our Common Good': Genital Modification and the Somatechnologies of Cultural (In)Difference." *Social Semiotics*, 17, 395–409.

Terry, J. 1999. "Anxious Slippages between 'Us' and 'Them': A Brief History of the Scientific Search for Homosexual Bodies," in *Deviant Bodies: Critical Perspectives on Difference in Science and Popular Culture* edited by J. Terry and J. Urla. Bloomington, IN: Indiana University Press, 129–69.

Tiefer, L. 1995. *Sex Is Not a Natural Act and Other Essays*. Boulder, CO: Westview Press.

Tiefer, L. 2008. "Female Cosmetic Genital Surgery: Freakish or Inevitable? Analysis from Medical Marketing, Bioethics, and Feminist Theory." *Feminism & Psychology*, 18(4), 466–79.

Tracy, E. E. 2007. "Elective Vulvoplasty: A Bandage That Might Hurt." *Obstetrics & Gynaecology*, 109, 1179–80.

Walsh, F. 2005. "The Arrival of the Designer Vagina." *Metro*, September, 54–9.

PART 3
Boundaries and Networks

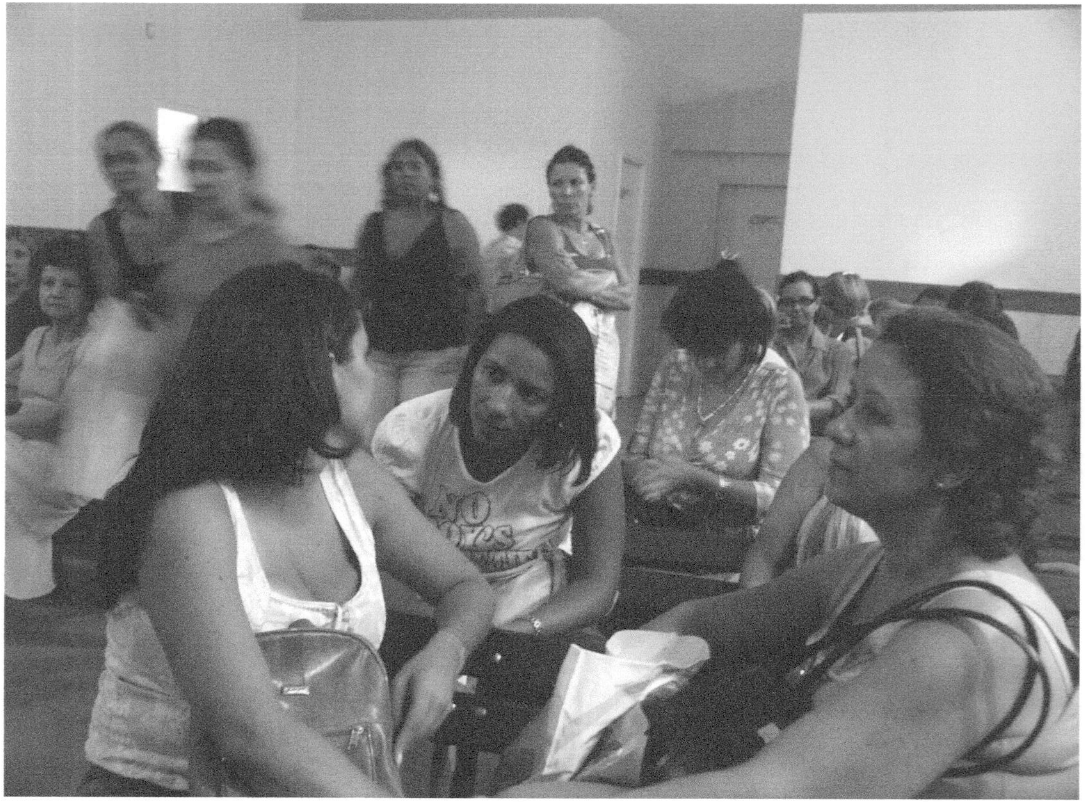

Figure 9.1 "Rio de Janeiro plastic surgery clinic" 2006

Source: © Alexander Edmonds

Chapter 9

"Engineering the Erotic": Aesthetic Medicine and Modernization in Brazil

Alexander Edmonds

Introduction

Brazil's democratization has been fraught with contradiction since it began in the 1980s. The end of military dictatorship brought not only free elections but also corruption scandals, increasing income concentration, and escalating cycles of violence (Caldeira 2000). An ambitious 1989 constitution guaranteed a universal right to healthcare while the gap between public and private care deepened as federal spending has plunged (Biehl 2005). And shantytowns sprawling next to luxury complexes have become icons of savage capitalism. A perhaps unexpected area of growth during these dire circumstances occurred in Brazil's beauty industry, with national media heralding a "democratization" of plastic surgery, or *plástica* as it is called.

Lower prices and new credit plans brought cosmetic surgery—once an elite practice—within reach of the middle class. And Brazil has become one of the only countries in the world to offer free cosmetic surgeries within a public health system to a population described by surgeons as the *povão*, the common people (Edmonds 2007a). Brazil's largest news magazine, *Veja*, ran a cover article titled, "Brazil: Empire of the Scalpel," which proclaimed the nation "champion" of plastic surgery in 2001.[1] As if to celebrate the "victory" a Rio samba school designed a Carnival allegory, titled "In Universe of Beauty," which paid homage to Brazil's leading plastic surgeon, Ivo Pitanguy. Why is one of the world's most unequal nations experiencing rapid growth in demand for cosmetic surgery?

Long before the birth of the discipline of anthropology, explorers, missionaries, and traders noted the remarkable diversity of bodily adornment they encountered in their travels. Whether denounced as barbaric, or appreciated for their potential for satire, exotic beauty practices became in the Western imagination potent signs of cultural difference. But the rise of practices such as cosmetic surgery, which

1 In fact, the US has more operations, but per capita rates in Brazil are higher than in much wealthier European nations ("Brasil, Império do Bisturi" 2001). A survey of 3,200 women in ten countries found that 54 percent of Brazilians (compared to 30 percent of Americans) had "considered having cosmetic surgery," the highest of the countries surveyed and more than double the average (Etcoff et al. 2004).

depend on commercial high-tech medicine and marketing, has prompted more critical views of the social *function* of beauty (e.g. Bartky 1990, Bordo 1993, Chernin 1981, Wolf 1991, Jeffreys 2005, Rankin 2005). These critiques argue the beauty industry is a gendered example of a modern disciplinary institution. Despite differences in theoretical orientation, from Marxist to Foucauldian, most of these arguments converge on the point that more extreme beauty practices function as a means for the social control of the female body within patriarchy.

In this chapter, I argue that this analytic frame needs to be re-conceptualized when moving to different cultural and economic contexts in the developing world (and if the jet-setting Brazilian elite do not represent sufficient cultural difference, the *povão* among whom plástica is now making inroads certainly do). As plastic surgery becomes staple fare on reality television, and "routinized," it may seem to us, unlike tribal body modification, all too familiar. Nevertheless, I would like to invite readers to view plástica in the same spirit of cultural (but not moral) relativism that ethnographers adopt in trying to understand, say, the scarification of the Nuba: to view it, that is, as a social practice grounded in a local context of meaning.

At least at first. Of course, plástica is also part of a global beauty industry. While tribal body modifications often enlist the help of experts, medicalized cosmetic surgery is different in its dependence on international expert knowledge and technology. Indeed, its status as medicine—or rather its ability to straddle boundaries between medical and consumer worlds—is crucial for understanding its particular appeal. But I argue that such global systems are transformed as workers, consumers, and medical practitioners take them up in different cultural and economic conditions.

Rio de Janeiro often signifies in the global and national imagination beauty and sensuality—from the grace of Tupinambá Indians to mulata *sambistas* to the luxuriant rainforests and white sand beaches of the Bay of Guanabara (the tradition of slippage between the beauty of nature and women dates to the founding of the colony). How then did it become a center as well for plastic surgery, a practice often equated with alienation, artificiality, and body-hatred? To answer this question I argue plástica should be seen as a "localized" form. While surgical techniques and marketing resemble those of the global specialty, they acquire a new significance as they are adapted to Brazil's particular bureaucratic rationality of the health system, political economy of reproduction, and cultural notions of sexuality and beauty. Tacking between analysis of structural change and local meanings, I show how the culture of beauty is intertwined with changes in the experience and "management" of motherhood and sexuality in a rapidly modernizing nation. Medical beauty practices reflect traditional corporeal aesthetics as well as the market inequalities of a highly stratified nation, but they also respond to new desires incited by the transformations of capitalist development.

The Scalpel and the Psyche: Plástica in the Public Health System

While private clinics emulate the hygienic comfort or even luxury of a health spa, in public hospitals I find a hectic atmosphere, with lines sprawling through dark, cramped corridors, dirty bathrooms, and formidable bureaucratic obstacles. Candidates for cosmetic operations wait alongside the severely disfigured, provoking crises of conscience for some: are there other cases needier than mine? The wards operate on a shoestring budget. Patients recuperate in shared rooms and at some hospitals, nurses instruct patients to bring their own sheets, painkillers, and a bottle of juice for when they wake up from anesthesia. In public hospitals, there are also different standards of privacy. In exchange for the free or discounted operation, the patient is also expected to make her body available for pedagogical discussion. After a wait lasting anywhere from a few months to a few years, patients must pass through one final hurdle before getting their operation scheduled: the *plano cirurgico*, a discussion of surgical technique where patients are examined (partially disrobed) in a lecture hall.

Despite these conditions, the povão has enthusiastically embraced plastic surgery. During the 1990s, patients camped out overnight to secure a place in line at Santa Casa hospital. Those who successfully navigate hospital procedures often come back for new operations. Some patients react with tears when told they are ineligible for their planned operation—or else keep their place in line by electing to have a different procedure. Tereza, who works as an elevator operator in a busy office building a few blocks from Santa Casa, was told after a year-long wait that her abdominoplasty would have to be deferred due to the discovery of a myeloma. She decided to have a *lifting* instead so as "not to lose this opportunity." One candidate for a cosmetic mammoplasty frustrated by the long line resorted to a more drastic strategy of burning her breasts (as reconstructive cases have priority). The popularity of plástica among the poor has not gone unnoticed by credit companies that offer medical financing plans. MasterHealth, which allows patients to divide their bill into 18 monthly payments, has begun marketing to the "long line of secretaries, office assistants, and maids waiting for cosmetic surgery at public hospitals."

But there are many patients who still cannot afford such credit plans, such as Dona Firmina, who was raised in a family of subsistence farmers in the state of Minas Gerais and moved to Rio de Janeiro in search of a better life. Like many migrants she worked for years as a domestic maid and now sells snacks at a working-class beach near the city center. "My face was awful," she told me, "because I was in the sun so much." Though she was disappointed with the results of the face-lift (and is now planning to have a *retoque*, a touch-up), she counts herself lucky to be able to have plástica.

It is true that some surgeons have privately questioned whether the "popular classes" are suitable candidates for cosmetic procedures. Dr. Eugenio, a resident, confessed his doubts: "You have patients who can't speak Portuguese well, who can't afford 25 dollars for a crème that helps heal the scars, who haven't been to the dentist. If I were poor I would take care of my teeth before having cosmetic surgery." Ana Regina, a psychologist who performs a required psychological evaluation of all patients in one plastic surgery ward, told me she thought that "the majority of patients are contra-indicated for surgery." Many of the patients she sees are low-paid service workers with anxieties about their jobs, officially not a "good motive" for plástica. Like Dr. Eugenio, though, "she rarely turns one away so as not to disappoint them." But most surgeons who work in public hospitals and their patients seem to agree with Pitanguy's vision, who declared that he never believed that "plastic surgery was only for the rich. The poor have the right to be beautiful."

Brazil's liberal 1988 constitution included an ambitious "universal right to health."[2] But since the 1990s there has been a marked deterioration of the public health system. From 1989 to 1993, per capita federal spending dropped from 83 to 37 dollars (Biehl 2005: 47). Middle-class Brazilians who can afford health insurance are fleeing the public sector creating a system of "excluding universalism": in which the elite and the middle class are excluded from the constitutional right to publicly provided health care (Faveret and Oliveira 1990 in Biehl 1999: 55). How is a cash-strapped public health system able to extend "the right to health" to cosmetic surgery?

Plastic surgery wards in public hospitals provide unique "opportunities" not just for the poor, but also for residents in surgery. Offering the chance to get valuable practice in cosmetic procedures, Brazilian residency programs attract applicants from around the world, particularly Latin America and Europe. In the United States, plastic surgeons generally do only reconstructive surgery during their residency, and must acquire experience in cosmetic procedures through a lengthy apprenticeship in a private practice. But in Brazil, residents perform cosmetic surgeries beginning in their first year. A European resident at Santa Casa told me he had performed 96 surgeries during his third year of residency, of which 90 percent were cosmetic. "There is nowhere else in the world," he said, "I could have gotten that kind of experience in so short a time."

By providing residents with valuable training in cosmetic procedures, public hospitals effectively subsidize the private sector (most graduates go on to work at lucrative private clinics). And in fact, prices in the private sector have been falling as large numbers of surgeons enter the market, attracting both poorer patients as well as foreigners and overseas Brazilians seeking a "cosmetic vacation." Since the 1960s, Pitanguy claims to have trained more than 500 surgeons. But this pedagogical rationale for offering cosmetic surgery in the public health sector would perhaps never have been accepted were it not for a parallel "therapeutic

2 The Constitution states: "Health is a right of every individual and a duty of the state, guaranteed by social and economic policies that seek to reduce the risk of disease and other injuries, and by universal and equal access to services designed to promote, protect, and recover health."

rationale," which views cosmetic surgery as a treatment for psychological suffering caused by a perceived aesthetic defect.

Cosmetic surgery was of course not always considered to be legitimate medicine (Haiken 1997, Gilman 1999). To gain acceptance by surgeons and the larger public, it had to be seen as a species of healing. The legitimization of plastic surgery in the West then depended on shifts in moral attitudes towards appearance as it was transformed from a "destiny" into a changeable index of psychic health and, especially in the United States, socio-economic success. However, in most of the Western world cosmetic surgery is still considered to be a medico-consumer service, not an aspect of a basic right to health. But in Brazil, the therapeutic rationale for cosmetic surgery has been pushed into new territory as it is applied in a public health system serving a population described by surgeons simply as *carente*, "needy."

A member of the first cohort of students trained by Pitanguy in the 1960s, Dr. Claudio founded a plastic surgery ward in a municipal hospital in Rio over 35 years ago. I asked him how he convinced the public health system to fund cosmetic surgery.

> You have to reach health by being happy. We were able to show this, that plástica has psychological effects, for the poor as well as the rich. And so estética was gradually accepted as having a social purpose. We operate on the poor who have the chance to improve their appearance and it's a necessity not a vanity.

When I began fieldwork I tended to see my field sites as almost saturated with irony. Patients disfigured by industrial fires, traffic accidents, untreated disease—which occur in the developing world at higher rates—wait in the same hallways along with candidates for *lipoescultura*. Funds from a faltering public health system are used to train residents in cosmetic procedures, enabling them to open lucrative private practices. And the poor are granted a right to beauty in a country where other rights are neglected. But the proximity of reconstructive and cosmetic surgery in public hospitals raises the question of where to draw the line between "necessity" and "vanity," as Dr. Claudio put it.

One of the only other attempts to systematically provide cosmetic surgery in a public health system—in the Netherlands—faltered on exactly this point (Davis 1995). Dutch health officials realized they would have to develop objective criteria to determine eligibility. They began experimenting with various measurements of aesthetic defects (for example, a difference of four clothing sizes between top and bottom). But such criteria proved impossible to implement fairly and the program was abandoned. The reasoning of the Brazilian surgeons is ingenious because it circumvents the problem of objectively measuring aesthetic defects, shifting the burden of diagnosis from doctor to patient. In Pitanguy's vision the surgeon becomes not an artist realizing his vision of beauty, but a "psychologist with a scalpel in his hand" (Pitanguy 1976: 125). The surgeon's task is not to judge beauty and normality, but merely "follow patient desires." But the therapeutic rationale has not only helped justify the provision of cosmetic surgery within a reforming public health system, but also opened the door to a radically expansive and flexible notion of "health" requiring new management regimes of female reproduction and sexuality.

The Aesthetic Management of Female Reproductive Health and Sexuality

Plastic surgery has been popularized in Brazil in part through a language of rights that blurs health with notions of happiness and beauty. But this newly emerging definition of health is also, of course, a highly gendered one.[3] In 2004, 69 percent of plastic surgery operations were performed on women in Brazil (SBCP 2005).[4] But this percentage is even higher in public hospitals where male cosmetic patients, aside from a few borderline reconstructive cases, are particularly rare. Gender is present not only in patient demographics but also in the links between plastic surgery and female life cycle events. Most of these—puberty, pregnancy, breast-feeding, menopause—are viewed as essential to "female nature." Plástica can also be associated with events of the *social* order: initiations into adulthood, marriage, and divorce. At 15, Tais receives a nose job as her coming out present (in place of the traditional debutante party or less traditional trip to Disneyland). Menstruation becomes the ground zero for plástica: the minimum age for surgery is calculated from the time of the patient's first period. After menopause a face-lift boosts the self-esteem. Body contouring is combined with sterilization, *after the factory has been shut down*, as Dani puts it. These events, some of the natural, some of the social order, punctuate the temporal unfolding of the life cycle. They divide the social experience of female nature into various "before and afters" that structure the proper timing of interventions.

But the transformative events by far the most often mentioned at public hospitals in connection with plástica are pregnancy and breast-feeding. Rosa, 36 years old, described why she needed a breast lift. "I was young when I had a kid, 19. My breasts were small and they grew too much. The breast is made of glands that secure the flesh (*carne*). But mine had too much flesh, and so it ended up falling, and was full of stretch marks." Other patients similarly blamed pregnancy and breast feeding for thickened waists, cesarean scars, localized fat, and bellies, breasts, and buttocks that were *caido* (fallen) and *murcha* (shrivelled). Patients and surgeons see plástica as a tool that corrects such "aesthetic defects." As a popular lay manual puts it, "During pregnancy the breasts grow, and then eventually become smaller than their initial size, losing their projection" (Ribeiro

3 I build here on my earlier analysis (Edmonds 2007a).

4 The surgeon patient interaction is also gendered, as senior surgeons are typically male, though rising numbers of women are now entering plastic surgery residency programs.

and Aboudib 1997: 125).[5] Breast lifts and reductions create a breast that is "higher, firmer, and smaller; totally different than that sluggish and dispersed breast" (69). Both patients and surgeons view several (but certainly not all) operations as a kind of "post-partum correction," even if they followed the patient's last pregnancy by three decades or more.

Plástica, however, is only one tool in a larger field, sometimes called *medicina estética* ("aesthetic medicine") that manages women's reproductive, sexual, and psychic health. Medicina estética draws from a broad range of medical specialties, including ObGyn, dermatology, geriatrics, nutrition, psychotherapy, and plastic surgery. The tone of educational and marketing materials almost recalls nineteenth-century positivism, in its appeal to notions of progress, hygiene, and development.[6] A bewildering proliferation of high-tech procedures on the fringes of medicine, often with foreign or foreign-sounding terminology, creates an aura of continual progress driven by technological innovation.[7] But what is perhaps most remarkable about medicina estética is its ability to forge links between diverse medical and non-medical specialties and merge notions of female health and beauty. For example, plastic surgeons combine tubal ligations with liposuction, while ObGyns refer their patients to plastic surgeons, or else perform "elective" cesarean deliveries motivated by sexual-aesthetic concerns. And national news media discuss technical advances, such as smaller liposuction needles that minimize bleeding, along with improved methods for diagnosing breast cancer and osteoporosis. This new experimental and hybrid field aims at the "positive" notion of health used by Dr. Claudio in arguing for a right to beauty. Instead of being negatively defined as the absence of disease, health becomes a qualitatively defined state that can be actively—and continuously—cultivated in which notions of physical, social, mental, and sexual well-being mingle.

More intensive medico-cosmetic management of the female body is emerging in other parts of the world as well. But I argue that in Brazil it takes on a pronounced, localized form in a context where family relationships, and female sexual and reproductive health are being "modernized" in a collapsed time frame. The growth of biomedicine in twentieth-century Brazil was intricately bound up

5 In fact the commonest procedure for performing a reduction—the "inverted T" technique, so named for the scar it leaves—was invented by Pitanguy in the 1960s.

6 E.g.: "Essential points in its field of activity: The treatment of physical, constitutional and aesthetic alterations … and 'unaesthetic' sequelae of illness and trauma. The postponement of aging and principally of … its physical and psychological repercussions. The reeducation of the individual to make him realize the possibility of preserving his biological patrimony through the development of mental, physical, and nutritional hygiene programs."

7 To cite just a few of dozens collected from the pages of consumer magazines: aesthetic ultrasound treatment, "instant plástica," Form Skin, isometria (bandages with electric current), micropigmentation treatments (to delineate lips or reconstruct the areola), sculpteur, and the "Russian Treatment" (developed for Soviet astronauts to prevent muscular atrophy).

with the hopes and anxieties of the modernization project. In the first decades of the century, "social and mental hygiene" movements combined a positivist faith in scientific progress with fears that cultural and racial barriers blocked the people's march to modernity (Stepan 1991). During this period, public health officials saw the *povão* as indolent and sick, who responded in turn with riots to government vaccination campaigns (Meade 1996). In the postwar period, populations once too remote or poor to have access to biomedicine have been encompassed by the growing structures of medical governance (Scheper-Hughes 1992).

In the area of reproductive health, the state retreated from a pro-natalist position in the 1970s, making cheap medical forms of contraception widely available within the public health system. The expansion of health care thus helped to institutionalize and secularize reproductive practices. State involvement in the area of family planning perhaps reduced the "psychological costs" of fertility control for Catholics (Martine 1996). And a rational, scientific understanding of sex and reproduction has been promulgated in educational shows on television and radio featuring doctors, sexologists, and psychologists (Parker 1991: 87). The dual processes of modernization and medicalization of reproduction contributed to a spectacular decline in Brazil's fertility rate, from six children per woman in 1960 to below 2.5 in the mid 1990s (Martine 1996). The spread of modern birth control helped culturally legitimate interference in biological processes, rational control over the body, and the separation of reproduction from sexuality, all factors which have prepared the cultural ground, as it were, for the acceptance of cosmetic surgery.

Many of these changes expanded women's reproductive and sexual autonomy during a time when traditional patriarchal family structures were declining (Castells 1997). But the expansion of biomedicine has not only profoundly changed patterns of fertility, mortality, and morbidity, but also masked or reproduced enduring economic inequalities. In her ethnography of a Northeastern shantytown, Nancy Scheper-Hughes (1992) shows how the symptoms of hunger are "treated" with pharmaceuticals while underlying social causes are ignored. She argues that not only are forms of social suffering like hunger medicalized, but medicine itself is invested with a powerful mystique of the modern. A piece of radioactive medical waste can be consumed as a magical panacea, while breast-feeding is rejected in favor of fortified infant formula, a commodity with prestige value. The "modernization" of female reproduction is especially important for understanding two linked surgeries with high rates in Brazil: cesarean deliveries and female sterilization. I discuss these two operations here because they shed light on the interlocking economic and cultural factors fuelling the growth of plástica as well.

It is perhaps not coincidental that Brazil has some of the world's highest per capita rates of cosmetic surgery as well as c-sections and tubal ligations. The national sterilization rate for women in union in 1996 was 37 percent, accounting for half of all contraceptive use in Brazil (Caetano and Potter 2004). Cesareans accounted for 36 percent of all deliveries in the 1990s, but can reach 70 percent or more in hospitals that have a policy to perform a cesarean unless the mother requests otherwise (Hopkins 2000). According to the WHO, rates above 10 to 15 percent indicate the operation is being used for "non-clinical reasons." A "culture of cesareans and sterilization" began with the expansion of the public health system in the 1970s and, like plástica, rapidly spread from rich to poor.

These elevated rates have complex causes but together point to some disturbing aspects of demand for biomedicine in conditions of scarcity. The health care system has built-in economic incentives to perform c-sections.[8] Economic pressures—along with lack of access to other options—can also lead to the abuse of sterilization.[9] But there is also considerable demand for sterilization, leading to a situation where the operation can be traded for political votes in regions with a long tradition of clientalistic politics (Caetano and Potter 2004). Sterilizations also feed cesarean rates as they are piggybacked onto a c-section for free in the public health system (as plástica is often linked to other operations to reduce costs by "taking advantage" of the anesthesia). But cesareans are also seen by some women and doctors as desirable in themselves: modern, convenient, pain-free, and even safer. As the Director of a São Paulo Clinic put it, "We have evolved. I think the cesarean is an improvement, and nobody can halt progress" (Downie 2000). Demand for medical care seen as "progress" is magnified by a health care system with deep inequities. The fact that wealthier women have higher rates of c-sections reinforces a notion of technological intervention as a "medical good." Conversely, poorer women see denial of a c-section as a form of negligence or even medical incompetence, to which they respond by employing a range of informal tactics—including "making a scandal"—to force ObGyns to perform the procedure (Béhague 2002). In this situation, even slight inequalities can create a "market for unnecessary interventions among women who feel marginalized from access to medical technology" (Béhague et al. 2002).

Cesareans and tubal ligations are very different procedures than cosmetic surgery. While all surgery carries health risks, estética (by definition) has no physical health benefit, while cesareans can be life saving, and tubal ligations expand contraceptive choice. But I argue that the procedures are linked in a management regime of reproduction and sexuality. Cesareans and tubal ligations familiarize women with surgical interventions (and resultant scarring) as a "normal" part of female reproductive health. And like plástica, cesareans may themselves be chosen for "sexual-aesthetic" motives. Maria Carranza (1994: 113–14) points to a "popular belief" (shared by some ObGyns) that a cesarean birth is not only safer for the baby, but is "also capable of preserving the vaginal and perineal anatomy of the woman, while a vaginal birth would produce distensions making sexual relations more difficult." While cesareans can be used as a pre-emptive measure against the

8 A Brazilian law tried to remove the incentive in the 1980s, equalizing reimbursement for cesarean and vaginal birth, but was not completely successful as c-sections take less time to perform.

9 A Parliamentary Commission presented evidence in 1992 that some employers were demanding "sterilization certificates" from female job seekers (Carranza 1994).

sexually unappealing body, cosmetic genital surgery is chosen as a corrective. The consumer magazine *Plástica & Beleza* reports on a rise in "intimate plásticas," claiming that "cosmetic surgery on the genitals offers the modern woman the freedom to improve her performance." I am not arguing here that natural birth is preferable to surgical intervention, but that a hunger for modern consumer and technological wonders in conditions of scarcity produces medical and corporeal fetishism. I find the figure of the fetish useful here to understand how the magic of the modern can work both in the dream worlds of consumption and medicine. Linking Marxist and Freudian ideas of "displaced desire" in the interplay between objects and persons, the fetish can suggest emotional relationships to medicine, commodities, and body parts. I use it here to indicate the mingling of economic and erotic desire, the embrace of high-tech medical services, and the division of the body into pathologized fragments.

The field of medicina estética, with its focus on technological progress and management of reproduction and sexuality, complexly shapes patient subjectivities. Lídia related how she had first discovered plástica soon after giving birth to her first child:

> I went to see my gynecologist and I asked him in the consultation about my belly. And he said that I could exercise, but that my belly would never go away with exercise, that I could only get rid of it with plastic surgery, and that's when I began to think about it ...

At first Lídia hesitated, but then decided to see a plastic surgeon.

> He gave me a lot of support. He said, "You are really young ... no way. You have to have a surgery. If your husband can't pay for your breast [surgery], I'll do it for free, because it's absurd, a young woman of your age having to look like that."

The offer was unnecessary because, not surprisingly, Lídia's husband agreed to pay for both operations when she recounted the surgeon's remarks. After the operation, Lídia recalled that she "felt *mais mulher*, more of a woman."

While Lídia linked her plástica to childbirth, other patients delay operations until the symbolic end of reproductive work, i.e. after a tubal ligation. They reason that sterilization is a guarantee that an unplanned birth won't "spoil" the aesthetic effects of plástica. But some women also associate the two operations because they signal a move from the duties of motherhood and towards the assertion of rights to self-care. Maria José argues that women suffer from the

> guilt of interfering with that sacred thing, the body. But women interfere with it in any case, with cesareans, hysterectomies, many times, mastectomy. But when it comes time to do a plastic surgery they themselves hesitate. In truth, it's because women have difficulty living out their own sexuality. As if after becoming a

> mother, the role of woman becomes secondary. (Ribeiro and Aboudib 1997: 155, my emphasis)

Maria José goes on to urge other women to have plástica, because after the sacrifices of motherhood, "plástica is good for the self."

Surgeons often ask, does the surgery compensate the scar, i.e. is the aesthetic benefit of the improvement greater than the unaesthetic result of scarring? But there are other "compensations" at work. The right to beauty compensates for all the rights that have not been "actualized," as political scientists put it. And plástica compensates for other events and interventions like breast-feeding, cesareans, and hysterectomies that take their toll on the body. This explains the eagerness, even cunning, with which patients approach plástica. Patient-consumers working in volatile informal and service economies, who have limited access to municipal services and some citizenship goods, nevertheless find they can tap into state resources in the form of pap smears, cesareans, tubal ligations, HIV tests, pharmaceuticals, and cosmetic surgery—many of these offered for free or at subsidized rates (Biehl 2005, Gregg 2003). Those who have not fully realized their citizenship can still remake themselves as "aesthetic citizens" experimentally employing medical technology and expansive notions of health as they negotiate new markets of work and sex.

The More Perfect Body

Many analyses of plastic surgery have stressed how it normalizes, medicalizes, and disciplines the female body (e.g. Morgan 1991, Bordo 1993). But one problem with this analytic framework is that it minimizes the aspirational and class dimensions of beauty practices. In Brazil, many patients do aim to correct traits they believe make them fall outside norms. But plástica does not only work through a negative logic of pathologization and body alienation. Rather, the body and medicine exist in a libidinal economy in which patient demand is effectively stimulated by forms of "positive incitement." Surgeons claim that they are merely following the desire of the patient. But such desires are mobilized by diverse economic and cultural factors: new expansive notions of health, the mystique of modern medicine, and—as I now discuss—a nationalist beauty myth.

Paula is the first patient I meet, introduced to me by Pitanguy. "She is pretty and young," he says, "and I expect we'll have excellent results." I meet Paula on the eve of her operation at his clinic, where she will stay the night accompanied by her mother, Bete. Paula has waited to have plástica since having a child at age 17 because a new pregnancy might ruin the results. Now sure she doesn't want more children, she is having a combined liposuction and breast lift. When I first met Paula she had told me this would be her first plástica. But during a later interview she reveals that she had once had liquid silicone injected into her buttocks in a beauty parlor. Now banned by the Brazilian government due to serious health risks, this procedure was more commonly performed in the 1980s, before plastic surgery become widely available. While medical cosmetic surgery is modern, prestigious, and even glamorous, *liquid* silicone is looked upon as a kind of "plástica of the people"—cheap, dangerous, and a little vulgar.[10] When I asked her why she had the procedure, she says it was in order to "better fit the Brazilian *padrão*, pattern."

Paula's comments point to how a cultural logic of the erotic body is being deployed in the commercial and medical beauty industry. In the twentieth century, the racially mixed body (infused with sensuality, grace, and eroticism) became a trope in the ongoing re-imagination of hybridity (*mestiçagem*) as crucial to modern Brazilian identity (Freyre 1986, Edmonds 2007b). Once feared as a cause of degeneration, the historical mixing of the "three sad races"—Portuguese, Africans, and Indians—was re-envisioned as a national patrimony: a cultural condition of creative hybridity, with erotic and aesthetic dimensions. While multiculturalism posits an official equality of racial types, the paradigm of mestiçagem posits one national corporeal type, but which officially encompasses all.[11] This type, or as Paula said, *padrão*, is often defined for women as "large hips, thighs, and buttocks, a narrow waist, with little attention to breast size" (Hanchard 1999: 78, Kulick 1998).[12] The view of female beauty is partly a legacy of the patriarchal relationships of slave plantations and points to a disturbing tradition of eroticizing racial domination. But it is also celebrated in popular culture, and embraced by some women across social classes (Goldstein 2003). We can see it thus as a nationalist and populist "beauty myth" (Edmonds 2007b).

Media and marketing materials make reference to this tradition in order to incite demand for beauty practices. Consumer magazines with names like *Corpo & Plástica* ("Body & Plástica"), which are sold in newsstands next to fashion monthlies, often interpolate their readers as *brasileiras*, Brazilian women: "We live in a tropical country, where the women are among the most beautiful in the world" (*Corpo & Plástica IV, 73).* Readers will find in their pages not only images of Brazilian models and *artistas*, celebrities, in seductive poses and environments, but also detailed technical advice from "world renowned experts" about how to acquire a "Brazilian *bumbum*" ("bottom"). Many operations make minor changes that are said to contour the body; for example, breast reductions that would not be "indicated" in North America's aesthetic culture. Paula chose to enlarge her buttocks with liquid silicone, but she could have achieved a similar—and safer, if

10 Many male transvestites though continue to use silicone, injecting several liters of the oil in the hips and buttocks.

11 Such encompassment also coexists with hierarchy where comparatively whiter facial features and hair are preferred.

12 The concept of beauty as national patrimony is of course gendered in Brazil. The image of the male body as athletic, graceful, but also playfully dangerous (represented in the samba dancer, the footballer, and capoeira player for example) is also a key symbol in *brasilidade*.

more expensive—effect with a silicone prosthesis, a procedure that was invented in Latin America and is "rare in other parts of the world," a surgeon said. Plastic surgeons and patient discussions of national identity can also explicitly mention Brazilian "miscegenation." Body contouring operations that aim to redistribute fat from the waist to the hips and buttocks, surgeons say, aim to emulate "African-European racial mixing." Plastic surgery should thus not be seen only as an exercise in "medical imperialism" that inscribes Western beauty standards on the female body. As the practice is adapted to Brazil, it also reflects a historical tradition of the body in which sensuality and racial mixture became a key symbol in a modern, proudly tropical, national identity.

These "body-contouring operations" though also indicate changes in gender and sexuality for different generations of women. In the last two decades, plastic surgery has begun attracting younger patients. Dr. Luciana (one of a growing number of female plastic surgeons) said she frequently sees patients in their twenties or teens. "I say to them, look, if I had your body, I wouldn't do surgery because it's more beautiful than mine. They have these marvelous waists and breasts and yet still want to be *more perfect*." (She rarely turns away such patients however as "they would simply go to another clinic.") The popularization of plástica has, in fact, been accompanied by a steep drop in the average age of the patient, from 55 in 1980 to 35 in 2000 ("Brasil, Império do Bisturi" 2001). The rate of plástica among teens is growing particularly rapidly, with 21 percent of patients in 2004 under the age of 19 (SBCP 2005).[13] In part, the trend stems from a shift towards "preventive" cosmetic surgery. But the younger patient profile also reflects the rising number of patients using plástica to enhance sexual allure, or as a Brazilian journalist put it, "engineer the erotic" (Denizart 1998).[14]

The growth of aesthetic medicine occurred during a period when family structures and sexual norms were rapidly changing. The right to sex as well as the duty to manage sexual allure have been legitimized for new groups of women defined in both consumer or medical worlds: the middle-aged, the divorced, the adolescent (Goldenberg 2004, Bassenezi 1996). Rising divorce rates have made new domestic arrangements more common: single mothers living with their single daughters dating at the same time (Castells 1997, Figueira 1996). "Liberated" in the not so recent past from patriarchal control over female sexuality, the teenager has

13 "If the girl is organically ready for plastic surgery," Dr. Froes argues, "there is no reason to wait. If you're offering a benefit to the patient, it should be done as soon as possible."

14 He used the phrase to refer to the body-sculpting methods of *travestis* (male transvestites), who use liquid silicone and female hormones, as well as cosmetic surgery, to acquire feminine forms. The women I met in public hospitals are very different in many ways from travestis, not least in their sexuality, but I also was struck by their sheer determination to "improve," willingness to undergo multiple operations, and in some cases, desires for minor changes that aimed at heightening sexual allure, rather than blending in, or looking "normal."

emerged as a central subject and object in Brazil's perhaps particularly eroticized consumer culture. But middle age is also being sexualized through mingling consumer, medical and psychotherapeutic discourses, as well as changing work and family patterns (Parker 1991). National media debate "Sex after 40," middle-age *artistas* define new models of femininity, and health experts "manage" the aesthetic-sexual dimensions of aging. In this new social environment, cosmetic surgery can be a means to "remain competitive." "In the past," Paula said, "a 40 year-old woman felt old and ugly. And she was traded for a younger one. But not these days. A 40-year-old is in the market competing with a 20-year-old because of the technology of plastic surgery. She can stretch [her skin], do a lift, put in silicone, do a lipo, and become as good as a 20-year-old."

Paula's comment suggests how plástica responds to—and generates—a competitive logic in diverse spheres of healthcare, work, and sexual relationships. In an expanding service economy and "markets" of sexual relationships, modifying appearance confers a competitive edge. Inequalities in healthcare contribute to demand for the fetishized high-tech services of medicina estética. And a populist beauty myth fuels a competitive mimesis articulated in relation to an idealized *national* body. In this context, the goal can become not a onetime passage into "normality" but rather an active and ongoing pursuit of the redundantly more perfect body.

The rapid growth and popularization of plástica can be seen as a "symptom" of diverse market anxieties and aspirations as consumers and workers in the peripheries of capitalism are exposed to the hazards—and opportunities—of generalized exchange. But despite its rhetoric of healing and freedom, it is difficult to see plástica as a liberatory practice. When I speak of freedom I refer to a negative freedom from older structures of domination. Still, it is important to recognize historical ruptures and the decline of ancient forms of male power. Scholarship on the Anglo or European worlds where the middle class is an implicit norm often neglects the competitive and class dimensions of beauty practices in "emerging markets."

On the face of it, we might think that beauty is just another realm for encoding class domination, a function that so many aspects of the body perform. But it is not because the poor are ugly that they suffer social exclusion. Physical beauty often impetuously disregards social hierarchy. It is quite obvious that the socially dominant are not always good-looking, even when their privilege thoroughly pervades others aspects of their habitus, from taste in photography to table manners. Beauty hierarchies do not simply mirror other forms of inequality. Rather it is precisely the gap between aesthetic and other scales of social position that make beauty such an essential form of value and all too often imaginary vehicle of assent for those blocked from more formal routes of social mobility (Edmonds 2007a).

And so while beauty work is not "resistance," it may be useful to view it as a "tactic," in de Certeau's (2002) terms: a maneuver performed by the weak on terrain defined by the strong. Such a tactic is a response to a social contradiction: motherhood is socially valorized and often essential to femininity, but the body visibly marked by motherhood is stigmatized. Patients embrace plástica as a solution to this conflict; in doing so, they expose the contradictory demands of normative femininity. And so despite the apolitical nature of beauty work perhaps it does in this sense, to use Paul Willis's (1977) term, "penetrate the mystifications of capitalism."

Acknowledgments

I am grateful to the Social Science Research Council and Princeton University for funding this research. The Museu Nacional in Rio de Janeiro, Princeton's Woodrow Wilson Society of Fellows, and a Woodrow Wilson Postdoctoral Fellowship at UCLA's Center for Modern Studies also provided financial and institutional support for this project. I would also like to thank the editors of this volume as well as many colleagues who have provided helpful comments: João Biehl, Vinçanne Adams, James Boon, Niko Besnier, Mirian Goldenberg, Hermano Vianna, Gilberto Velho, Thomas Strong, Kirsten Bell, Pál Nyíri, Chris Huston, Kalpana Ram, Kirsty McClure, Vince Pecora, Cristina Rocha, Tamara Griggs, and Julie Park.

References

Bartky, S. 1990. *Femininity and Domination: Studies in the Phenomenology of Oppression*. New York: Routledge.

Bassenezi, C. 1996. *Virando as Páginas, Revendo as Mulheres: Revistas Femininas e Relações Homen-Mulher, 1945–1964*. Rio de Janeiro: Civilização Brasileira.

Béhague, D. 2002. "Beyond the Simple Economics of Cesarean Section Birthing: Women's Resistance to Social Inequality." *Culture, Medicine and Psychiatry*, 26, 473–507.

Béhague, D., Victora, C., and Barros, F. 2002. "Consumer Demand for Caesarean Sections in Brazil: Informed Decision Making, Patient Choice, or Social Inequality?" *BMJ*, 324, 942.

Biehl, J. 1999. "Other Life: AIDS, Biopolitics, and Subjectivity in Brazil's Zones of Social Abandonment." Ph.D. dissertation, University of California, Berkeley.

Biehl, J. 2005. *Vita: Life in a Zone of Social Abandonment*. Berkeley: University of California Press.

Bordo, S. 1993. *Unbearable Weight: Feminism, Western Culture, and the Body*. Berkeley: University of California Press.

"Brasil, Império do Bisturi" 2001. *Veja*, January 10.

Caetano, A. and Potter, J. 2004. "Politics and Female Sterilization in Northeast Brazil." *Population and Development Review*, 30(1), 79–109.

Caldeira, T. 2000. *City of Walls: Crime, Segregation, and Citizenship in São Paulo*. Berkeley: University of California Press.

Carranza, M. 1994. "Saúde Reprodutiva da Mulher Brasileira," in *Mulher Brasileira É Assim* edited by H. I. B. Saffioti and M. Muñoz-Vargas. Rio de Janeiro: Rosa dos Tempos.

Castells, M. 1997. *The Information Age: Economy, Society and Culture, Vol. II. The Power of Identity*, Cambridge, MA; Oxford, UK: Blackwell.

Chernin, K. 1981. *The Obsession: Reflections on the Tyranny of Slenderness*. New York: Harper and Row.

Corpo & Plástica. No date. Ano IV, Edicão 18, 73.

Davis, K. 1995. *Reshaping the Female Body: The Dilemma of Cosmetic Surgery*. New York: Routledge.

Denizart, H. 1998. *Engenharia Erotica: Travestis no Rio de Janeiro*. Rio de Janeiro: Jorge Zahar.

de Certeau, M. 2002. *The Practice of Everyday Life*. Berkeley: University of California Press.

Downie, A. 2000. "Brazil Reexamines Birth Options." *Christian Science Monitor*. Available at: http://www.csmonitor.com/2000/1107/p6s1.html.

Edmonds, A. 2007a. "'The Poor Have the Right to be Beautiful': Cosmetic Surgery in Neoliberal Brazil." *Journal of the Royal Anthropological Institute*, 13(2), 363–81.

Edmonds, A. 2007b. "'Triumphant Miscegenation: Reflections on Race and Beauty in Brazil." *Journal of Intercultural Studies*, 28(1), 83–97.

Etcoff, N, Orbach, S, Scott, J, and D'Agostino, H. 2004. "The Real Truth About Beauty: A Global Report." Available at: http://www.campaignforrealbeauty.com.

Faveret F. and Oliveira, P. J. 1990. "A Universalização Excludente: Reflexões sobre as Tendências do Sistema de Saúde." *Dados*, 33(2), 257–83.

Figueira, S. 1996. "O 'Moderno' e o 'Arcaico' na Nova Família Brasileira: Notas sobre a Dimensão Invisível da Mudança Social," in *Uma Nova Família?* edited by S. Figueira. Rio de Janeiro: Jorge Zahar.

Freyre, G. 1986. *Modos de Homen & Modas de Mulher*. Rio de Janeiro: Record.

Gilman, S. 1999. *Making the Body Beautiful: A Cultural History of Aesthetic Surgery*. Princeton: Princeton University Press.

Goldenberg, M. 2004. *De Perto Ninguém É Normal: estudos sobre corpo, sexualidade, gênero e desvio na cultura brasileira*. Rio de Janeiro: Record.

Goldstein, D. 2003. *Laughter Out of Place: Race, Class, Violence, and Sexuality in a Rio Shantytown*. Berkeley: University of California Press.

Gregg, J. 2003. *Virtually Virgins: Sexual Strategies and Cervical Cancer in Recife, Brazil*. Stanford: Stanford University Press.

Haiken, E. 1997. *Venus Envy: A History of Cosmetic Surgery*. Baltimore: Johns Hopkins University Press.

Hanchard, M. 1999. "Black Cinderella? Race and the Public Sphere in Brazil," in *Racial Politics in Contemporary Brazil* edited by M. Hanchard. Durham, NC: Duke University Press.

Hopkins, K. 2000. "Are Brazilian Women Really Choosing to Deliver by Cesarean?" *Social Science and Medicine*, 51, 725–40.

Jeffreys, S. 2005. *Beauty and Misogyny: Harmful Cultural Practices in the West*. London and New York: Brunner/Routledge.

Kulick, D. 1998. *Travesti: Sex, Gender and Culture Among Brazilian Transgendered Prostitutes*. Chicago: University of Chicago Press.

Martine, G. 1996. "Brazil's Fertility Decline, 1965–1995." *Population and Development Review* 22(1), 47–75.

Meade. T. 1996. *"Civilizing" Rio: Reform and Resistance in a Brazilian City, 1889–1930*. University Park, PA: Penn State Press.

Morgan, K. P. 1991. "Women and the Knife: Cosmetic Surgery and the Colonization of Women's Bodies." *Hypatia*, 6, 25–53.

Parker, R. 1991. *Bodies, Pleasures, and Passions: Sexual Culture in Contemporary Brazil*. Boston: Beacon Press.

Pitanguy, I. 1976. "Evaluation of the Psychological and Psychiatric Aspects in Plastic Surgery." *Revista Brasileira de Cirurgia Plástica*, 66(3–4).

Rankin, C. 2005. "Prescribing Beauty: Women and Cosmetic Surgery in Postmodern Culture." *Body Modification: Mark II Conference*, April 21–23, Macquarie University, Sydney, Australia.

Ribeiro, C. and Aboudib, J. H. 1997. *Você e a cirurgia plástica: tudo o que você precisa saber sobre cirurgia plástica*. Rio de Janeiro: Record.

Scheper-Hughes, N. 1992. *Death Without Weeping: The Violence of Everyday Life in Brazil*. Berkeley: University of California Press.

SBCP 2005. Brazilian Society of Plastic Surgery, press release obtained by personal communication.

Stepan, N. 1991. *The Hour of Eugenics: Race, Gender, and Nation in Latin America*. Ithaca: Cornell University Press.

Willis, P. 1977. *Learning to Labour: How Working Class Kids Get Working Class Jobs*. Farnborough, Hants: Saxon House.

Wolf, N. 1991. *The Beauty Myth: How Images of Beauty Are Used Against Women*. New York: William Morrow and Company, Inc.

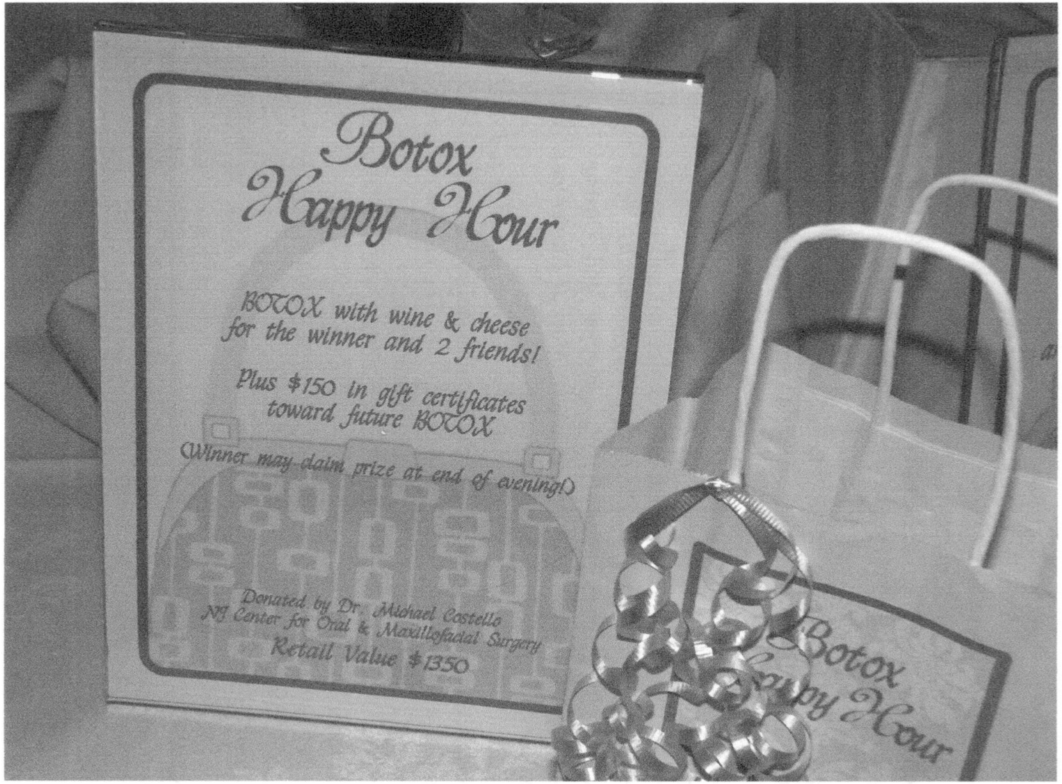
Botox
Happy Hour
BOTOX with wine & cheese
for the winner and 2 friends!
Plus $150 in gift certificates
toward future BOTOX
(Winner may claim prize at end of evening!)
Donated by Dr. Michael Costello
NJ Center for Oral & Maxillofacial Surgery
Retail Value $1350
Botox
Happy Hour

Figure 10.1 "Botox Happy Hour" 2006, photo taken in Franklin Lakes, New Jersey, USA

Source: © Sara K. Tracey

Chapter 10
Pygmalion's Many Faces

Meredith Jones

My local butcher's shop has an extraordinary painting on its wall. A young bull frolics on his hind legs, grinning and salivating. A starched white bib is tied in a bow around his neck and in his hoof he holds a silvery meat cleaver. He is strangely twisted around on himself, like a dog chasing its tail. This is because he is chopping his own rump into a neat row of T-bone steaks. The bull is a comical and grotesque mix of hybrids, including provedore/consumer and victim/killer. Carole Spitzack describes a video of a cosmetic surgery operation:

> A staff of happy professionals surrounding a relaxed patient, the needles and knives almost beside the point, fading into the background, into the skin, the body. The patient appears happy about the prospect of her own effacement. (1988: 44)

The patient is relaxed, the doomed bull is gleeful and neither of them feels pain. The bull literally chops at himself while the patient, aware and awake, metaphorically performs her own surgery as the medical professionals and surgical instruments fade into the background. In both of these images many important interlocutors are left out of the frame: the bovine body conflates butcher and customer while almost the entire meat industry including farms and abattoirs is obfuscated; the patient's body remains in the spotlight while surgeon and medical instruments fade into the background. It is what is often left out of the common frames of cosmetic surgery that I'm interested in here: both academic and popular discourse tend to focus most often on the patient, occasionally on the relationship she has with the surgeon, but quite rarely on other actors, many of whom are very powerful (for instance, pharmaceutical companies, prosthesis producers and developers of digital imaging devices).

I am focusing on the world of cosmetic surgeons, which is complex, multifaceted, and rapidly changing and should be of deep interesting to feminist scholars. These practitioners are intricately and intimately connected with the recipients of cosmetic surgery, sharing with them surgical and consulting spaces and—to a degree—the unique phenomenologies and temporalities of metamorphosis that they undergo. Cosmetic surgeons have institutional and ontological connections with ancient medical and surgical practices; they also negotiate the modern world with its ubiquitous media (much of it about cosmetic surgery in some way or another), new technologies, highly informed patients, and hostility from various quarters. They have been the anchor characters of fictional television dramas (*Nip/Tuck*) and reality television (*Dr 90210*), in which their personal lives are shown to be deeply interwoven with their chosen profession.[1] They are the supporting stars on cosmetic surgery reality TV programs like *Extreme Makeover* and *The Swan.* Some contemporary cosmetic surgeons also hold celebrity status: Ivo Pitanguy, the world's most famous cosmetic surgeon, is fêted in Brazil as a national hero (see Edmonds in this volume) while Vicky Belo is popularly known as the "Ambassadress of Beauty" in The Philippines.[2]

This chapter sets out to think about cosmetic surgeons, to outline some of the main issues around this group that feminists might be interested in, and to flag some theoretical ways forward in thinking about them. I suggest two interlinked ways of analyzing them: firstly as Pygmalion figures (covering roles of father/creator, lover, and artist), and secondly as figures within the complex world of cosmetic surgery who must negotiate within webs far larger than the simple surgeon/patient dyad.

Surgeons as Fathers/Creators

The mythical Ancient Greek sculptor Pygmalion is disillusioned with the women around him. He shuns them all. The problem is he still wants sex:

> Pygmalion loathing their lascivious Life,
> Abhorred all Womankind, but most a Wife:
> So single chose to live, and shunned to wed,
> Well pleased to want a Consort of his Bed.
> (Ovid: *Metamorphoses, Book X*)

---

1 Televisual depictions of cosmetic surgeons are not without their detractors in the medical profession: Leigh Turner, writing about *Extreme Makeover* in the *American Medical Association Journal of Ethics*, notes that such "... programs ignore the consequences of characterizing surgeons as amoral technicians guided only by aesthetic preferences and the desires of their patients. There is no examination of whether the provision of multiple cosmetic surgery procedures in a televised context violates professional norms, poses a challenge to notions of professional integrity, and makes cosmetic surgeons complicit in promoting narrow, damaging notions of beauty ... Every first year medical student is introduced to the notion of respect for patient autonomy. However, situated within market constraints, advertising, and attenuated notions of 'ideal' body types, the ethic of personal autonomy leads to the strangest of outcomes" (Turner 2004).

2 The connection between cosmetic surgery and celebrity is not unique to our era: Elizabeth Haiken describes Dr. Howard Crum, who was, to the United States general public, "plastic surgery personified" in the 1930s. Crum declared after a public operation performed with live music "You see I'm an artist rather than a surgeon. I model in human flesh" (1997: 80).

To distract himself from lust Pygmalion carves a marble woman, Galatea, but then inconveniently falls in love with her. He prays to Venus to bring her to life: finally, after some false starts and several negotiations, his wish is granted and the statue becomes his wife. We all know this legend of the man-made woman in one form or another: it has been the inspiration for *My Fair Lady*, *Pretty Woman*, and countless other entertainments. Although the tale is about a woman created from scratch rather than one simply restored, renovated, or improved, it nevertheless resonates strongly with cosmetic surgery texts and has been variously used to inform psychological analyses (see Goin and Goin 1981: 115), journalistic accounts (see Bankard 2004), and feminist critiques (see Blum 2003: 92–6, Davis 1998, and O'Connor 2000). *Pygmalion* is, perhaps predictably, also deployed by surgeons in their promotional material. For example, an article written by a surgeon in the popular Indian women's magazine *Femina* states that

> A Greek myth tells the story of Pygmalion, a sculptor who made such a beautiful statue of a woman that he fell in love with it ... Cosmetic surgeons tell this story to illustrate what they call the Pygmalion complex—the desire to create perfection, not out of marble but out of human flesh. In reality, cosmetic surgery aims at what is possible—a better profile, a younger—looking face, and larger or smaller breasts. (Talwar 2002)

Similarly, a 2007 featured report in *The Cosmetic Surgery Times* about cosmetic surgery for people who have undergone massive weight loss (MWL) is titled "Channeling Pygmalion":

> In perhaps no other surgical venue does the aesthetic practitioner more literally serve as sculptor ... Sculptors since Michelangelo have written of their vision—not of sculpting a figure in marble—but rather, of releasing the figure trapped within the massive block. This seems the perfect analogy for how the cosmetic surgeon liberates the MWL patient through his science and his sculpting art. Perhaps the most apt metaphor for this Special Report topic is that of the mythological sculptor Pygmalion, whose ivory sculpture of Galatea was so realistic that it actually came to life. (McNulty 2007)

Occasionally the *Pygmalion* story is used by surgeons less positively, but with equally strong effect. For example, when asked by a journalist why so few women become plastic surgeons, Jane Petro, a professor of plastic surgery, said it was partly due to "the Pygmalion angle ... Just look at the number of male plastic surgeons whose second wife was once their patient. It's unbelievable" (quoted in Kuczynski 1998).

Clearly, the myth is versatile: detractors often couple it with the Frankenstein story to emphasize cosmetic surgery's monstrous "unnaturalness" while others mobilize it to lend cosmetic surgery dignity by aligning it with an "eternal" artistic theme.

Importantly, what many of these diverse texts have in common is the way they deploy *Pygmalion* to support a view of cosmetic surgery as happening inside a simple binary relationship between doctor and patient. This is problematic for two reasons. Firstly, because cosmetic surgery industries are part of an increasingly complex, media-saturated set of global flows and there are far more entities and actors involved in its matrix than just doctors and patients. And secondly, because versions of the *Pygmalion* myth rarely afford Galatea, the statue/wife, any power. As raw material to be worked upon she remains voiceless, totally under the surgeon's control. This is in stark contrast to the ways in which contemporary cosmetic surgery recipients[3] have described themselves to me and to other researchers in interviews.[4] Further, as I have argued elsewhere (2008a), there is an important element of parthenogenesis—where woman gives birth to herself—in symbolic readings of cosmetic surgery that is not present in *Pygmalion*.

So while I deploy the Pygmalion narrative here myself, this is in order to open up what is often characterized as a closed relationship between doctors and patients. I ask, firstly, to what extent are contemporary cosmetic surgeons Pygmalion figures, while cosmetic surgery recipients are Galateas, and secondly, what or who are the other players involved in the cosmetic surgery matrix?

Pygmalion the Lover

Like a lover, the surgeon has intimate access to the woman's naked body: he penetrates with scalpel and implants while she is prostrate; he is her caregiver and confidante. Virginia Blum notes in *Flesh Wounds* that "insofar as conventional heterosexual male and female sexualities are experienced psychically and represented culturewide as the relationship between the one who penetrates and the one penetrated, surgical interventions can function as very eroticized versions of the sexual act" (2003: 45). The surgeon-lover connection also echoes through cosmetic surgery's promotional rhetoric: "I can easily push my 'aesthetic' button. It takes little for a male surgeon to appreciate female beauty. But to go beyond lust,

3 In this chapter I refer to surgeons as "he" and recipients as "she." While there are certainly female (even perhaps feminist) cosmetic surgeons who deserve attention, as do male recipients of cosmetic surgery, my generalizations merely highlight the gendered state of contemporary cosmetic surgery. Most cosmetic surgeons are men (one in nine is a woman) and most cosmetic surgery recipients (91%) are women (Davis 2003: 41). Suzanne Fraser says that in popular culture surgeons are nearly always presented as male and recipients as female. She argues that this is not merely indicative of how things are but that such discourse is also materially productive, helping to create the conditions that it represents: "the representation [in popular magazines] of surgeons as male and recipients as female is both the 'product and process' of cosmetic surgery as a technology of gender; here gender stereotypes emerge from and help produce asymmetrical patterns in surgical practice" (2003: 63).

4 See Davis 1995, Gimlin 2007, and Jones 2008.

to define physical beauty, and to struggle to bring it forth through operation, is a different matter, requiring study and training" (Robert Goldwyn, quoted in Adams 1997: 60). For this surgeon, artistic surgical skill is tied to heterosexual attraction. He describes the surgeon–patient relationship in terms of sex and gender: the act of cosmetic surgery may go "beyond lust" but it remains an extension of heterosexual desire. Thus cosmetic surgery is positioned as a "natural" extension of "natural" impulses—in the operating theater beauty meets medicine, sex meets surgery, and lust meets artistry.

In a lecture I gave in 2007 to an Australasian convention of cosmetic surgeons, I told them I thought their public image was one of "glamorous semi-criminality." Interestingly, they did not dispute this descriptor but rather laughed about it. Alex Kuczynski, writing about the time before Restylane was approved for human use by the US Food and Drug Administration, quotes her dermatologist, Patricia Wexler (New York's "dermatologist to the stars"):

> Nobody will say they are using it, but believe me, there are lots of little moles bringing it into the country … you go to your doctor and they will go to the cabinet and unlock it and tell you not to tell anyone. Nobody is going to admit to it. (2006: 224)

Cosmetic surgeons' willingness to ship non-approved drugs from abroad—and inject them into patients—is part of how they are characterized, and part of how many of them like to be seen: as cutting-edge, ahead of the bureaucrats, willing to take risks, the adventurous "bad boys" of the medical world. This story is also connected to surgery in general: Anthropologist Joan Cassell writes that surgeons "display a specific and recognizable temperament, or ethos … that differs from that of members of other medical specialities" (1991: 33). Several of the surgeons she interviewed compared themselves to astronauts; she notes that "the successful surgeon takes risks, defies death, comes close to the edge, and carries it off" (1991: 34).

Two decades ago feminist academic Carole Spitzack visited a cosmetic surgery clinic and underwent a "diagnosis" and consultation. She describes the visit's "subtle splitting and jarring that prompts intense self-scrutiny, leading to an externalization and internalization of disease" (1988: 41). Spitzack's inquiry about a rhinoplasty ended in unwanted advice about skin resurfacing. She experienced intense embarrassment when she was placed in front of three brightly lit mirrors and asked to describe her "problem." Then, once her deficiencies had been properly identified—and she had accepted that two operations instead of one were not elective but necessary—the physician offered to help deceive her insurance company by stating they were necessary medical procedures. Spitzack surmised that she and the surgeon would be "cohorts in deception, like lovers committing a crime" (1988: 46–7). During the consultation he sat close to her, his hand on her back gently adjusting her position (1988: 46). He skillfully undermined her confidence, using the power of diagnostic language to make her "see" that her skin needed resurfacing. Then, heroically, he offered a "solution"—one bound up in secrecy, in the closed heterosexual dyad, and in the promise of beauty.

Spitzack's interpretation of "surgeon as lover" positioned him as a dishonest exploiter. And certainly the dirty tactics she experienced still exist. But they're differently manifested in the early twenty-first century: notably, power relations around cosmetic surgery now occur in an information-saturated mediascape. Everyday consumers of popular media are mightily, perhaps overly, informed about cosmetic surgery (often whether they want to be or not) while active knowledge-seekers have access to techno-medical databases and thousands of informative cosmetic surgery websites and chat rooms. Crucially, there was very little of this kind of media available when Spitzack had her consultation. The surgeon was almost her sole information provider. His role as medical, psychological, and aesthetic expert was active, multiple, and transcendent while she describes hers, for the period she is in the consulting room, as singular and passive—"the female patient is promised beauty and re-form in exchange for confession, which is predicated on an admission of a diseased appearance that points to a diseased (powerless) character" (1988: 39). Twenty years later, feminists rail against and despair about cosmetic surgery having become ubiquitous, even obligatory, via media and celebrity culture. However, one powerful side effect of this media saturation is that recipients are no longer dependent on surgeons for information and expertise. The surgeon–patient relationship now occurs within a mediascape that extends way beyond the consulting room. The interviews I conducted showed that surgeons are now often the end-point of recipients' research about cosmetic surgery rather than the starting-point, and surgeons are acutely aware of this. This means that the controlling, patriarchal relationship between surgeons and patients has been softened: if we stick with a romantic heterosexual metaphor, then they must now be suitors rather than lovers: they must woo clients, win them, and then work hard to keep them.

Another, darker, side to the eroticism of cosmetic surgery is connected to the fact that many cosmetic surgeries are violent. Some, like blepharoplasties, require meticulous work but most do not. The precision of the brain or heart procedure is a far cry from the physical brutality of breast augmentation or liposuction. Slits in the breast are prized apart with instruments that look like shoe horns, implants are shoved up between fat and muscle: the surgeon has to exert a fair amount of leverage and force. Liposuction cannulas look like long metal straws. They are jabbed in and then rotated rapidly, the surgeon moving his arms rhythmically as if he's stirring a big tin of paint. This is surgeon as abusive lover. Spitzack's surgeon "blandly" told her how he would dislocate or break her nose before carving it into a more "feminine" shape. Horrified, she writes "having one's nose broken calls forth violent imagery: physician as bodily harm, as villain" (1988: 46) and her subsequent analysis works partly as a cathartic retaliation. But again, the victim/abuser framework is problematized by the new media saturated world of cosmetic surgery wherein patient has become "client." Instead of doctors using their medical arsenals to bully women into having cosmetic surgery they must now *sell* the procedures to discerning and knowledgeable clients. Elizabeth Haiken points out throughout her excellent *Venus Envy* (1997) that the profession of plastic surgery began to incorporate cosmetic surgery procedures largely because of consumer demand. Thus contemporary cosmetic surgery has its roots in a capitalist market driven partly by consumers. Cassell too describes how social attitudes towards surgeons began to change from the 1980s: in a newly emerging model of doctor–patient relationships "rather than 'surrendering' to the prophet-healer's powers, the patient seeks agency, alliance, parity" (1991: 194). I have argued in earlier work that redefining a patient as a client partly de-stigmatizes the cosmetic surgery recipient (2008b). It replaces the diseased body that Spitzack was made to "see" in her doctor's cruel three-sided mirror with a consumer body—a body with spending power.

Surgeon as lover rhetoric is also found in relation to cosmetic surgery that yields less-than-perfect outcomes:

> if there is a problem, that's when the doctor-patient relationship needs to be strongest. Some patients you have big relationships with are the ones who had little problems. We [have to] be partners, go through it together ... Some problems have to be fine-tuned. That's when it's important to have a good relationship with your doctor. You have to stick together, and if a revision is needed for the final result, be prepared to go for it. (Dr. Michael Powell quoted in Lerche Davis, 2003)

The doctor's voice portrays the doctor–patient relationship like a marriage where couples must "stick together" through difficult times. This manipulative rhetoric aims to discourage the unhappy patient from seeking compensation or making formal complaint, and instead to return to him and him only for further treatments. It sternly enlists her courage and audacity—"be prepared to go for it"—and her ability to maintain strong relationships. But alongside the calculating language there is an important acknowledgment of her as a "partner." This rhetoric acknowledges patient and doctor as *collaborators* rather than as active creator and passive receiver. It may have been cynically written to minimize lawsuits but it also inadvertently highlights the woman's powerful position as a critical and potentially litigious consumer. The surgeon wishes to counteract the potential promiscuity of the shopper: he wants commitment and monogamy while she wants to leave her options open, and to litigate if the project fails to live up to its promises. As one surgeon said, we "sit down with patients in consultation, but we're both obviously interviewing each other" (quoted in Rosen 2004: 5).

"I Made Her for You"—Cosmetic Surgery and the Erotic Triangle

There is a silent partner standing in the shadows of the operating theater who further complicates the sexual dynamics between surgeon and patient. The patient's boyfriend or husband, or simply a more general male gaze, may well play a key role if we are to theorize cosmetic surgery in terms of heterosexual romantic love. As the surgeon works he may consider, consciously, unconsciously, or at a cultural level, the sexual interest of another man (this is not without precedent in other surgery—think of obstetricians performing episiotomies and then putting in an extra stitch "for your husband"). Such dynamics enact the erotic triangle that Eve Sedgwick describes in *Between Men* (1985), in which women are intermediaries deployed to allow men to bond intimately with each other at a "homosocial" level. Sedgwick explores, *pace* Gayle Rubin, what she calls a paradigm of "male traffic in women" (1985: 16), arguing that patriarchal heterosexuality uses "women as exchangeable, perhaps symbolic, property for the primary purpose of cementing the bonds of men with men" (25–6). I do not have room here to explore this idea more, but I flag it as a potentially fruitful way in which to examine cosmetic surgery, especially in terms of how and why the triangle is always carefully elided in discourse about cosmetic surgery (for example, does the triangular constellation potentially work as a disruption or disturbance to established order?). Without reifying a heteronormative framework for thinking about cosmetic surgery, or imposing a simple triangular formation on a set of deeply complicated interlocking networks, we could ask for example: What of the woman surgeon in this triangle? What of the male patient? Certainly if, as Sedgwick argues, the erotic triangle can be used as "a sensitive register precisely for delineating relationships of power and meaning, and for making graphically intelligible the play of desire and identification by which individuals negotiate with their societies for empowerment" (27), then it is a potentially powerful tool for feminist analysis of cosmetic surgery.

Surgeon as Artist, Recipient as Impostor

Haiken has shown how plastic surgery has always been considered both an art and a profession: post World War One surgeons, keen to distinguish themselves from quackery and so-called "beauty doctors," placed themselves within a "classical context" anchored in traditional art (1997: 5). They argued they were governed by an "abstract, artistic ideal of beauty rather than one that is culturally defined" (221).

I asked a plastic surgeon how he learned the aesthetic (rather than medical) skills necessary to change faces:

> All plastic surgery is about that. … And you train in it. That's what training's all about, it's not picked up like cosmetic surgeons at a "weekend workshop"

> [said with contempt, making quote marks in the air] or observing someone, it is actually working with [an experienced specialist] in hospitals, seeing the patients before the surgery, being operated on, doing the operations, seeing them in an outpatient clinic, and eventually doing your training, being examined in it—you've gotta learn aesthetic proportions, its all been done for thousands of years. (Dr. Young)

My interpretation of this wordy answer is simply that there is no formal training or examination for surgeons in terms of artistic skills. It is picked up on the job, by watching others, through experience and via the intriguing "thousands of years" of aesthetics. It is very much a cultural training, then, based upon social judgments, individual taste, and contemporary notions of beauty. Cosmetic surgeons develop aesthetic sensibilities not only through the mysterious "thousands of years" of history but also through the ideals of visual beauty, often expressed within popular media, cultures in which they are embedded. Thus, desirable aesthetics are always based on contemporary ideals of beauty and these are slippery ideals that are far from stable:

> Dr. Palmer can help you achieve the look that you've always desired through a combination of surgical mastery with a blending of artistic vision and sound aesthetic judgement that's taken years to cull [*sic*]. But, aesthetic vision and expertise vary among surgeons—so be sure that you're in the hands of someone who is highly skilled, well experienced and aesthetically gifted … like Dr. Palmer. (http://www.beverlyhillsplasticsur.com/procedures.html)

Despite its intangibility the "aesthetic gift" is something that many cosmetic surgeons try to sell. Contemporary cosmetic surgeons' websites range from simple pages with contact details to detailed textual and pictorial resources with hundreds of links. The grander sites have some interesting characteristics in common. There is often a self-professed devotion to "good" (read morally commendable) work (for example, performing pro-rata operations for underprivileged children with cleft palates), sometimes with a charity named after the doctor himself. There are usually some flattering portrait-style photos of the doctor. There are invariably before and after photos of his patients. Surprisingly, many surgeons display their own works of art. It seems that cosmetic surgeons are also painters, photographers, sculptors, and even musicians.[5] Many professionals have artistic hobbies, but why do cosmetic surgeons actively include theirs as part of their advertising? I suggest that a characteristic of contemporary cosmetic surgeons is that loss of

5 For example, Dr. Francis R. Palmer III at http://www.beverlyhillsplasticsur.com/art.html is a painter; Dr. Michael Evan Sachs at http://www.michaelevansachs.com/artgallery.htm is a photographer; Dr. A. Chasby Sacks at http://www.azcossurg.com/aboutus.htm is a sculptor; Dr. Tony Prochazka at http://www.finecosmeticsurgery.com/our_doctor.htm is a musician.

status as sole expert is compensated by the deployment of a new kind of artistic expertise. The most vivid claims about artistry I came across are on the website of Francis Rogers Palmer: "As an artist in watercolor, oil and acrylic mediums who's [*sic*] style can best be described as photorealism, he considers himself a modern day soft tissue sculptor adding his artistic flair to every aspect of his surgery" (http://www.beverlyhillsplasticsur.com/index2.html). It is worth noting that such representations of cosmetic surgery are laughed at by some others in the profession:

> All this business about artistry and that, it's—you know, it's part of the commercial patter. It more or less trivialises the whole thing, and, you know, this [breast augmentation] is real surgery … you can end up in the chest cavity if you don't know what you're doing … if you've had a proper surgical training, you can deal with that complication. (Dr. Peter Haertsch, plastic surgeon, in *Buyer of Beauty, Beware*, 2006)

Spitzack suggests, *pace* Foucault, that the eye/gaze of the surgeon is part of the powerful set of knowledges and disciplines that construct a woman's body as pathological and a potential threat to the dominant order. She felt inspected by a series of experts, most of them housed in the body of the doctor: "all around me, one who does not know, the eyes of judgment, from persons who know" (1988: 43). But now, in our media-saturated visual culture, those visual and aesthetic experts are dispersed and are no longer coagulated in the figure of the doctor. Hence, my suggestion that surgeons' attempts to promote artistic skills are connected to having lost control over an area of cosmetic surgery that they once dominated. One plastic surgeon I interviewed was contemptuous of women doing their own research. He disagreed with their aesthetic choices and saw himself as an expert whose opinions were being ignored:

> … some people are already fairly savvy, they're on the Internet, they're scanning, they're looking at pre and post [surgical photographs], reading it, even younger people coming in, eighteen- or nineteen-year old ladies, they're already onto it, they know what I'll tell them on statistics … they're researched, and if they come to me I've usually got a letter from their GP saying "Sharon wants to have her breasts augmented, I've suggested strongly against it but she still insists so please assess." She'll come in and say, "He's a schmuck, what's he know, I've got the right to vote, I live with my boyfriend, I'm 19, I'm going to uni next year, I want to go on vacation, what's wrong with having large breasts?" What can I say? What can I say? (Dr. Young)

He felt bombarded by young women wanting breast implants that he thought were too large. He wasn't against implants per se—far from it—but *he knew* what looked good: "someone who doesn't look like they're augmented, but rather just having nice breasts—perky—cleavage."

Like the other surgeons I spoke to, Dr. Young was less concerned about medical issues to do with large breast implants—for example he didn't mention that encapsulation (painful internal scarring that can make the breasts hard and lumpy) is more likely to occur with larger implants—and more concerned with aesthetic issues and matters of power. In fact, I got the strange impression that he viewed these new "knowing" clients as trespassers on his territory, bossy and opinionated impostors who were deluded about both their surgical and aesthetic choices. They were simultaneously welcome (as patients) and unwelcome (as informed consumers) in his clinic. While Spitzack was fearful that she "... might not identify [her] problem correctly" (1988: 45), the women Dr. Young described to me were confidently self-describing. They certainly didn't see the surgeon as an omniscient seer and knower but rather as a means to an end and as a technician rather than an aesthetic expert. The surgeon's status as expert and his role as artist, which at the time of Spitzack's writing were intertwined and almost unquestionable, have become somewhat separated and must now be managed alongside clients' own self-determined needs, expectations, knowledges, and aesthetic sensibilities.

Botox and the Hidden Networks of Cosmetic Surgery

> Your social appointments are escalating as the festive season nears. End the year looking rejuvenated and fresh. *Smooth, Youthful, Beautiful.* Spend fifteen minutes having BOTOX wrinkle treatment and reap the rewards through the party season and New Year. *Rejuvenate, Refresh, Revitalise.* (Botox brochure, inVIVO communications, collected July 2004, italics and capitals in original)

Surgeons' roles are changing in relation to their clients. In addition to this, they must also now negotiate with powerfully marketed products such as brand-name implants and injectibles like Botox. Botox is one brand name for a neuromuscular blocking agent called botulinum toxin. Botulinum toxins paralyze or weaken the muscles they are injected into, and they have been used therapeutically since the 1960s to treat eye muscle disorders such as uncontrollable blinking. Doctors using them for these purposes soon noticed that the frown lines and crows' feet of patients who had been treated for eye disorders were diminished or "softened." By the 2000s the toxin was being aggressively sold as a wrinkle treatment.

The brochure in which the quote above appears states "It's not magic, it's Botox," but in fact it does invoke a strong impression of magic and work. Botox is aligned with transmogrification and offered as a medical wonder. It is even allied with penicillin, arguably the twentieth century's real wonder drug: "Botox is a highly purified protein that is extracted from bacteria, in a similar way that penicillin comes from a mould." It is thus framed as simultaneously magical and mundane—desirable and transformative but not frightening or dangerous. The main protagonist in the brochure is not a recipient or a surgeon but Botox itself:

"to … ensure a safe and effective treatment, ask for Botox by name." And in fact the product *is alive*: it is a living toxin made from the same bacteria that cause the food-poisoning botulism. In this glossy pamphlet Botox is the star, cosmetic surgery recipients are both audience and stage, and doctors play mere supporting roles. The back page advises: "to find out if Botox might work well for you, please consult a cosmetic specialist who is a trained professional and can judge the optimum treatment to enhance your appearance." The procedure, the decision, the recipient, and the doctor take second place to the registered, branded, marketed product. A surgeon told me:

> … the various plastic surgical supply companies, [the suppliers of] prostheses, or the suppliers of injectables, market directly to the public. And the surgeon becomes an intermediary in this, so that the public become the customer of the surgical supplier rather than what in the ordinary course of events would be the correct way, that the doctor is the customer and the controller of the product. (Dr. Fred)

In his view the "correct way"—where doctor is main protagonist—is compromised by the power of the brand. Doctor is recast as mere middleman. Botox is only a brand name but has been marketed so strongly that all the cosmetic surgery recipients I spoke to thought of it as "the product." The surgeon continued:

> It's a great name, very hard to break, its like being called Hoover instead of vacuum cleaner or something like that, … it's like that, it's something that's clear in the public's minds. And they've managed to link their name to the product so accurately that it will be very hard to break. (Dr. Fred)

Botox further disrupts conventional medical practices because it can be injected in non-medical spaces: "Botox parties" held in private homes, mainly in order to save on cost, are notorious (and have a reputation for being far more glamorous than they often are). It may also be injected in medi-spas, by para-medical practitioners such as nurses, and by GPs (get your Botox at the same time as your flu shot). It is thus part of a set of social and industrial power-relations that are more fluid and flexible than traditional doctor–patient relationships.

Botox then, has an agential presence that appears in the cosmetic surgery world and exists somewhat independently of patients, clinics, or doctors. It is active as a *moral actor* in the deployment of cosmetic surgery. Through texts like this brochure it positions itself as a middle-class and desirable accoutrement, a sign of deserved, worked-for wealth and comfort: your Botoxed face says that you are part of a deserving group that has worked hard and can afford to choose to look "better." While Botox may be designed to minimize wrinkles I argue it is not intended to give the illusion of having led a leisurely life. Rather, it is part of a new style of management of the self where working—no matter how hard—must never leave us looking exhausted because "tired is ugly." Having Botox is now part of the presentation of a *successful* hardworking self: being a person who can afford the treatments, being a person who "looks after herself." "Botox. A simple, non-surgical procedure that can dramatically reduce even your toughest wrinkle within days. **So it's really up to you. You can choose to live with wrinkles or you can choose to live without them**" (inVIVOcommunications, Botox brochure, bold in original). Here, agency is superficially located in the hands of the consumer, who has the "choice" to live either with or without wrinkles in the same way that she has the choice to live with or without a cracked vase. This brochure text acknowledges the hard-earned status of the middle-aged woman who leads a busy life. Serenity is not an option or a desire for her, but its illusion is. Her feelings might include stress or anger but her face must present a smooth consistency. Like the four-wheel drive that she might buy for herself, or a skiing holiday, Botox is presented as a reward for hard work, as a treat, but also as part of the correct management of a certain kind of public image, part of the staging of enterprise and success.

Surgical Encounters, Surgical Stories

Forms of interpersonal discourse, especially the conversations that happen between patients, surgeons, and other medical practitioners, are waiting to be analyzed in studies of cosmetic surgery. Feminists know that discourse is in constant productive relation with material and semiotic worlds and that women are "active in positioning themselves within discourses and in investing a commitment to a subject position" (Ormrod 1995: 31). Keeping this in mind it is interesting to hear stories about recipient–surgeon encounters and to consider how certain kinds of conversations show how the cosmetic surgery experience may have changed over time. For example, some of the women I interviewed described, like Spitzack, being intimidated in their consultations. However, the general reaction to this wasn't the "internalization of disease" and sense of dejection that Spitzack describes, but instead a quick dismissal of that particular doctor.

> When I went to talk to the surgeon about general appearance I asked him what he would do if he were me and he said apart from taking the fat pads out [from under my eyes] or having this procedure [blepharoplasty] he would … inject fat [into my face]—you know how you can take fat cultures from your thighs and put them into your face? Because he looked at my face and thought it was thin. And he thought I would look better with that procedure. And I thought about that and I thought mmmm, no. (Simone)

This interviewee attended a consultation wanting to fix her putty eyelids and also actively sought the doctor's opinion about the rest of her face. When he told her that he thought she should have fat injected into her cheeks, she rejected his suggestion (interestingly, she told me that it was partly because she had dieted for years to be thin and the last thing she wanted now was a fatter face, even if it did make her look younger). She then saw photos of women who had had the fat-injecting procedure, and thought they looked like chipmunks.

Most of the women I interviewed had shopped around for surgeons and procedures. Some had taken intense dislikes to certain surgeons. One who was seriously considering a face-lift told me:

> I already went and spoke to one surgeon … who was recommended by my GP … it was a woman … I didn't like her, I really didn't like her. I didn't like the consultation, I found it, although it was highly informative, and fact-giving, it was … I found her a bit Margaret Thatcher—"you will do this and you will do that"—she was a bit kind of authoritative … I came away shaking … I put it on the back burner after that consultation so maybe it was quite good, because it made me really think about it. I just didn't like her. (Donna)

Another said, "I went along and he just made me feel really at ease" (Judith). Both connected or disconnected with their doctors on a level more to do with trust (or lack of it), empathy, and understanding than medical expertise. Liking the doctor was important and had a direct impact on the decision to have surgery or not. Another interviewee had thought about breast enlargement for a long time but didn't pursue it until she met a surgeon socially. He was the father of her young daughter's school friend and she had many informal chats with him before making her first appointment.

Anthropologist Rebecca Huss-Ashmore has found that for most patients cosmetic surgery is a positive experience described in terms of "transformation" or "healing" (2000: 29). However, she argues, seemingly counter intuitively, that this transformative and healing process does not come about because of the surgery. Rather, she suggests it is formed through language, via patients' and medical practitioners' narratives before and after operations. She finds that the *processes* of cosmetic surgery—the events and interactions that happen around, before, and after the surgery itself—are described by recipients as having had restorative effects between self and psyche, and body and body-image:

> I think that it occurs through the creation and acting out of a therapeutic narrative, a lived story in which the "me I want to be" or the "me I really am" is brought into being through the linguistic, emotional, and physical experience of surgery and recovery. (2000: 32)

Spitzack describes this relation in a much more dystopic way: "the highly *material* 'illness' of physical/aesthetic imperfection is 'cured' through complex and overlapping mechanisms of confession and surveillance" (1988: 38). Similarly, for contemporary commentator Virginia Blum there is still little negotiation or leeway in the encounter with the surgeon. She tells of a surgeon she was interviewing for her book "turning on" her, demanding to know about her nose job, reassigning her from academic professional to "defective female plastic flesh" (2003: 21–2):

> There is no choice involved in this relationship. If his effect happens only through my response, I can at the same time argue that my response wells up uncontrollably to the positional power he commands over my body ... This institutional power is inextricably tethered to the degree to which women are the perfect subjects of and for cosmetic surgery. (2003: 22)

All three viewpoints show the importance of narrative in the surgical process, especially as it is constructed through particular surgical or medical moments. Interestingly, this somewhat belies the power of the surgery itself, suggesting that if there is therapeutic value to be gained through cosmetic surgery it could be more to do with social encounters and shared narratives than with physical changes wrought by the scalpel.

Beyond Pygmalion and Galatea

The power that surgeons yield, like all power, is based in the networks in which they are embedded—in this way they don't exactly "hold" power, instead certain networks converge to exalt them. Traditionally these networks have been made up of elite schooling, professional organizations, universities, hospitals, medical journals, and those less visible networks that include supportive wives, hardworking nurses, cleaners, and receptionists. However, as Haiken points out, "authority derives as much from the patient (and, more broadly, from the realm of the consumer culture the patient both inhabits and embodies) as from the surgeon" (1997: 7).

Perhaps the most influential institution supporting and justifying cosmetic surgeons is the global mediascape, which influences purchase of equipment, doctor–patient relations, considerations of what is beautiful, and even diagnoses. Some of a contemporary cosmetic surgeon's power comes from his ability to decipher media trends and decide to what extent he should become involved in them. The doctor's eye, once the primary diagnostic and aesthetic tool in cosmetic surgery now competes with the patient's increasingly critical and knowledgeable eye and an all-encompassing media eye. Surgeons express both pleasure and dissatisfaction with this state of affairs: they mourn loss of autonomy and status but acknowledge that stronger patient knowledge and wider dissemination of information about cosmetic surgery equals more business and larger profits. This change perhaps also means that responsibility for shady practitioners is now more broadly spread—the onus is very much on the consumer to research the expertise of her practitioner—as the title of an Australian television documentary about cosmetic surgery states, "Buyer of Beauty, Beware" (2006).

The Internet and other media have created new landscapes for cosmetic surgery. The vast amount of free information available to those in the over-developed world means that the distribution of agency and the human actors within cosmetic surgery have been dramatically altered in the last ten years. Further, the growth of powerful brand names such as Botox complicates networks of actors who may negotiate, co-opt, and undermine each other. These cultural shifts show that feminist analyses of cosmetic surgery undertaken largely in terms of patient agency or simple doctor–patient power relations are no longer adequate. Not only do these lines of analysis risk recreating the dichotomy that they describe, they also keep the action focused on the simple dyad of doctor/patient: there is a closed, two-handed relationship here at best, and at worst the patient is also obscured, leaving only the heroic doctor standing, sweating and laboring for his own glory (Davis 2003: 41–57). The doctors I interviewed were acutely, painfully, and sometimes angrily aware that there were networks larger than themselves at play, that theirs was an industry being recreated by other industries, particularly by the popular media, and that the cosmetic surgery business was morphing at a rate they found difficult to keep up with. One said, when I asked him whether he had a computer imaging system so that clients could see digitally created "after" photos of themselves before surgery, "[I don't, but] I'll end up doing it, because that's what the market wants, everyone wants it, and we're unfortunately driven by what the media tell us we've got to tell our patients" (Dr. Young).

The making of Galatea occurs in the real world and in the mythical one, out of material stuff, out of discourse, and out of magic. Pygmalion and Galatea are actors inside a network of materiality, myth, and misogyny. The contemporary cosmetic surgeon is a Pygmalion figure who operates as a decentralized figure in a web where he plays lover, father, salesman, aesthete, medical expert, competitor, artist, advertiser, and technician. Galateas of the contemporary world may be unfaithful to their origins, may turn on their creators, or may actively employ doctors' expertise to their own ends. They are likely to be discerning shoppers, canny ingestors of research, and knowing consumers. Cosmetic surgery is a complex world where agency is negotiated and movable through doctor–patient relationships and interactions, where human and non-human players such as Botox have roles of high importance, and where various stakeholders constantly redefine each other. Pygmalion and Galatea still exist, but they share a crowded and multilayered stage with many, many other players.

Cassell describes a colleague's reaction to hearing about her fieldwork on general surgeons: "when she learned that I had been funded to study the morality of surgeons, she assumed without question that I was investigating their *immorality*" (1991: xiv). In medicine, notions of morality and immorality are perhaps nowhere more apparent than in the cosmetic surgery world—indeed, the play between them is what makes *Nip/Tuck*, in which cosmetic surgeons are depicted as charlatans, heroes, capitalists, mutilators, artists, and playboys, so brilliantly operatic. Stereotypes of general surgeons as knife-happy butchers are magnified tenfold for cosmetic surgeons. Cassell spent 33 months behind the scenes with surgeons to research her *Expected Miracles: Surgeons at Work.* She begins the book with a quote from Spinoza's *Ethica*: "Non ridere, non lugere, neque detestari, sed intelligere"—*Not to ridicule, not to deplore, not to denounce, but to understand.* I imagine that this attitude wasn't too difficult for her to maintain when observing surgeons performing life-saving operations, but it is a far greater challenge for the feminist studying *cosmetic* surgeons. It is more or less accepted practice for us to denounce, ridicule, and distrust these practitioners. We tend to see them as the baddies of the cosmetic surgery world—their features remain for the large part blurry as we focus on the agency, motives, and desires of the (mostly) women that they operate upon. And yet there is much to be gained from looking closely at cosmetic surgeons. They may be the ultimate pin-up boys of a culture in which negotiations and understandings of morality and immorality are undergoing significant change: examining their desires, values, and positions may well provide unique insights about our contemporary worlds.

Acknowledgments

Parts of this chapter have been drawn from "Morphing Industries: Surgeons, Patients and Consumers", chapter three in my book *Skintight: An Anatomy of Cosmetic Surgery* (Berg 2008).

References

Adams, A. 1997. "Molding Women's Bodies: The Surgeon as Sculptor," in *Bodily Discursions: Genders, Representations, Technologies*. Albany, NY: State University of New York Press, 59–80.

Bankard, B. 2004. "Ugly Women." *Phillyburbs Insider*, April 13. Available at: http://www.phillyburbs.com/pb-dyn/news/212-04132004-281113.html.

Blum, V. 2003. *Flesh Wounds: The Culture of Cosmetic Surgery*. Berkeley, Los Angeles, London: University of California Press.

"Buyer of Beauty, Beware" 2006. Four Corners Television Documentary, Australian Broadcasting Corporation, aired 23 October. Available at: http://www.abc.net.au/4corners/special_eds/20061023/.

Cassell, Joan. 1991. *Expected Miracles: Surgeons at Work*. Philadelphia: Temple University Press.

Davis, K. 1995. *Reshaping the Female Body: the Dilemma of Cosmetic Surgery*. New York: Routledge.

Davis, K. 1998. "Pygmalions in Plastic Surgery: Medical Stories, Masculine Stories." *Health: An Interdisciplinary Journal for Health, Illness, and Medicine*, 2(1), 23–40.

Davis, K. 2003. *Dubious Equalities and Embodied Differences: Cultural Studies on Cosmetic Surgery*. Oxford: Rowman & Littlefield.

Fraser, S. 2003. *Cosmetic Surgery, Gender and Culture*. London and New York: Palgrave Macmillan.

Gimlin, D. 2007. "Accounting for Cosmetic Surgery in the US and UK: A Cross-Cultural Analysis of Women's Narratives." *Body & Society*, 13(1), 43–62.

Goin, J. and Goin, M. 1981. *Changing the Body: Psychological Effects of Plastic Surgery*. Baltimore: Williams & Wilkins.

Haiken, E. 1997. *Venus Envy: A History of Cosmetic Surgery*. Baltimore: Johns Hopkins University Press.

Huss-Ashmore, R. 2000. "'The Real Me': Therapeutic Narrative in Cosmetic Surgery." *Expedition*, 42(3), 26–38.

Jones, M. 2008a. "Media-bodies and Screen-births: Cosmetic Surgery Reality Television." *Continuum*, 22(4), 515–24.

Jones, M. 2008b. *Skintight: An Anatomy of Cosmetic Surgery*. Oxford: Berg.

Kuczynski, A. 1998. "Plastic Surgeons: Why So Few Women?" *The New York Times*, July 12.

Kuczynski. A. 2006. *Beauty Junkies: Under the Skin of the Cosmetic Surgery Industry*. London: Vermilion.

Lerche Davis, J. 2003. "10 tips for a successful face lift." Available at: http://www.msnbc.msn.com/id/3076544/.

McNulty, T. A. 2007, "Channeling Pygmalion." *Cosmetic Surgery Times*, September 1. Available at: http://www.cosmeticsurgerytimes.com/cosmeticsurgerytimes/Cover+Story/Channeling-Pygmalion/ArticleStandard/Article/detail/457698.

O'Connor, E. 2000. "Part Seven," *The Love Song of Plastic Surgery: a meditation in eight little parts*. Available at: http://www.erinoconnor.org/writing/plastics7.shtml.

Ormrod, S. 1995. "Feminist Sociology and Methodology: Leaky Black Boxes in Gender/Technology Relations," in *The Gender-Technology Relation: Contemporary Theory and Research* edited by K. Grint and R. Gill. London and Bristol: Taylor & Francis, 31–47.

Ovid 2004. *Metamorphoses, Book X* edited by H. Günther. Available at: http://www.latein-pagina.de/ovid/ovid_m10.htm#5.

Palmer, F. R. No date. "Beverly Hills-Plastic Surgery.Com". http://www.beverlyhillsplasticsur.com.

Rosen, C. 2004. "The Democratization of Beauty." *The New Atlantis: A Journal of Technology and Society*, Spring. Available at: http://www.thenewatlantis.com/archive/5/rosen.

Sedgwick, E. K. 1985. *Between Men: English Literature and Male Homosocial Desire*. New York: Columbia University Press.

Spitzack, C. 1988. "The Confession Mirror: Plastic Images for Surgery." *Canadian Journal of Political and Social Theory*, 12(1–2), 38–50.

Talwar, P. K. 2002. "Scalpel Pretty." *Femina*, October 15. Available at: http://www.clsci.net/scalpel_pretty_femina_october_15_2002_issue.htm.

Turner, L. 2004. "Television on the Cutting Edge: Cosmetic Surgery Goes Prime-Time." *Virtual Mentor*, 6(10). Available at: http://virtualmentor.ama-assn.org/2004/10/msoc1-0410.html.

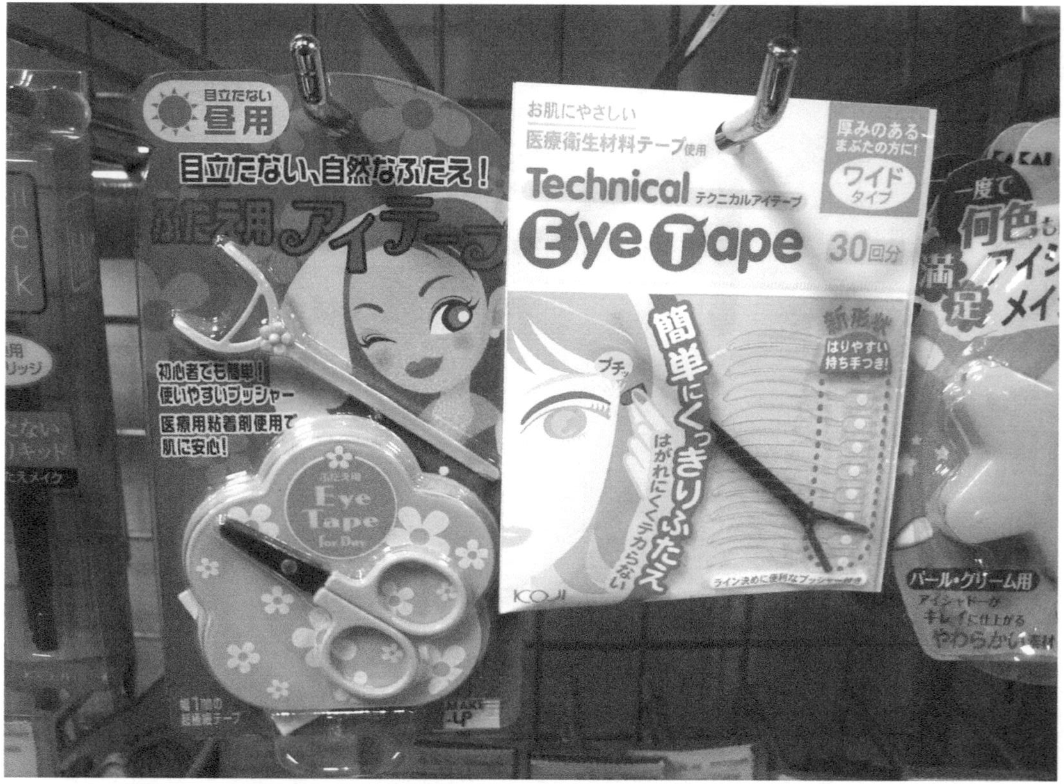

Figure 11.1 “Eyelid Tape” 2006, photo taken in Hong Kong

Source: © Andria Lam

Chapter 11
All Cosmetic Surgery is "Ethnic": Asian Eyelids, Feminist Indignation, and the Politics of Whiteness

Cressida J. Heyes

In the short-lived but much-dissected TV series *Extreme Makeover*, the monotonous parade of white women (and a few token white men) undertaking total surgical transformation is upset in series two by the introduction of "ethnic cosmetic surgery" (ECS). The mainly white cast is interrupted by the introduction of an African American woman seeking surgery to narrow her wide nose and reduce her prominent lips. The surgeon selected to undertake her procedures is African American cosmetic surgeon Anthony C. Griffin, who assumes a new prominence in this episode. Suddenly, a show striking for its stubborn refusal to engage the political and ethical questions raised by cosmetic surgery turns self-questioning. Speaking earnestly to the camera, Griffin explains that of course all his patients of color want to retain their distinctively ethnic identity, as well (somewhat contradictorily) as their individuality. The task for the "ethnic" cosmetic surgeon, then (where "ethnic" simultaneously describes the surgeon, his patients, and the surgical practices), is to retain ethnic distinctiveness and enhance individual beauty without appearing to capitulate to the demands of normative whiteness. As long as procedures are fairly conservative (in kind if not in number), justified by the surgeon's measured and authoritative voice, and legitimized by his own presumed racial loyalty, it seems, the rationale of enhancement within a zone of ethnically marked normalcy can hold up.[1]

This rationale will likely not be very convincing to most feminist viewers. The balancing act is evidently fraught, and Griffin doesn't attempt to explain why none of his black or Latina patients are seeking to have their ethnic noses widened, or their lips made more pronounced. Indeed, the possibility of capitulation to racist norms is raised only to be evaded. In a previous analysis of *Extreme Makeover*, I puzzled over this inclusion in a show that so blatantly glamorizes the power of cosmetic surgery for positive transformation (Heyes 2007: 23). Why bother even implying that "ethnic cosmetic surgery" generates any distinctive ethical

1 Due to lack of space for a fuller exploration of the issue, throughout this essay (as in the texts it cites), the terms "racial" and "ethnic" and their cognates are used without explicit theoretical attention to the distinctions between the two.

dilemmas? The surgical propulsion of the white women makeover candidates towards normative femininity, by contrast, is celebrated, and certainly not problematized by the introduction of a female cosmetic surgeon who might assure us that they are not losing their individuality or capitulating to a misogynist norm of female appearance.

I am not the only cultural critic to identify a context where this double standard prevails. Kathy Davis recounts the reactions of her feminist colleagues to a comparison of cosmetic surgery's role in perpetuating ideals of femininity and of whiteness. Thinking about (implicitly, white) women's choices with regard to femininity-enhancing surgeries, "they did not believe in a blanket rejection of cosmetic surgery, but rather in taking a nuanced, critical stance: cosmetic surgery is acceptable in individual cases but should be treated in general with caution." In the case of cosmetic surgery "to eradicate signs of *ethnicity*," by contrast, they were "incensed" and thought Asian eyelid surgery (Davis's proffered example) "completely reprehensible" (2003: 87). Thus the double standard, with its greater moral anxiety about ECS, appears to prevail in some feminist responses as well as in popular representations of cosmetic surgery.

Davis points out that

> cosmetic surgery when undertaken by people of color or the ethnically marginalized is framed in a political discourse of race rather than beauty. Whether they are positioned in a narrative of racial passing or cultural assimilation, ethnic or "racial" minorities generally have less discursive space than their white counterparts for justifying their decisions to have cosmetic surgery. (2003: 94)

She reaches this claim via a brief discussion of the history of cosmetic surgery that draws heavily on Sander Gilman's work. Gilman is the best-known proponent of the view that the modern history of cosmetic surgery needs to be understood primarily as an intervention into racial psychology and ethnic belonging, rather than only as a form of gender normalization or beautification. His work has been very important in humanistic and historical understandings because it presents the larger institutional picture of cosmetic surgery's implication in emergent racial taxonomies and projects of diasporic ethnic integration and assimilation (see especially Gilman 1998; also 1999a, 1999b, 2000). In part because he focuses on historical periods when most recipients of cosmetic surgery were men (1999a: 32), however, his treatment of how gender structures the phenomena he identifies tends to be superficial and descriptive, and he pays little attention to the available feminist literature.[2] Elizabeth Haiken's history of cosmetic surgery includes an

2 See, for example, his bizarre and confusing description of "a generally accepted feminist reading of aesthetic surgery in the 1990s," which uses a student dissertation as its exemplary text and appears to conclude that the stark increase in women having cosmetic surgery cannot be attributed to greater unhappiness with physical appearance or low self-esteem because this would pathologize those women (Gilman 1999a: 33).

excellent chapter on race, ethnicity, and cosmetic surgery, but it too by definition examines the *longue durée* and larger institutional picture, rather than the ethical and political complexities of the contemporary world (Haiken 1997: 175–227). Although it might seem, on the other hand, as though there is a substantial feminist debate on contemporary cosmetic surgery, nationality and diaspora, racial norms, and ethnicity, in fact there is surprisingly little published work that directly takes up these issues—although there is plenty of discussion of Western white women's relation to cosmetic surgery.[3] Thus in some ways, the best-known humanistic writing on cosmetic surgery encourages a theoretical disjunction between race/ethnicity and gender in ways that structure both the "discursive spaces" available to individuals, and the larger ethical and political framing.

In this chapter I want to show how some of the most widely cited literature on ethnic cosmetic surgery starts from an example—Asian blepharoplasty—that supports a particularly blunt-edged reading of women recipients as dupes of internalized racism. I suggest that the dominant reading of this case study leads to an inability to take seriously the very ethnographic results that purport to motivate it, by repeatedly countermanding the self-interpretations of the women interviewed. It also hives off "ethnic" procedures from other kinds of cosmetic surgery, making these projects of self-transformation into the sole province of women whose bodies are already racialized. Rather than arguing that such procedures are *not* prima facie evidence of cosmetic surgery's implication in racist norms, I recognize the history of ethnocentrism and assimilation against which these choices are made, but suggest that a more fine-grained analysis of women's complicity, resistance, passivity, and agency is overdue. What feminist readings of ethnic cosmetic surgery need most, I conclude, is a critical approach that reads all bodies as ethnically marked—not just as differential sets of ethnic and non-ethnic parts—and understands white, Western people as also engaged in racial and ethnic projects of bodily conformity or appropriation.

3 The widely held impression that the feminist scholarly literature on "ethnic cosmetic surgery" is terribly large and diverse may come from the plethora of popular commentaries on the topic, including articles in women's magazines, or from the fact that many feminist analyses of body politics make tangential reference to surgery and ethnicity or race without actually discussing it in any great detail. For such allusions see e.g. Dull and West 1991: 58–9, Balsamo 1996: 62–3, Little 2000: esp. 166–7. For an original and insightful analysis of national differences in the justifications used for having cosmetic surgery in the US and the UK, see Gimlin 2007.

Asian Eyelid Surgery: Beyond the Archetype

Kaw and Her Inheritors

The most discussed politically controversial contemporary ECS procedure is Asian blepharoplasty (eyelid surgery), which is performed on patients with east or southeast Asian heritage who have a single upper eyelid—i.e. one without a visible crease in it. Any attempt to describe the physiognomy of different racial group members risks reifying factitious categories, but the common story about this distinctive anatomical feature is that most non-Asians start off with a double eyelid (one with a crease), although as the skin around the eye droops with age, for example, the crease is quite commonly obscured. Many Asian people (including many Japanese, Koreans, and Chinese) do have a naturally occurring eyelid crease, but it is often less arched and closer to the lash line than in young non-Asians. The surgery involves making an incision in the upper eyelid, removing some fat and skin, and suturing the wound closed in such a way that when the eye is pulled open by the tendons attaching to the lid, a crease forms. Blepharoplasty is also routinely performed on non-Asians, of course, to create similar effects, but the anatomical structures involved and hence the surgical techniques used are subtly different, and the procedure is associated more closely with aging than with ethnicity. The aesthetic effect of the surgery (for all groups) is to create the impression of a more wide-open, rounder eye.

I raise this example because for many commentators (including Davis), Asian eyelid surgery is the archetype of ECS: it is the first example raised, the object of the most aggressive critique, and the stand-in for the whole (contested) array of "ethnic" procedures. The most widely cited feminist text on ECS is probably Eugenia Kaw's 1993 article, "Medicalization of Racial Features: Asian American Women and Cosmetic Surgery," which won an annual prize for best essay in *Medical Anthropology Quarterly*.[4] It is very widely reprinted in textbooks on body politics and still—15 years after it was first published, which is eons in cosmetic surgery scholarship—features on numerous reading lists as exemplary of how to interpret race and body modification from a critical, feminist perspective. Kaw interviewed 11 Asian American women in California for her study, of whom nine had had either eyelid or nose surgery, while two were considering double-eyelid surgery; she also interviewed five plastic surgeons in the Bay Area, and conducted reviews of clinical, promotional, and popular literatures. Kaw argues to the conclusion that

> Asian American women's decision to undergo cosmetic surgery is an attempt to escape persisting racial prejudice that correlates their stereotyped genetic physical features ("small, slanty" eyes, and a "flat" nose) with negative

4 A different version of the article was also published as Kaw 1994, and in turn reprinted in at least three other collections.

> behavioral characteristics, such as passivity, dullness, and a lack of sociability. … Through the subtle and often unconscious manipulation of racial and gender ideologies, medicine, as a producer of norms, and the larger consumer society of which it is a part encourage Asian American women to mutilate their bodies to conform to an ethnocentric norm. (1993: 75)

Two features of Kaw's work are particularly noteworthy in light of subsequent debates in the wider feminist literature on cosmetic surgery. First, she quotes her interviewees only to reject the descriptions and justifications they offer, countermanding their interpretations with her own:

> Although the women in my study do not view their cosmetic surgeries as acts of mutilation, an examination of the cultural and institutional forces that influence them to modify their bodies so radically reveals a rejection of their "given" bodies and feelings of marginality. On the one hand, they feel they are exercising their Americanness in their use of the freedom of individual choice. Some deny that they are conforming to any standard—feminist, Western, or otherwise—and others express the idea that they are, in fact, molding their own standards of beauty. Most agreed however, that their decision to alter their features was primarily a result of their awareness that as women they are expected to look their best, and that this meant, in a certain sense, less stereotypically Asian. (1993: 77–8)

Later Kaw stresses that "all of the women said that they are 'proud to be Asian American' and that they 'do not want to look white,'" (1993: 79) while almost all the women "stated that their unhappiness with their eyes and nose was individually motivated and that they really did not desire Caucasian features" (1994: 248). Some went further. For example, "Nina" "stated she was not satisfied with the results of her surgery from three years ago because her doctor made her eyes 'too round' like that [*sic*] of Caucasians" (1994: 248). Kaw doesn't explore this particular response, returning instead to her generic feminist interpretation: after quoting the women's desire to avoid appearing sleepy, dull, or passive, she concludes that "Clearly, the Asian American women in my study seek cosmetic surgery for double eyelids and nose bridges because they associate the features considered characteristic of their race with negative traits" (1993: 79). Kaw sums up her position with a remarkably broad statement akin to the radical feminist work of scholars such as Sheila Jeffreys or Janice Raymond: "Rather than celebrations of the body, [such practices as cosmetic surgery] are mutilations of the body, resulting from a devaluation of the self and induced by historically determined relationships among social groups and between the individual and society" (78).

Kaw anticipates the objection that she may be "undermining the thoughts and decisions of women who opt for [cosmetic surgery]," citing Davis's first published article on cosmetic surgery and women's agency (Davis 1991). Her engagement with this ethnographic quandary is to state, in a paragraph that fits poorly with the rest of the argument, that:

> the decision of the women in my study to undergo cosmetic surgery is often carefully thought out. Such a decision is usually made only after a long period of weighing the psychological pain of feeling inadequate prior to surgery against the possible social advantages a new set of features may bring. Several of the women were aware of complex power structures that construct their bodies as inferior and in need of change, even while they simultaneously reproduced these structures by deciding to undergo surgery. (1994: 245)

This uncomfortable awareness of the politics of aesthetic norms and ambivalence about capitulating to them—what Davis would later call "the dilemma of cosmetic surgery"—can always be reduced, however, if the woman eventually chooses ECS, to the expression of an overdetermined ideology of racial inferiority caused by internalized racist stereotypes (1993: 80) and the concomitant alienated desire to mutilate oneself.

Second, Kaw several times emphasizes that Asian American women who seek a double eyelid or a more prominent nose (she says much less about the latter) are choosing the procedures for racially motivated reasons in a way that white people modifying their bodies never are. As she puts it, the desire of Asian American women "to look more spirited and energetic through the surgical creation of folds above each eye is of a different quality from the motivation of many Anglo Americans seeking facelifts and liposuction for a fresher, more youthful appearance" (1994: 250). Most strikingly, Kaw argues that:

> the constraints many Asian Americans feel with regard to the shape of their eyes and nose are clearly of a different quality from almost every American's discontent with weight or signs of aging; it is also different from the dissatisfaction many women, white and nonwhite alike, feel about the smallness or largeness of their breasts. Because the features (eyes and nose) Asian Americans are most concerned about are conventional markers of their racial identity, a rejection of these markers entails, in some sense, a devaluation of not only oneself but also other Asian Americans. It requires having to imitate, if not admire, the characteristics of another group more culturally dominant than one's own (i.e. Anglo Americans) in order that one can at least try to distinguish oneself from one's own group. (1994: 254)

Subsequent authors writing about the ethics and politics of ethnic cosmetic surgery have largely taken on board Kaw's model without further comment, and she is frequently cited in ways that make her work seem something of an orthodoxy. For example, in her powerful reading of the racialized history of cosmetic surgery in America, Haiken cites Kaw and states that "despite surgeons' and patients' protestations to the contrary, cosmetic surgery among Asian Americans is about more than objective aesthetic standards … [D]ecoding the terminology used to discuss eyelid surgery among Asians suggests that here race (and the meanings attributed to it) is … the central issue" (1997: 208). In "Significant Flesh: Cosmetic Surgery, Physiognomy, and the Erasure of Visual Difference(s)," Catherine Padmore's "key question" is "how the examples of facial transformation that appear in these discourses might affect lived, embodied subject(ivitie)s" (1998, following note 5). Padmore focuses on Asian blepharoplasty, and cites Kaw liberally. Finally, Sara Goering (in "Conformity through Cosmetic Surgery: The Medical Erasure of Race and Disability") likewise rehearses Kaw's position in aid of her conclusion that cosmetic surgery is "a pernicious practice that threatens diversity" (2003: 172). It is not clear, however, why the quite generic arguments that frame her case studies of "racial" cosmetic surgeries and those designed to erase the markers of disability (for which facial surgery on children with Down syndrome is her archetypal example) do not apply to *all* cosmetic surgery, or why peculiar moral outrage should apply to this rather than any other body modification practice implicated in aesthetic norms.

Challenging the Orthodoxy

One easy lesson we can derive from these readings is that the limited feminist literature on ECS is strongly committed to the structural overdetermination of individual action—at least where "ethnic" women are involved. Kaw provides ethnographic data and an insider's voice that provides accessible and straightforward analytical tools to those who follow her that are politically intuitive from any feminist perspective—but perhaps thereby less interesting. These analyses are responding, in part, to the banality of magazine articles, TV shows, and surgeons' promotional materials that often simply state—rather than show—that for ethnic minority women, changing their ethnically marked features never indicates complicity with white ideals. A rhetoric of individual freedom, in which we are each urged to do whatever we "choose" in the aid of our own individuality without any second order evaluation of why we make the choices we do, is so self-evidently facile from any feminist perspective that the question of why our choices are so relentlessly patterned takes on a particular urgency (Bordo 1997).[5] In this context, Kaw's work has a politically useful role to play.

However, Kaw and her inheritors tend to generalize from what was at best a large, theoretically driven political conclusion drawn from a very small set of

5 Frustration with this position also motivates some popular "feminist" representations of ECS. It is quite common to see soul-searching features on whether having eyelid surgery means young Asian women want to look white that castigate those women for their race treachery. For an extreme example, see a recent episode of *The Tyra Banks Show* where Banks lambasts Liz—a 23-year-old Korean American woman guest—with extraordinary vigor for being deceitful about her own participation in racist norms. The segment can be viewed at: http://www.youtube.com/watch?v=L8C5ZnQA08c&feature=related.

interview data. The feminist literature on ECS has thus become somewhat stymied by a narrow analysis of internalized racism and the desire on the part of ethnic minority women in developed, multicultural countries to "look white." When this is the a priori conclusion there is little call to investigate further or draw more nuanced conclusions—just as, in the early days of white women writing about cosmetic surgery, cosmetic surgery was perceived to be so blatantly and univocally oppressive as to be barely worth theorizing. Is there any feminist perspective other than the assumption that those procedures taken to be readily identifiable as "ethnic" are evidence of false consciousness in a white supremacist world?

In "Reflections on a Yellow Eye: Asian I(\Eye/)Cons and Cosmetic Surgery," Kathleen Zane begins to articulate an internal feminist critique of the dominant orthodoxy on Asian blepharoplasty (see also Davis 2003: esp. 92–100). This article is tucked away in an obscure collection, and rarely cited; Zane herself implies that her research met with opposition from academic feminism (1998: 163–4). Articulating the discomfort that my own reading of Kaw points towards, Zane argues that

> The totalizing and dismissive assumption that Asian women who elect [to have double eyelid] surgery obviously desire to look/be Western has seemed too readily to essentialize Asians as degraded imitations and mimics. Labeling Asian surgical clients as mere victims of internalized racism resulting from their enthrallment with the patriarchal gaze of Western cultural imperialism seems to further a divide between enlightened or true feminists and these "other" less privileged "natives." (164)

Zane suggests that the insistence on attributing Asian blepharoplasty to internalized racial self-hatred rests on a prior assumption that the single eyelid is "normal, 'natural', and proper in an Asian's face"—although when it appears on the face of a non-Asian it properly denotes the undesirable signs of tiredness, age, and passivity. Thus the Asian's transgression of racial boundaries becomes a "moral issue—as denying her 'natural' body, origins, and authenticity—in the manner of anti-miscegenation rhetoric" (166). Zane argues that even Asian cultural products designed to challenge eyelid surgery can be drawn back into the same discourse: "Within the process of acknowledging institutional racism, the viewer [of the films analyzed] is encouraged to see these others only as unwitting victims or as unenlightened collaborators who reproduce the system" (171).

Zane does not deny that ethnocentrism is a significant driving force in the history and contemporary practice of Asian eyelid surgery. However, she points out various nuances in the way different Asian communities understand the surgery, as well as the surgical options they choose or reject. She also points out that the surgeries are not only a means of escape from racial identity "but also from the traditionally limited options within a specific culture's gender-coded relationships" (174). Arguing against the view that Asian women who have eyelid surgery are necessarily engaged in projects of capitulation to the exclusion of resistance, Zane hopes for social criticism that attaches greater epistemic significance to the position of the critic in relation to those whose actions she judges. She concludes:

> Understanding how, for non-privileged classes of women, forms of personal power or ways to manipulate disadvantageous social circumstances can be creatively engaged, we may confront the power and privilege that accrues from our espousal of our particular oppositional strategies. As multicultural feminists, in sum, we have to interrogate received notions of racialized and gendered subjects without conflating uses of power with issues of agency. From a less defensive posture, we may better see the power of an ethnic communality without regarding it as essentialist or essentially anti-feminist. (180)

Zane's writing is full of equivocation, and she must balance the desire not to appear politically naive with her evident frustration that dominant explanations of Asian eyelid surgery are so dismissive of the complexity of recipients' narratives. My goal in juxtaposing these texts is not to suggest that Zane has offered a better feminist interpretation and Kaw a weaker one; Kaw writes with clarity and conviction, as well as being, in my opinion, right on a number of key points. Rather I've stressed the self-proving nature of Kaw's position, as well as the reception of her work, to contrast with the difficulties that beset Zane in making a compelling representation of her view. What are the convincing aspects of Zane's argument, and how might they be developed?

"Ethnic Cosmetic Surgery"

Asian blepharoplasty, I've pointed out, is very often the example of choice for critics of ECS. Whatever critical arguments can be made about the complicity of cosmetic surgery with normative whiteness and ethnic conformity seem to start most compellingly from this case study, and then slide into theoretical claims about a much broader range of practices. Asian blepharoplasty provokes particular moral attention, I suggest, because it has three features that are not so straightforwardly present with any other procedure:

a. In the popular imagination it actually creates an ethnic feature that is not otherwise present rather than modifying one that is already there. This assumption is, of course, simplistic. Many Asian people already have a double eyelid, and indeed a common version of the surgery is the refinement of an existing crease. Some non-Asian people do not have an eyelid crease, or have lost it. Therefore on one level the exercise of sorting kinds of eyes into "Asian" and "non-Asian" types begs the question. Furthermore, Asian blepharoplasty is commonly represented using an ontology of "creating" the eyelid crease, while anti-aging blepharoplasty on non-Asians is presented as "restoring" it. As Zane points out, Asian blepharoplasty is actually done by *removing* tissue (167), so the ontology is, in a descriptive sense, inaccurate. More importantly, however, it makes it seem as though candidates for Asian blepharoplasty are appropriating a proprietary bodily feature that somehow rightly belongs to European people, and are thereby complicitous with racist norms. If the example we started from were rhinoplasty (and Kaw makes little of this, although some of her interviewees have had nose jobs), then discussion would center not on the generation of a novel feature, but rather on the shades of gray involved in reshaping a bodily feature—or even the constituent parts of one (bridge, nostrils, etc.)—that virtually everyone has.

b. Asian blepharoplasty is undertaken by a group of ethnic Others who are already closely associated with controversial and conflicting stereotypes surrounding assimilation. East and southeast Asian immigrant groups in Western countries are notoriously labeled "model minorities"—high-achieving and upwardly mobile new citizens, who succeed by dint of a strong work ethic and willingness to conform to the standards required for success under capitalism. An existing tacit (racist) discourse thus encourages a view of such immigrant groups as, on the one hand, hyperbolically competitive strivers for upward mobility and professional achievement. On the other hand, popular stereotypes of Asian women represent them as passive, prone to conventionality, and subservient to patriarchal values in their cultures of origin. The intersection between these two sets of potent stereotypes creates a double bind for Asian women, especially a younger second (or more) generation: gestures of assimilation are easily read through a quasi-feminist lens of disdain for those who "want to be white," while the refusal to participate in Westernization can throw Asian women back onto the charge that they are the passive victims of a male-dominant minority culture. I have a suspicion that Kaw's work has been well received by feminist scholars and teachers in part because it feeds on this contradictory set of racist stereotypes in ways that have not been adequately explored. Of course, this is in a way Kaw's original point—that recipients of Asian blepharoplasty have internalized stereotypes that originate outside themselves in white-dominant societies. She walks a fine line, however (which the reception of her work is likely to cross), between describing this dynamic and reinforcing the very stereotypes that the surgery is, on her own account, an effort to undermine.

c. Asian eyelid surgery has been effectively marketed by cosmetic surgeons as a distinctively ethnic procedure with its own anatomical, technical, and cultural challenges, rendering it peculiarly visible and available for political critique. Because surgeons want to open up new niche markets and distinguish their services from those of less qualified or skilled competitors, the idea that "the Asian eyelid" has a distinctive anatomy and requires the development of special skills and techniques has a currency beyond its medical truth. The large clinical literature on Asian blepharoplasty is written by specialist surgeons who are at pains to represent themselves as skilled in understanding both the technical and cultural needs of their patients. Surgeries to breasts or noses, by contrast, while they have racial meanings, are much less often specialized in the same way, and tend to be grouped together under the blanket heading of "cosmetic surgery for people of color." Thus Asian blepharoplasty is peculiarly isolable as an "ethnic" procedure not only because of the motives of the individuals who have it, but because of its institutional location.

These three observations help to explain why Asian blepharoplasty functions so neatly as the case study for an analysis of racism in cosmetic surgery, while at the same time showing that any critique must tread carefully in explaining this surgery's rhetorical appeal. Beyond her choice of primary example, however, there are some more general problems with Kaw's analysis. As I showed, she is committed to the view that ethnic cosmetic surgeries can be separated from those that have no particular ethnic meaning, in two ways. First, in addition to the quotes above, she opines that "the features that white women primarily seek to alter through cosmetic surgery (i.e., the breasts, fatty areas of the body, and facial wrinkles) do not correspond to conventional markers of racial identity" (1993: 75). It is not clear to me that all these body parts are not racially indexed: large breasts and fleshy hips have long been associated with African heritage, for example. Gilman claims that "beginning with the expansion of European colonial exploration, describing the form and size of the buttocks became a means of describing and classifying the races. The more prominent, the more primitive." Citing notorious historical representations of the southern African Koikhoi people (of whom the most famous was Saartjie Baartman—a Dutch given name commonly replaced with the offensive term the "Hottentot Venus"), Gilman argues that "the fascination with the body of the black woman was evidenced by white scientists from the nineteenth-century French anatomist Cuvier to Weimar Germany's Magnus Hirschfeld, who analyzed the black woman's body in relation to the range of 'normal' body shapes" (1999a: 212–13). Gilman offers a parallel history of the shape of the female breast, invoking various sources to suggest that the overall size and shape, and the size, color, and form of the areola and nipple, were widely represented through racial taxonomies (220–225). These "racial" projects have contemporary currency; breast reduction continues to be disproportionately popular among African American women, as is liposuction, while breast augmentation is disproportionately popular among Asian American women.[6] This reflects, among other things, the current ideal "Western" breast, which is large but not sagging or drooping, high on the chest, prominent,

6 For African American patients in 2007 in North America the three most popular surgical procedures were nose reshaping, liposuction, and breast reduction, while for Asian Americans they were nose-reshaping, breast augmentation, and eyelid surgery. Source: http://www.plasticsurgery.org/media/statistics/loader.cfm?url=/commonspot/security/getfile.cfm&PageID=29435.

and more spherical than in previous fashions, and has a "proportionate" areola diameter and nipple projection.[7]

Of course, Kaw could simply accept that she underestimated the number of body parts that can be considered "markers of racial identity." When black women use various means to reduce the size of their breasts and hips, perhaps they are simply engaging in another kind of internalized racism perfectly analogous to the Asian woman who has double eyelid surgery. However, once we see that bodies can be racially marked in unanticipated and pervasive ways, the project of hiving off "ethnic" cosmetic surgeries for a certain kind of ethical disapprobation is thrown into question. Thus a second and more important difficulty with Kaw's ontology is that it assumes that the only people undertaking cosmetic surgery with a racial ideology in play are those with ethnically marked bodies—that is, that white people who have cosmetic surgery are *not* having "ethnic" cosmetic surgery. Despite her extensive approving citation of Kaw, Padmore approaches this point when she says that "the blepharoplasty procedures discussed in this essay do not erase signifiers of race; they erase the ideological underpinnings of an aesthetic apparatus through which one type of ethnicity becomes invisible and 'other' ethnicities become hyper-visible. It is a system in which certain flesh is perceived to be 'ethnic' while other flesh is not" (1998, prior to note 18). Of course cosmetic surgery is implicated in numerous projects of ethnic marking, but privileged people also participate in these projects when they have cosmetic surgery. For example, Gilman comments that "in Brazil today breast reduction has become commonplace among upper-middle-class families, so as to distinguish their daughters from the lower classes, who are imagined as black" (1999a: 225; see also Yalom 1997: 236). Kaw alludes to "facial wrinkles" being devoid of ethnic meaning, but face-lifts (and related techniques) may be a particularly pointed example of the obscured racial currency of surgeries favored by white people. Cosmetic surgery promotional materials as well as the popular wisdom of the mediascape stress that members of different ethnic groups age differently—a claim that is also supported by a clinical literature (e.g. Odunze, Rosenberg, and Few 2008). In a curious racial inversion, Northern Europeans purportedly age "worst" due to thinner facial skin that is also more vulnerable to sun damage, and hence to wrinkling and "falling," while Asian women in particular (and to some extent African women) are often lauded for their youthful faces. Thus when pale-skinned women lift their faces to erase lines and folds, they may be working against their ethnic heritage in a way that goes unremarked and untheorized.

---

7 For historical discussion of ideal breasts see Gilman 1999a: esp. 218–31. Gilman also contrasts the large-breast fashion with older Asian norms that understood a flat-chested woman as desirably modest and discreet (Gilman 1999b: 54). Marilyn Yalom's history of the breast includes a discussion of the political role of breasts in promoting European nationalisms (see Yalom 1997: 105–45), although next to no discussion of the racial politics of breasts (but see 123–5, 236), and none at all of their racialized aesthetics.

Given that cosmetic surgery invokes norms that almost no white, Western people can actually live up to, its projects might furthermore be understood as fantasy constructions as much as attempts to literalize "the" white, Western body. Perhaps this is why Michael Jackson provokes so much controversy: his popularly perceived objective of becoming white has been enacted in a way so grotesque, parodic, and extreme that he has revealed the absurdity of whitened norms to a predominantly white general public consoled by the more conventional language of moderation and moral "clean hands" in cosmetic surgery (see Davis 2003: 95–7, and Sullivan 2004). He thereby complicates the disingenuity of conventional explanations. This is the same anxiety that is assuaged by *Extreme Makeover*'s surprise problematization of "ethnic cosmetic surgery": it speaks to a white audience by assuring them of the racial loyalty (and hence racial "place") of their sisters of color. Stressing that cosmetic surgery in fact preserves and enhances ethnic difference reassures white people that they are not being deceived by "passing" post-surgical tricksters (as well as mitigating any lingering white guilt about the very existence of ECS) (Heyes 2007: 23). When feminists take the opposite tack and argue that ethnic differences are being erased by ECS they do not really undermine this dynamic: although in this critique surgical candidates may successfully become less ethnic in order to gain social advantage, this move is interpreted as a gesture of racial disloyalty or internalized racism, in a way that upholds the authenticity of originary ethnic identities, as well as obscuring the ethnic projects in which "white" people may be engaged. The whole debate is permeated with the assumption that whiteness really is desirable and that all people of color would look more white if they possibly could. To point this out is not to deny the power of white norms for bodily appearance; rather it is to suggest that the more complex psychologies of hugely diverse ethnic minorities in Western countries, as well as the visual cultures they have produced, may actually have had some effect in changing norms and expectations. To deny this possibility seems to be to deny the possibility of actively combating racism.

The basic premise underlying all of my arguments is that feminist analysis of ethnic cosmetic surgery badly needs to learn the lessons of critical whiteness studies that are already widely integrated into feminist work on other topics (e.g. Frankenburg 1993; Cuomo and Hall 1999). These lessons might direct us to investigate how cosmetic surgery enables white women to appropriate pieces of "ethnic" physicality for their exoticism and eroticism, without risking the oppression that more marked bodies are vulnerable to (Haiken 1997: 225). When post-surgical white people emerge with pouty, bee-stung lips, or "Latin" buttocks modeled after Jennifer Lopez, they presumably do not intend to pass as racially transformed. But their choices have a racial inflection that Kaw's model simply denies. Even when surgeries arguably aim to make already white people whiter (refining a nose that carries the implication of Mediterranean or Middle Eastern ancestry, for example), there is something to be said about their ethical implications. In the absence of such an analysis, Kaw's model perpetuates the dynamic that Davis initially identified: it makes already ethnically marked people peculiarly guilty for their complicity in racist norms, and enables critics to project moral culpability for cosmetic surgery unequally onto people of color. Although the authors I've discussed include analysis of a larger industry and mediascape that is held loosely to blame for perpetuating racist norms, it is those individuals who choose ethnic procedures whose race treachery is most available for scrutiny. This move evades examination of the putative roles of other systems and actors in perpetuating racism—including white people who have cosmetic surgery.

References

Balsamo, Anne. 1996. *Technologies of the Gendered Body: Reading Cyborg Women.* Durham, NC: Duke University Press.

Bordo, Susan. 1997. "Braveheart, Babe, and the Contemporary Body," in *Twilight Zones: The Hidden Life of Cultural Images from Plato to O.J.* Berkeley: University of California Press 27–65.

Cuomo, Chris J. and Hall, Kim Q. 1999. *Whiteness: Feminist Philosophical Reflections*. Lanham, MD: Rowman and Littlefield.

Davis, Kathy. 1991. "Remaking the She-Devil: A Critical Look at Feminist Approaches to Beauty." *Hypatia*, 6(2), 21–43.

Davis, Kathy. 2003. "Surgical Passing: Why Michael Jackson's Nose Makes 'Us' Uneasy," in *Dubious Equalities and Embodied Differences: Cultural Studies on Cosmetic Surgery*. Lanham, MD: Rowman and Littlefield.

Dull, Diana and West, Candace. 1991. "Accounting for Cosmetic Surgery: The Accomplishment of Gender." *Social Problems*, 38(1), 54–70.

Frankenburg, Ruth. 1993. *White Women, Race Matters: The Social Construction of Whiteness*. Minneapolis: University of Minnesota Press.

Gilman, Sander. 1998. *Creating Beauty to Cure the Soul: Race and Psychology in the Shaping of Aesthetic Surgery*. Durham, NC: Duke University Press.

Gilman, Sander. 1999a. *Making the Body Beautiful: A Cultural History of Aesthetic Surgery*. Princeton: Princeton University Press.

Gilman, Sander. 1999b. "By a Nose: On The Construction of 'Foreign Bodies.'" *Social Epistemology*, 13(1), 49–58.

Gilman, Sander. 2000. "Proust's Nose." *Social Research*, 67(1), 61–79.

Gimlin, Debra. 2007. "Accounting for Cosmetic Surgery in the USA and Great Britain: A Cross-cultural Analysis of Women's Narratives." *Body and Society*, 13(1), 41–60.

Goering, Sara. 2003. "Conformity through Cosmetic Surgery: The Medical Erasure of Race and Disability," in *Science and Other Cultures* edited by Robert Figueroa and Sandra Harding. New York: Routledge, 172–88.

Haiken, Elizabeth. 1997. *Venus Envy: A History of Cosmetic Surgery*. New York: Johns Hopkins University Press.

Heyes, Cressida J. 2007. "Cosmetic Surgery and the Televisual Makeover: A Foucauldian Feminist Reading." *Feminist Media Studies*, 7(1), 17–32.

Kaw, Eugenia. 1993. "Medicalization of Racial Features: Asian American Women and Cosmetic Surgery," *Medical Anthropology Quarterly*, 7(1), 74–89.

Kaw, Eugenia. 1994. "'Opening' Faces:' The Politics of Cosmetic Surgery and Asian American Women," in *Many Mirrors: Body Image and Social Relations* edited by Nicole Sault. New Brunswick, NJ: Rutgers University Press, 241–65.

Little, Margaret Olivia. 2000. "Cosmetic Surgery, Suspect Norms, and the Ethics of Complicity," in *Enhancing Human Traits* edited by Erik Parens. Washington DC: Georgetown University Press, 162–76.

Odunze, Millicent, David Rosenberg, and Julius Few. 2008. "Periorbital Aging and Ethnic Considerations: A Focus on the Lateral Canthal Complex." *Plastic and Reconstructive Surgery*, 121(3), 1002–8.

Padmore, Catherine. 1998. "Significant Flesh: Cosmetic Surgery, Physiognomy, and the Erasure of Visual Difference(s)." *Lateral: A Journal of Textual and Cultural Studies* 1. Available at: http://pandora.nla.gov.au/pan/10233/20010602-0000/www.latrobe.edu.au/www/english/lateral/Issue1998-1/index.html.

Sullivan, Nikki. 2004. "'It's as Plain as the Nose on His Face': Michael Jackson, Modificatory Practices, and the Question of Ethics." *Scan Journal*, 1(3). Available at: http://www.scan.net.au/scan/journal/display.php?journal_id=44.

Yalom, Marilyn. 1997. *A History of the Breast*. New York: Knopf.

Zane, Kathleen. 1998. "Reflections on a Yellow Eye: Asian I(\Eye/)Cons and Cosmetic Surgery," in *Talking Visions: Multicultural Feminism in a Transnational Age*, edited by Ella Shohat. Cambridge, MA: MIT Press, 161–92.

PART 4
Ambivalent Voices

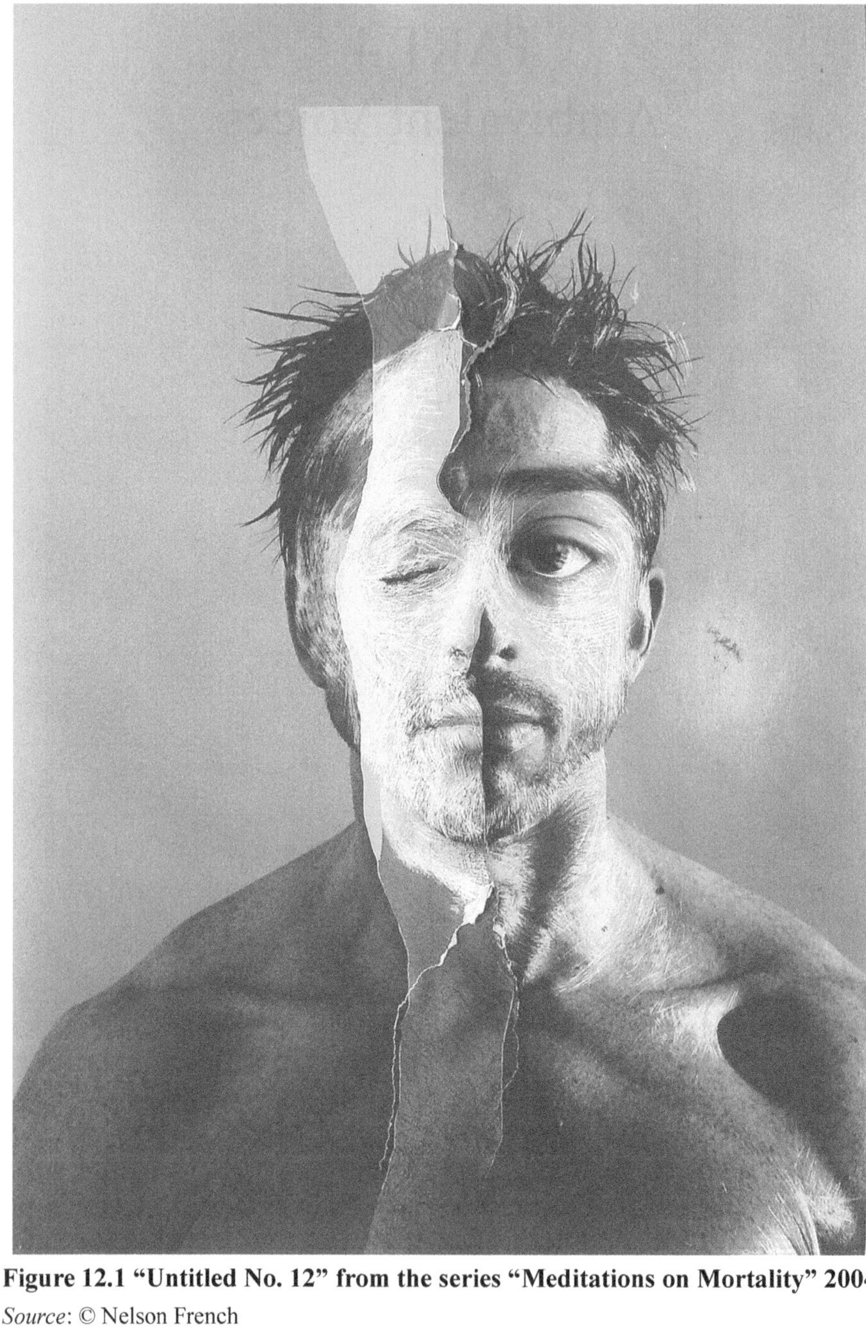

Figure 12.1 "Untitled No. 12" from the series "Meditations on Mortality" 2004

Source: © Nelson French

Chapter 12
In Your Face

Cindy Patton and John Liesch

> We have a right to feel bad about ourselves. We have the right to look the best we can or feel the best we can. I'm sort of lucky that I can try to look my best—if I wanted to. If I needed a face lift I think that I could have one but I don't think of that as something that's for me. But I have friends who've had it done, much younger than me and it makes them feel fantastic so hey go for it if it makes you feel great. I've been telling people I'm just going to age gracefully [laughs]. (GF01)[1]

> I was talking to a colleague who had not had the procedure done, and he was talking about one guy who looks as though his face has been shrink-wrapped with that hermetically sealed plastic, [a] vacuum packed look. And when he said that I almost had a visceral reaction because I remember what that was like for me and I remembered how much it hurt it physically hurt my face. In the shower in the morning when I would wash, my face would ache. It's not just a psychological and emotional impact, but there is physical pain associated with loss of facial fat. (GF05)

Despite the rejection of a "face-lift" by the first of the HIV-positive men quoted above, both have undergone surgery to fill out the voids in their cheeks that result from extreme loss of facial fat related to their illness. While the men share a diagnosis of HIV metabolic syndrome, their understanding of the cause and ramifications of their changing faces is quite different—from one another's, and again from those who undergo body modification surgeries that are framed as "personal" choices or the result of social prejudices. Women who change the shape of their breasts, and women and men who have "tucks" or "nose jobs," for example, frame their activities through discourses of beauty, ability to compete in the workplace, or aging. But HIV-positive men have been encouraged to think of their faces in medical, rather than social terms; they begin their journey to the cosmetic surgeon's suite after faces like theirs have been thoroughly medicalized by the clinicians who refer them for care outside of internal medicine. Only after

1 Instead of using the common convention of inventing pseudonyms for respondents, we have retained our own codes. Invention of names, while pleasing to the reader, creates a false sense of intimacy between the reader and the respondent, now many steps removed. For this reason, we use the code system "GF" for Good Face, the name of our project, followed by the number assigned to the subject.

their family practitioner, HIV doctor, or metabolic specialist's medicines have proven unfit for the task of undoing the damage to a ravaged face does the lowly discipline of cosmetic surgery find its place in the pantheon of HIV care.

Thus, men are invited from the outset to understand their face not as the thin membrane that connects inner and outer worlds, but as the parchment on which have been etched the marks of a disease (or its treatment). Elsewhere, we explore the specific, clinical dynamics of facial filling surgeries for HIV-positive persons. In this paper, we describe our research, then briefly trace the development of the HIV metabolic syndrome diagnosis. This history reveals how HIV clinicians have come to refer their patients for cosmetic surgery for facial lipoatrophy. If they otherwise view such surgery as frivolous, HIV clinicians' medicalized approach to facial lipoatrophy rests on the assumption that the procedures can improve patients' mental health. They've also come to view wasting as an iatrogenic condition caused by HIV medication, and hence, as something their prescribing practices are partly responsible for, making referral to the plastic surgeon more palatable. We next explore men's own beliefs about the cause and consequences of their condition and their rationale for seeking (or not seeking) surgery, highlighting the ways in which many men accept the medical frame, at least insofar as it permits them to go forward with the surgery, but also how they graft different discourses (aging, disability, empowerment, and combinations of these) onto this fundamentally medicalized HIV discourse. Along the way, we point to how these same competing narratives pose difficulties for those advocating for change, including public funding for surgeries, on behalf of people with HIV metabolic disorder.

The Good Face Project

The Good Face Project is a small study that extends two larger research projects we have conducted: a clinical ethnography on an HIV metabolic disorders clinic and a multi-partner collaboration focused on aging with HIV.[2] One of the authors of this paper, Cindy Patton, directs the Health Research and Methods Training Facility (HeRMeT), the qualitative research facility at Simon Fraser University, which has hosted all three projects. Co-author John Liesch is a member of HeRMeT's community-based research staff, working primarily on gay-community related projects. Cindy and John originally met through a gay and lesbian social group. John has been living with HIV for more than 20 years and has experienced several of the effects we are studying. Cindy has been involved in gay and AIDS

2 The Understanding Lipids Project operated from 2003 to 2005 with funding from the Small Institutional Grants Programme of the Social Science and Humanities Research Council (Canada) and the Steele Foundation. The Accidental Communities Project began in 2003 with funds from the Michael Smith Foundation for Health Research and has been funded for 2005–2008 through a Standard Grant from the Social Science and Humanities Research Council (Canada).

organizing since 1981 and has extensive knowledge of the medical aspects of the metabolic syndrome.

In the Good Face Project we interviewed ten politicized gay men who have severe facial wasting, seven of whom have undergone one or more filling procedures, and three of whom have chosen not to. As community-based researchers, we have a network of key informants through whom we recruited individuals willing to participate in the interview process and who could refer us to other men who fit our criteria. These men range in age from 42 to 59, with both an average and median age of 51. Of the ten men, six have stopped working or are retired and collect some form of disability insurance. One lived on disability income for some time, but recently returned to work to teach in his former profession, a change that reflects his understanding that he might indeed live a longer life than was originally predicted for him. The subjects are or have been professionals in government, corporate, or educational settings, and all ten men are active in gay community and HIV/AIDS organizations. The retired civil servants see their work as "volunteer" opportunities to utilize their skills on behalf of their community, while two of the other men define themselves as community activists rather than volunteers. All but one of the men have participated in gay community political organizations as well as social and artistic groups for as long as 20 years. All subjects live in the greater Vancouver area and socialize frequently in the "gayborhood." They have formed extensive networks of friends and colleagues there, but also nationally and internationally, and been exposed to the diversity of North American gay culture. Thus, we carefully chose men who have a wide range of discourses of beauty, gender, medicine, and community to draw upon as they craft their understanding of their faces.

Our interviews with these men were open-ended, unstructured conversations designed to maximize participants' freedom to define for themselves the important dimensions of their experience of facial wasting and how they have grappled with the question of seeking facial reconstruction/cosmetic surgery or not. We asked a range of questions concerning participation in the gay community: their degree of "outness" and to whom, when they first noticed changes in their face, how they feel about their bodies, how they feel others perceive them, and how the changes in their face affect their sense of masculinity and participation in social, professional, and sexual settings, particularly with respect to the differences between gay and non-gay spaces. We asked them what they believe is the underlying cause of facial lipoatrophy (and theirs in particular), what procedures they are aware of for "filling," and how they have decided for or against undergoing one of these. The interviews were about an hour long (the first two conducted by both of us, the remainder by John), and all identifying information was removed in the transcription.

Theoretical Context

In this and our other medical service related projects, we view our interview subjects as situated in a world where medical ideas, mainstream social mores, and subcultural values intermingle to produce beliefs and practices of bodily care, an approach generally aligned with social studies in medicine. For this project, we take that general approach and engage with feminist literature on cosmetic surgery and the gender studies work on body modification. While very interesting work exists about men, masculinity, and other forms of body modification—such as phalloplasty, use of steroids, and use of implants to enhance masculine appearance—there is no attention to use of facial implants. Nor has the work on metabolic side effects in HIV-positive men considered the social construction of gender and emotion that makes the feminist work on women's quest to negotiate their bodies in the context of patriarchy values so revealing.

There are two reasons why men's facial surgery has been neglected in both feminist and gender studies. First, the face is not as clearly the domain of masculine gendering as the penis or pectoral muscles, and so not immediately an interesting topic for work on men, masculinity, and body modification. Second, as Haiken (2000b) has shown, the line between cosmetic surgery and reconstructive surgery has been gendered from the very beginning of modern body modification surgeries. While there have long been attempts to repair bodies damaged in combat, reconstructive surgery made huge strides as a surgical sub-discipline after World War I, when the practice was applied to male veterans with severe battle wounds. Such reconstructive surgery was understood as serious business practiced on deserving men who sought a return to their former state of "normal looks" (Haiken 2000b). By contrast, "cosmetic" surgery has been seen as developing in relation to cultural demands for women to achieve certain beauty norms; that is, it does not return them to a state of normalcy, but helps them exceed the perceived limitations of being ordinary or even ugly (Haiken 2000a). Once established as a kind of battle scar in the war against AIDS, facial surgery for men with HIV was easily projected as "reconstructive" rather than enhancing.[3] We are suggesting,

3 Women with HIV may also seek facial reconstruction. However, men and women have different proportions of hormones, and thus, there are sex-linked differences in how HIV metabolic syndrome expresses, as well as social codings that make particular signs more troublesome to men or to women. There are also marked differences in the proportion of women versus men who receive early HIV treatment. For example, both men and women experience breast enlargement. However, while some women experience this as painful and difficult to manage, for men, it becomes an embarrassing gender crisis. In a parallel part of the original study of the lipids clinic, women we interviewed perceived their wasting, until it became extreme, as an ironic benefit of their illness; that is, they claimed to be happy that they could now eat whatever they wanted without gaining weight. They were generally less knowledgeable about HIV metabolic syndrome and did not immediately register wasting limbs and trunk thickening as related to HIV or HIV medications. For a full discussion of these issues, see Patton (2008).

then, that the ancillary medicalization of the HIV lipoatrophic face tipped the understanding of the nature and value of facial filling surgery away from perceived frivolous acquiescence to beauty and toward a perceived serious return to normal in cosmetic/plastic surgery debates.

Our work here also challenges the emerging body of qualitative research on the psychological effects of HIV metabolic syndrome, which is almost exclusively the domain of clinical and psychological literatures, areas that have yet to recognize feminist theory, and especially the work on body modification, as conceptual resources. In general, this research examines men who have presented to counselors with concerns about their body and a focus on their "depression," which is said to be identified with a cascade of poor HIV treatment outcomes. While our own interviewees talked of discomfort, depression, and isolation related to their changing bodies, these were not so clearly related to any particular health outcomes and were also intermingled with issues of aging and anxiety about whether it is morally acceptable to be concerned about one's appearance. Our sample of largely healthy and happy gay men aging with HIV presents a very different picture than studies that draw their research subjects from clinical settings. Like the feminist cosmetic surgery work that focuses on ordinary women outside counseling contexts, we have sought to place our subjects, their body perception, and their body agency in the larger social and cultural context. We add to the recent feminist work on cosmetic surgery that has tried to understand the complex reasons why women undergo procedures, suggesting that it is not done to match a cultural norm or to accede to others' demands, nor even to seek beauty, but rather to bring their bodies to a state they view as "normal," albeit one that, from an objective standpoint, is clearly a social product.

Medicalizing the Face of AIDS

Since the introduction of protease inhibitors in the mid 1990s, people with HIV have been surviving longer. This unexpected longevity has brought with it new issues, including coping with aging and living with long-term effects of both the virus and the drugs that suppress it. Although all of the generations of anti-HIV drugs have had serious side effects, the significance of these has paled in comparison to adding years to the HIV-positive person's life. After the mid 1990s, with the dramatic increase in success of subsequent combination therapies, dealing with side effects became a new priority for patients, clinicians, and researchers, whose new task was to sort out the relative contribution of HIV, HIV drugs, aging, and genetics in the overall metabolic picture of people with HIV. Side effects related to changes in lipids profile came to the attention of patients, clinicians, and researchers on the heels of the success of the first generation of combination therapies in the mid 1990s. Lipodystrophy refers to the redistribution of fat deposits in the body, one aspect of what is now called HIV metabolic syndrome.[4] In HIV-related lipodystrophy, this includes the disappearance of body fat from the face and extremities, and the accumulation of body fat in "buffalo humps" on the cervical spine or around the internal organs, resulting in a prominent belly. The reduction of body fat in the feet and buttocks can be quite painful and can disrupt simple activities like walking and sitting, while the buffalo humps impair neck mobility and constrict blood vessels that supply the face and brain. These changes also cause a certain amount of embarrassment, which requires adjustments to one's social relationships.

But perhaps the most troubling morphological change is the extreme thinning of the face that results from loss of fat in the cheeks. Facial lipoatrophy, the focus of our investigation here, is physically painful and emotionally draining. Since we all "face" the world, for people with this condition, managing self-perception and coping with other's reactions become chores that often lead to decreased social activity and depression. Many activists have also argued that the distinctive "look" of facial lipoatrophy identifies a person as having AIDS and makes them a potential target for prejudice and discrimination. Such claims have medicalized and politicized the lipoatrophied "face." Those with lipoatrophy are increasingly seeking facial surgery to "fill" the voids left by their fat loss, and activists argue that such surgeries should be covered by medical insurance.

Historically speaking, HIV metabolic syndrome was first recognized by AIDS physicians and the affected persons who were their patients in the late 1990s, especially within that first generation of people who had availed themselves of the promising new anti-HIV combination therapies, called Highly Active Anti-Retroviral Treatment (HAART, colloquially, the "AIDS Cocktail") after 1996. Like the early moments of the AIDS epidemic, when clinicians began to circulate information about the unexpected deaths among their gay patients, lipodystrophy and an apparent increase in heart attacks appeared as a conundrum for clinicians writing letters to the editors of medical journals like *The Lancet*. Researchers—especially clinician-researchers—quickly moved to investigate the prevalence, associated factors, and hence, potential causes of these unexpected side effects of what were hoped were lifesaving medicines.

Meanwhile, within gay male urban centers, a new nomenclature arose to describe the look of men who expressed unusual bodily changes. These folk terms suggest that gay men, already accustomed to sharing information about HIV and engaging in folk epidemiology, had already made up their minds that the source of these bodily changes was the new drugs. "Crix belly," the distended paunch that is as clear an identifier of HIV positivity as the hard, tight female belly is

4 The defining criteria for HIV metabolic syndrome include visible physical changes (wasting at the periphery, fat massing subcutaneously in the neck and viscerally in the torso) and clinical measures (cholesterol and blood sugar values indicative of cardiovascular prodromes and diabetes). In addition, and controversially, there are dips in testosterone and human growth hormone in some persons who have HIV metabolic syndrome.

of pregnancy, linked the new drug Crixivan with the emergent syndrome of side effects. While grateful for lifesaving drugs, HIV-positive gay men experienced "crix belly" with an ironic attitude: the price of a longer life now included a kind of low-slung scar of shame. The announcement that the new drugs might be exacerbating or even causing serious cardiovascular disease was greeted with far less irony; however unhappy gay men were about their lumpy middles and stick-figure arms, complaints about this "look" ranked low, and HIV clinicians, trained to kill a virus, not improve the metabolic status of their patients, devoted their attention to the new possibility of cardiovascular and metabolic complications. Even among treatment activists, militating for treatments that spared body shape gave way to demanding research into anti-HIV drug combinations with fewer cardiovascular side effects. For the most part, physicians now apply an algorithm of treatments that favors less metabolically demanding drugs, and they only recommend combinations known to cause or exacerbate cardiovascular problems when first-line regimens fail. There was a quickly emerging consensus that HIV drugs were the main culprit in the range of symptoms that were now being investigated as HIV metabolic syndrome, although research would ultimately show that the particular patterns of fat loss or redistribution and biochemical changes were caused by a combination of specific anti-HIV drug combinations, length of time of infection, aging in general, and genetically determined composition of fat-storing cells.

The complexity of HIV metabolic syndrome engendered a new medical subspecialty, further medicalizing the bodies of people living with HIV. The "lipids guys," as our research subjects call them, merged their background in endocrinology with their clinical experience of HIV (see Patton 2007 for a closer discussion of HIV endocrinology). These clinicians prescribed diet, exercise, and conventional drugs already in use among non-HIV patients to improve cardiovascular status and delay the progression of diabetic signs and symptoms. Although fenofibrates in some cases helped the body sufficiently soften the fat accumulated in the neck for successful liposuction, it did not work alone. And, for reasons that no one can yet explain, the buffalo humps seemed to recur. Unable to control the metabolic problems of their patients through their usual strategies, the HIV endocrinologists—a lower status set of practitioners than clinical virologists—turned to another struggling subspecialty, cosmetic surgery, in hopes of changing the appearance of their lipoatrophic patients.

It is important to understand the significance that this chain of referrals—from the space of terminal illness to the suite of the cosmetic surgeon—has had for medicalizing the face of those with fat loss: not only were men, from the beginning, positioned as worthy patients harmed by a serious illness and its treatment, but cosmetic surgeons, perpetually asked to justify their aesthetic practice as real medicine, also benefited by having a new role in the fight against the most sensational disease of the twentieth and twenty-first centuries. Not only did "cheek jobs" for these patients seem nobler than similar work undertaken for ordinary reasons, but the assertion that the cause of the facial wasting was iatrogenic suggested that it might be possible to have these surgeries covered by medical insurance plans. (To date, in Canada, only liposuction of buffalo humps is covered, since it is understood to cause a mechanical impingement and nerve or circulatory impairment.) Thus, from the beginning, our research subjects were asked to understand their presenting complaint (their face) as the proper domain of serious medical practice. But, as we'll show, they came to their encounters with a wider range of understandings about both the cause of their condition and the justification for having surgery.[5]

Aging

While, on one hand, the men quickly agreed that their facial wasting was caused by their HIV antiretroviral medication, they also engaged in very complicated discussions about which drugs were most associated with the range of problems linked to HIV metabolic syndrome. Six of the men who had facial filling viewed the procedure as a repair job to fix a side effect of their medication. However, one of these men (aged 60 and living with HIV for more than 20 years) believed that it was not medication but having HIV for a long time that caused his facial wasting. He also suggested that aging in general also played a role; indeed, there is scientific support for both of these views. Aging in general results in incremental fat loss in the face, and HIV seems to attack the mitochondria, the energy production component of each cell, which theoretically could result in widespread and selective over-utilization of fat cells for fuel.

> I don't think it's the medications that caused the wasting, I think it's just the HIV that causes the wasting because if you look at Africa, where they're not on any medication, you know they have the severe wasting. I think it's just a progression of the disease over the years. Although as [partner] said, "you know you're not a 20-year-old anymore [everyone laughs!] you can expect this at your age." (GF01)

Initially rejecting the other men's view of lipoatrophy as an iatrogenic disorder that entitled them to medical procedures to "fix" it, this man utilized discourses associated with "healthy aging" to contextualize his wasting. He believed that repair of facial lipoatrophy should be covered, but because it is part of a disease, not the consequence of treatment for disease. In his comments, he juxtaposed

5 The men in our study used one or more of the following compounds for their facial filling, often as part of a research/product study: calcium hydroxylapatite (Radiance, Radiesse), hyaluronic acid (Restylane, Perlane, Hylaform), silicone oil (Silikon 1000, VitreSil 1000), expanded polytetrafluoroethylene (ePTFE) implants (Gore-Tex, Gore S.A.M., SoftForm), and polyalkylimide (Bio-Alcamid). These substances are injected or sliced into the face using a range of surgical techniques, depending on the compound, to fill the subcutaneous space from which the fat has been lost.

facial surgery that might undo the signs of age with facial filling for lipoatrophy, arguing that "aging is a natural process," but that his facial wasting is the result of a "disease ... so the government should pay for that." But, in effect, his facial surgery accomplished both a "filling" that resulted from a disease and a "lift" that resulted from aging. As a long-term survivor, for this man aging was completely intertwined with being HIV-positive, and his playful interrelating of the two blurs the line between reparative and cosmetic surgery. He joked several times about his age and the longevity in his family and said that if he lived to be a hundred he might need "a little tuck," but his mannerism while mentioning the tuck, as well as his equivocation about the status of his own facial wasting, suggest that he holds a basic view that worrying about one's appearance constitutes frivolous vanity. In the end, when pressed on the matter, he conceded that for younger men facial wasting is both physical disability and an iatrogenic disorder, but he also felt that the *effects* of facial wasting are primarily psychological, and thus, something one might deal with without surgery.

Not all of the men were concerned about looking and being older. There was a strong sense that the general condition of facial atrophy—except in extreme cases—was congruent with a kind of chiseled masculinity: "I like my—I like my older—grayer—gaunter—older man look" (GF10). Others conveyed how associated changes in body fat distribution and exercise undertaken to offset them can result in a highly prized muscular look:

> You know I've had other people admire the veininess and stuff they think that's amazing. "How do you get your body fat down that low?' and you go, you don't really want to know so [its kind of cool], it is, yeah. (GF08)

One man discussed the social power that can accompany aging male faces and how this can be enhanced by more age, gray hair, and the lines that facial lipoatrophy mimics.

> You know what when I had a really hard time as an immigrant here [20 years ago]. When I started teaching—when I started doing research—people would not take me seriously. The moment I started getting gray hair, I stopped having problems, even to cross the border. It's that male thing that we all have engrained and I can see it in my students. If I teach with a younger colleague or a female colleague, [the students will] turn to me and to ask questions until you. (GF03)

Disability

The men in our study were also very conscious that their management of a thinning face had social repercussions. In the interviews, they reported that workmates either had not noticed or had ignored their thinning face. Meanwhile, they felt strongly that strangers responded actively to their facial wasting. Some thought strangers viewed them as ill, but most said they themselves actually triggered awkward social situations because strangers picked up on the men's growing difficulty in negotiating the somatics of their atrophied faces, especially in the simple and usually spontaneous act of smiling, a newly difficult muscle movement for men with severely atrophied faces. Several men noted that before they had their faces "fixed," they'd been increasingly reluctant to go out into social spaces, not so much because they felt others would react to their gauntness, but because they had lost control over the most basic of social signifiers. One man found this interactional change more troubling than the change in his appearance. He describes his philosophy about putting on a good face and how getting his procedure enabled him to return to a much-loved activity of walking in the park:

> When [I see] people on the street of course you know I smile at them. I think if you're not scowling when you're walking down the street people don't scowl back at you. When you're walking in the park and you're seeing people walking their dogs or they're taking their kids for a walk or pushing a stroller … I find myself—especially with people with pets because I'm a dog person—you recognize them more, you smile and say hi, or "nice dog" or "what kind of a dog" and you know you just—you make a communication where you may not have before [the procedure]. (GF02)

The incremental decline in smiling is complicated. Men both noticed that they looked different, and the skin and muscles actually felt different when they smiled. Over time, the men's facial atrophy before surgery caused a change in their psychic disposition and in their sense of the fit between their inner feelings and their ability to express them. Some men said that at a certain point they began to carefully guard their emotions in order to avoid having to use their faces to signify their feelings. Incrementally, men simply stopped smiling, sometimes because of the discomfort, but often also because they came to hate the appearance of their smile, which some men described as feeling like joy but looking like a grimace:

> Ugh—that looks awful so then you just stopped [smiling]. It—it probably wasn't a conscious decision, but you saw these pictures and ugh that doesn't look very good I don't want to do that anymore.
>
> [*Interviewer*: do you remember feeling sort of joyful and wanting to smile and sort of stopping yourself?]
>
> I think so—yeah—I mean if it was just a very close group of people then it would probably wouldn't have bothered me but when I was with a group of coworkers or clients I probably would have just refrained a little bit just to—to eliminate the problem … (GF02)

If they experienced a certain level of anxiety about their ability to present themselves in public spaces, they felt a kind of comfort in the company of other men whose bodies were also obviously undergoing complex changes in shape. They describe a knowing look exchanged among men with wasting and "crix belly" as sometimes acting as a tribal marker, sometimes as a sexual mechanism, and sometimes as simple recognition of the reality of others in the same situation.

Empowerment

Contra the social assumption that gay men are vain and scrutinize each other for blemishes, many of the men described post-surgery faces with the phrase, "he looks very much himself again" (GF10). This was echoed in one man's recollection of his mother's reaction to his surgery.

> Probably the biggest comment of course would be my mom when she saw me a couple of months later. [She said] it's like having my old son back—cause of the difference in my face I looked like I used to look. (GF06)

But this attention to self-sameness is in tension with an obvious attention to gay male beauty norms. This contradiction between the right to be returned to a former state of normal looks and the imperative to look one's best is important both in shoring up the medicalization of facial lipoatrophy and underwriting activist politics in support of getting the procedure covered by public health funding bodies. We therefore pressed the question by explicitly asking men whether, whatever the cause of their wasting, concern over appearance isn't mainly a form of vanity. From the responses we received, there appears to be a fine line between reconceptualizing the body as it is and remaking it. One of the men who had chosen not to have surgery eroticized his "ugliness," describing himself as a "gargoyle":

> We tend to start looking like gargoyles which are very powerful mythical figures. They're ugly figures but they're the protectors and they're very strong and they have these very strange bodies, right? They're winged and they're kind of devils but they're not vampires. It's interesting in the gay community: in a way we're creatures of adoration and disgust at the same time and it's a very interesting place to be as a man alive after 20 years. I'm very open about my HIV status and many people run the other way. They run—and then they stay watching in awe of what happens. (GF03)

This man asserts his gnarly face as a challenge to the presumed beauty standards of younger men, and he feels this enables him to gain sexual power over them. He was quite disdainful about getting facial filling, which he views as a waste of money and an acquiescence to gay male and larger cultural stereotypes about male beauty and youthfulness. At the same time, he was steeped in an aging narrative.

Much like the interviewee whose view of surgery was balanced between its value in terms of repairing the effects of long-term illness and staving off aging, this man also maintained an implicit hierarchy of "corrections" versus "modifications," and he recognized that the concept of vanity is applied differentially to various forms of body modification and how these are perceived by younger and older men. In the following passage, we see him struggle to define the line between acceptable forms of body modification, which are roughly designed to smooth over the process of aging with HIV, and those that are quick fixes, perhaps no work or commitment on the part of the person modifying their body:

> I thought really hard about certain things: I go to the gym, I work out, I do a lot of yoga and stuff like that but I'm fighting age, right? And I feel very good about doing those things. But would I consider [surgery]? For example if it was a hump … for me [that disfigurement] would be a problem. I always think okay, I'll deal with [choosing surgery] when I get there, but I wouldn't have Botox. (GF03)

Indeed, he went on to make some fairly derisive comments about facial procedures, but then wryly acknowledged that individuals adhere to different forms of vanity, finally dismissing some as "cultural" and unrelated to the question of HIV within the gay community.

> I mean I'm ready to drop $10,000 this very minute to have my teeth complete. I grew up with the idea from my mother that you should always take care of your teeth. But that's more cultural—it has nothing to do with any of this. (GF03)

Another subject also ordered the troubling aspects of his lipodystrophy using a cascading logic, pointing out that once he had his face filled, his worries shifted to "the stomach thing." But he too equivocated about whether the cause, and hence the solution, is biomedical or lifestyle-related. Like the gargoyle, he views surgery as a passive option, as opposed to exercise, which requires "work." Quite clearly, in his view, only if the cause of lipodystrophy is medical does he deserve to take the "passive" repair option, representing a return to the overarching medical narrative that was available to all the men in their assessment of their metabolic disorder and its repair. (At any rate, a passive fix for the enlarged belly is unavailable, since visceral abdominal fat cannot be removed through liposuction.)

> What bothers me the most now is the tummy thing. I'd like to say part of that is I just haven't been doing the exercising and as healthy eating and part of it is the lipodystrophy. The stomach bothers me more than the cheek thing in a way—but I haven't done anything about that actually [laughs] but then that involves more effort. (GF06)

A Complex of Narratives

There has been considerable discussion among gay men about the public representation of lipodystrophy, and treatment activists have struggled to position themselves in relation to both wasting and the surgeries that can treat it. Drawing on discourses of disability and stigmatization, Australian activists have contested the practice of projecting giant pictures of case studies at medical conferences, an act that, they argue, verges on the carnivalesque and risks circulating an image that, if it were to become part of the mainstream semiotics, is seen by the activists as having the potential to reignite discrimination. These politics of anti-representation contrast (or better, are complemented by) a politics of visibility and empowerment in the form of actions by Montreal-based Lipo Action. Using the direct action style of 1980s' ACT UP, LIPO creates an "in your face" forum for those with lipodystrophy and their supporters to acknowledge the particular bodily experience of stigma associated with the visual manifestations of HIV metabolic syndrome. This project is an interesting inversion of the body politics that Kathryn Pauly Morgan (1991: 45) envisioned as a means to disrupt the link between cosmetic surgery and beauty culture by reappropriating (or making undecidable) the category "ugly," which she argues is not "parasitic on that of 'beauty," but rather opposed to "the plain and the ordinary." Through their theatrical use of the grotesque, LIPO underscores the reality of living with physically apparent signs of illness, which are easily represented in the masks and costumes used at direct action events. But they also advocate for changes in the medical system so that providers will also recognize the less discernable signs of HIV metabolic syndrome discussed earlier, including increased risk of cardiovascular disease and diabetes. LIPO's position paper argues for more research emphasis on developing HIV medications that will not result in these side effects; greater autonomy for patients who want to select combination therapies that will avoid the visible effects; and finally, greater access to health plan coverage for the two surgeries necessary to reduce the effects of the fat maldistributions that those affected view as most disfiguring: filling (for facial wasting), and liposuction (for buffalo humps).

While activists plot a difficult course through competing narratives towards better treatment options and financial support for facial filling, we found that our subjects have tended to blend narratives in a way that best suited their needs. For example, many of our subjects seemed comfortable acknowledging vanity in areas not touching on HIV or wasting. Even after his procedures, one man continued to navigate between vanity, normalcy, and illness, and thus between the competing narratives about his metabolic disorder, when talking about his face. In the interview, he revealed his mixed motives for getting his face filled and how "looking better" became intermingled with his hope to avoid AIDS-phobia and to retain his privacy about his HIV illness:

> I'm not a vain person. I don't give a shit. I mean if they don't like me that's fine. Well, I shouldn't say that. I [got the procedure] to look better but I think

> what really bothered me was when that guy said [to a neighbor] "you can't spray the garden because there's somebody upstairs on the third floor who's HIV positive." Number one I never say that [I was positive]. He knows I'm gay because he lives there. But I thought, "I guess I look pretty sick for him to say that." That was upsetting. Not from a vanity kind of perspective but just from privacy—it was like being tattooed on the forehead: HIV positive. I mean, when you see sunken cheeks—it's not even a vanity sort of thing that that prompted me to want to do something about it. I'm normal—or at least look normal, back in the mainstream. Such an importance is placed on looks in society, that it seems sad. But the [surgery to my] ears was strictly vanity. (GF07)

When men discuss their decision-making process regarding surgery it is clear that, like the activists who struggle over the best politics with regards to wasting and filling, they have been actively negotiating the somatics and meanings of a wasting body across spaces with different standards of beauty and different norms for appearing healthy. If they experience discomfort with how they are perceived (or were, before surgery) in general settings, it is/was within the discourse of illness and avoiding those who are ill, and not within the specific discourse of avoiding gay men or people living with AIDS. Inside the gay cultural setting, the issue is different: it's about revealing seropositive status or looking near death, both of which have been experienced by the men as incrementally resulting in withdrawal from that social contact. But even this is tempered by the discourse of aging: several of the men admitted that they have reached an age when it is simply less comfortable to circulate among young gay men.

Indeed (and this should probably go without saying), even within gay male culture there are multiple norms of attractiveness and beauty. One interviewee, who has not undergone filling and is very publicly involved in both HIV activism and the gay male sexual world, is especially articulate about his efforts to come to terms with his face.

> At one point I had KS and I was covered in lesions from head to toe. So this is—in the—the context of that this is not as shocking right? I mean from seeing yourself in the mirror with purple lesions, using makeup and seeing people's disgust. I'm in my 40s [now] and this is happening—as opposed to being in my 20s [when] you're using your sexuality. There's more vanity or there's a different kind of vanity. I think it might be very hard for young people experiencing lipodystrophy—or any body change—because it certainly was hard for me at 30—to be disfigured—but at 40—with that experience—sure it's hard, but I carry it. I understand it—I'm not saying I like it—I mean—but I understand it. (GF03)

Another gay man, who is also very publicly involved in HIV/AIDS work, and for whom an empowerment narrative was obviously available, articulated his experience in his community this way:

> I was kind of a late sero-converter—having worked in the HIV/AIDS field ... for a number of years before this happened to me. ... I kind of turned it around as I try to do most things that aren't working especially well and look at it from a new angle and see how it might work—work for me and I chalked it up to a badge of honor—you know a member of the tribe. (GF05)

Whether "fixing," coming to terms with, or mythologizing an HIV-ravaged face, we found a longing among these men to return to normal, tempered by a realistic view of life as aging gay men with HIV. In these cases cosmetic surgery *is* reconstructive and affords them a measure of normalcy and control in lives otherwise framed by HIV—lives in which they themselves otherwise must see AIDS each day, in their first glance in the mirror. One hope offered by the surgery then, and one that must be considered outside of the dominant, strictly medical narrative associated with it, is perhaps that it could "reconstruct" the experience of living with AIDS: could it become only the *second* thing one thinks of in the morning?

Our study has unfolded some of the complexities, as well as internal and social battles involved in deciding to undertake such a reconstruction. These insights point to the need for more research into the differing ways our bodies are "seen" in unique times and places and by particular individuals or groups, and how these perceptions are constructed and understood, particularly in the context of invasive surgical modifications. It remains to be determined whether greater knowledge of this complex of perceptions can quell the anxieties of individual men and women surrounding how they look. As the men's responses hint, there may be no surgery that can guarantee our face will be accepted everywhere it is seen.

References

Haiken, E. 2000a. "The making of the modern face: cosmetic surgery." *Social Research*, 67(1), 81–97.

Haiken, E. 2000b. "Virtual virility, or, does medicine make the man?" *Men and Masculinities*, 2(4), 388–409.

Morgan, K. P. 1991. "Women and the knife: cosmetic surgery and the colonization of women's bodies." *Hypatia* 6(3), 25–53.

Patton, C. K. 2007. "Bullets, balance, or both: medicalization in HIV treatment." *The Lancet* 369(9562), 706–7.

Patton, C. K. 2008. "Unexpected side-effects: Uncovering local impacts of knowledge proliferation about HIV metabolic disorder in two distinct populations," in *Global Science, Women's Health*, edited by C. Patton and H. Loshny. Amherst, NY: Teneo Press.

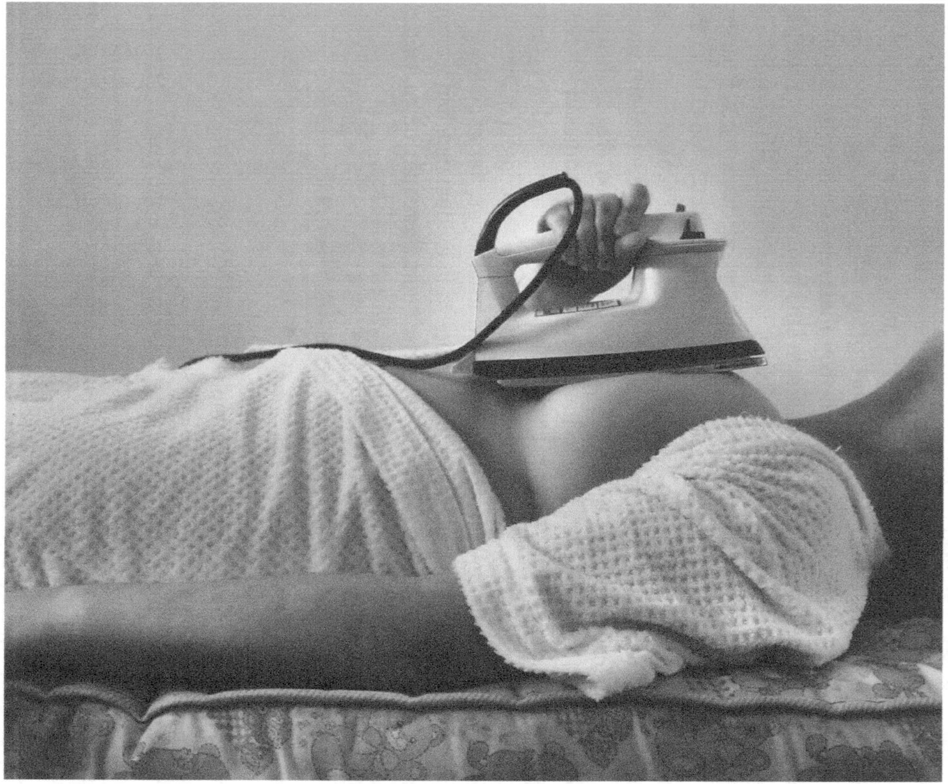

Figure 13.1“DIY Cosmetic Surgery/Breast Reduction” 2006

Source: © Janet Leadbeater

Chapter 13
Crossing the Cosmetic/Reconstructive Divide: The Instructive Situation of Breast Reduction Surgery

Diane Naugler

Introduction

According to studies conducted on behalf of the American Society of Plastic Surgeons, 39,639 breast reduction surgeries were performed in North America in 1992. This number rose to 97,637 in 2001, an increase of 146 percent in nine years. During 2001, these surgeons also performed 206,354 breast augmentations, 81,089 breast reconstructions, and 18,730 breast implant removals. Breast reductions, reconstructions, and implant removals are considered reconstructive procedures, while augmentation is considered cosmetic. Grouped together there were over 400,000 breast operations on patients who were culturally legible as female in North America during 2001. It is worth noting that in 1992, just a decade earlier, fewer than 110,000 of these various breast operations were performed (National Clearinghouse of Plastic Surgery Statistics 2001).[1] Among these surgeries breast reduction surgery has largely escaped significant attention by feminist scholars though its precarious situation as a "reconstructive" plastic surgical procedure provides interesting evidence of the interrelationship of discourses of gender and health as they are implicated in the delivery of plastic surgery.

> *Sharleen*: When I think cosmetic, I think oh, tucks and … [i]njections to make lips puffy or, you know. That's mostly what I think of as cosmetic even, I guess, at the same time as I think of [breast reduction surgery as] cosmetic but more as plastic surgery. I don't know why. It's just totally different, eh?

> *Emma*: I think I have consciously *not* considered it to be cosmetic surgery … At the same time, I don't think … that breast reduction surgery can just be understood … as a medical procedure …

1 There are no available Canadian statistics on reconstructive and/or plastic surgeries. These figures include both US and Canadian procedures.

> *Tonya*: I do see [breast reduction surgery] as cosmetic surgery … Because, for me, it was so much more cosmetic than medical … I think that our bodies are our own to … deal with as we please.[2]

These comments were made by Sharleen, Emma, and Tonya, Canadian women in their twenties who have had breast reduction surgery. Their statements demonstrate the instability of the popularly accepted boundary between "cosmetic" and "reconstructive" surgeries. Critical commentators, health care professionals, and everyday folks frequently invoke the difference between cosmetic and reconstructive surgeries but, when pressed, find the distinction hard to specify. Where should, or can, a line be drawn between the cosmetic and the reconstructive? What is at stake for feminists in using this dichotomy?

In the discourse of health professionals, the distinction between these cosmetic and reconstructive surgery focuses on a given procedure's relationship to the aesthetics of appearance. Reconstructive surgeries and procedures are "performed on *abnormal* structures of the body, caused by birth defects, developmental abnormalities, trauma, infection, tumors or disease" [emphasis mine] (American Society of Plastic Surgeons 2008), whereas cosmetic surgeries and procedures are those which "reshape[…] healthy anatomical structures, whose appearance falls within the *normal* range of variation" [emphasis mine] (Sullivan 2001: 13). The boundary between normal and abnormal, however, is always under contestation (Gilman 1999: 13). These definitions foreground ideas of "normal" and "abnormal" and have important ramifications for the acceptance, accessibility, and personal meanings of specific plastic surgery procedures.[3] Specifically these medical distinctions are grounded in everyday constructions and valuations of "normal" appearance.

Feminists have widely commented on the rising popularity and proliferation of cosmetic surgeries.[4] In particular, we have been critical of the focus of "popular critical consciousness" on "the pathological or extreme—on the unfortunate minority who become 'obsessed' or go 'too far'" (Bordo 1990: 85). This focus as Bordo also suggests, obscures the powerful normalizing forces that underlie all body management decisions, including gendered practices of diet and exercise as

2 All first person accounts excerpted from interviews conducted between 2001–02 as part of the research for "To Take a Load Off: A Contextual Analysis of Gendered Meanings(s) in Experiences of Breast Reduction Surgery," a dissertation completed through the Graduate Program in Women's Studies at York University, Toronto, Canada, September 2004.

3 In the case of breast reduction surgery, its situation as a reconstructive plastic surgical procedure has increased its popular acceptance and potential accessibility. It has also shaped the personal understandings of those who have chosen this operation (a point on which I elaborate elsewhere in this paper).

4 Some significant contributors in this area are: Bordo 1990, 1999, Brumberg 1998, Davis 1995, 1997, 2003, Furman 1997, Gimlin 2002, Morgan 1991, Sullivan 2001, Wolf 1990.

well as decisions regarding plastic surgery. Any decision to alter, reduce, display, conceal, tattoo, augment, or otherwise mark one's body is enacted in reference to the broader normalizing discourses of femininity and gender. The overwhelming focus of feminist criticism on cosmetic procedures such as breast augmentation has left the cultural understanding of the cosmetic/reconstructive divide unchallenged. This divide, and the contemporary situation of breast reduction surgery as a reconstructive plastic surgery, are enacted through the gendered politics of aesthetic normalcy. There, gendered norms of embodiment are embedded in the delivery of plastic surgeries and the politics of the contemporary division between reconstructive and cosmetic surgeries.

This chapter examines how these gendered aesthetic normalcies structure the discursive situation of breast reduction surgery as a reconstructive plastic surgery. In this analysis I specifically consider the limited available feminist discussions of breast reduction surgeries and patients' expectations and acceptance of postoperative scarring in order to examine how feminine norms of a smooth and unblemished form[5] function in relation to breast reduction surgery's reconstructive status. In the final section of the chapter I consider interviewees' reflections on how their experiences of breast reduction surgery relate to their understandings of cosmetic surgery and situate their understandings as evidence of breast reduction surgery's existence at the discursive tipping point between reconstructive and cosmetic surgeries.

The research for this chapter involved in-depth interviews with ten women who had breast reduction surgery. Interview subjects were located through word of mouth and the use of university campus email lists. Interviews were conducted in Toronto, Ontario between 2000 and 2001. Most interviews took place in interviewees' homes or offices and in one case in a local coffee shop. Interviews were tape recorded and transcribed. Interviewees were given a copy of the interview transcript to review before authorizing its use. The interviewees ranged in age from 20 to 40 years and had undergone the surgery as recently as six months prior to the interview to over ten years earlier. The women were all Caucasian-appearing, though their geographic backgrounds and ethnic heritages varied considerable and included First Nations and Jewish ancestries.

Valuing Normalcy

Despite the growing popularity of breast reduction surgery, and the relative lack of social stigma attached to it, this surgery remains a somewhat suspect challenge to the boundaries of the female body. This suspicion is also highlighted in the cautious, albeit limited, treatment of the operation by most feminist scholars of plastic and cosmetic surgery. Deborah A. Sullivan, for example, includes breast

5 These standards are discursively linked with concomitant masculine valorizing of "battle scars" in a manner which reproduces dichotomous gender norms.

reduction surgery in her 2001 examination of cosmetic surgery, noting: "Breast reduction is distinguished from augmentation because most physicians and patients argue that the primary motivation for the former is functional, not cosmetic. Breast reductions are included, nonetheless, because there is still debate over the need for this elective surgery" (Sullivan 2001: 160). The debate Sullivan refers to concerns the enhancement aspect of the operation. That is, breast reduction surgery can be said to improve the functioning or health of the patient (lessen pain, reduce the risk of further complications such as nerve damage), but it also potentially "improves" her approximation of the narrow norms of aesthetic femininity.

Sullivan's skepticism about the medical necessity of breast reduction surgery is quietly echoed in the work of other feminist theorists (Young 1990: 201, Bordo 1999: 42). Usually this skepticism is tentative, as in Kathryn Morgan's qualifying footnote from "Women and the Knife":

> This paper addresses only the issues generated out of elective cosmetic surgery which is sharply distinguished by practitioners, patients, and insurance plans from reconstructive cosmetic surgery which is usually performed in relation to some trauma or is viewed as necessary in relation to some pressing health care concern. This is not to say that the distinction is always clear in practice. (Morgan 1991: 280)

As these caveats demonstrate, feminist scholarship has generally been complicit in upholding this dubious divide as cosmetic procedures have been taken up as more obvious capitulations to the dictates of gendered normativity than those that are framed as reconstructive.

Despite its status as a reconstructive surgery (with all its attendant restorative connotations), the sexualized meanings of female breasts dictate that breast reduction surgery cannot be discursively reconciled with the more acceptable uses of plastic surgery techniques (e.g. surgery to correct a cleft palate, or burn reconstruction). The postoperative "advantage" produced within a heteronormatively presumptive discourse of femininity renders this surgery as always already suspect. As presently delivered in Canada, the United States, and Great Britain, plastic surgeons design their breast reducing interventions to produce greater breast symmetry and a more proportional breast size in relation to the patient's body. This entrenchment of the operation within broader norms of gendered embodiment insures a strong correlation with what are popularly understood as the "most" thoroughly "cosmetic" procedures (e.g. breast augmentation, face-lift, and liposuction). Thus breast reduction surgery can be a medially authorized strategy in the pursuit of more properly feminine proportionality. Through its situation within and reinforcement of culturally specific discourses of health, gender, and embodiment, breast reduction surgery exists in an uneasy and contested middle ground of contemporary plastic surgery. This middle ground is the most unstable as meanings of breast reduction surgery are contextually and simultaneously pulled in both directions in a reflection of the mutually constitutive nature of definitions of cosmetic and reconstructive (abnormal and normal).

Reflected in commonsense perceptions of the relative necessity of various plastic surgeries is an underlying (and under-examined) adherence to the aesthetic dictates of normalcy as they are inflected by gender, age, and race. Cosmetic and reconstructive procedures alike are premised on attaining (more) normal appearance. The delivery of breast reduction surgery is designed to meet this goal. Postoperative symmetry of the breasts, the cutting away of excess areola tissue to match the new breast size, and an overall insistence on the resulting breast(s) being in proportion to the rest of the patient's body are all central features of the surgery.

The tensions and interplay between the physical, emotional, and aesthetic considerations as they are exhibited in the project of breast reduction surgery attest to the intrinsic sociality of bodies and illnesses (Lorber 1997). What these operations come to mean and how they are delivered are products of social knowledge. The pursuit of (government or insurance industry paid) breast reduction surgery in Canada, the United States, and Britain is currently acted out under the rubric of illness. As such, emotional and aesthetic concerns are seen as secondary to physical complaints. As I will argue, this hierarchical valuation has a profound impact on patient's experiences of the surgery.

Popular Acceptance of Breast Reduction Surgery and Postoperative Scarring

Breast reduction surgery is generally seen as a reasonable measure for a woman to take to alleviate pain caused by the dragging weight of overly large breasts. Practitioners acknowledge that this pain is both physical and psychosocial (Haiken 1997: 233). But it is physical pain that figures most prominently among the diagnostic criteria. Commonly cited symptoms that may indicate breast hypertrophy requiring breast reduction surgery include: stooped posture, bra strap shoulder grooves causing pain and/or numbness, upper back pain, and pain of the neck and/or shoulders.

Physicians understand that their clients experience emotionally painful social situations due to people's reactions to, and perceptions of, their large breasts. However, an examination of popular literature on breast reduction surgery reveals clear distinctions drawn between physical and psychosocial pain. For example, the website of Dr Michael Bermant notes: "Women with very large, pendulous breasts may experience a variety of *medical problems* caused by the excessive weight … And unusually large breasts can make a woman—or a teenage girl—feel *extremely self-conscious*" [emphasis mine] (Bermant n.d.). In part because of the controversies surrounding cosmetic procedures, but also, in Canada, a government-mediated system which seeks to entice potential patients/clients, and controls payment, practitioners acknowledge aesthetic benefits but rule them out as insufficient justification for the surgery. These social factors are necessarily reflected in individuals' narratives of their surgeries (Gimlin 2007).

Medical literature on breast reduction surgery often exhibits a disavowal of cosmetic enhancement. More subtly, this literature offers potential breast reduction patients the possibility of cosmetic enhancement without actually promising its delivery. For example, the website for SurgiCare a consortium of health clinics in the United Kingdom reads, "All women are different and not everyone wants to think big. For many of you the physical discomfort associated with very large breasts can be the bane of your life. Small is beautiful." (SurgiCare 2008) A key component of this disavowal of cosmetic enhancement is an insistence—in the form of direct statements to potential patients during pre-operative consultation—on the occurrence of postoperative scarring. All materials published by surgeons and their advocates mention scarring. But even so, most downplay its significance:

> The procedure does leave noticeable, permanent scars, although they'll be covered by your bra or bathing suit. (False Creek Surgical Centre 2008)

> The incisions from the procedure should fade over time. Fortunately, the incisions for breast reduction are in locations easily concealed by clothing, even low-cut necklines. (SurgiCare 2008)

> Surgeons increasingly aim to reduce the amount of scarring after breast reduction. Ideally, scars should be placed in the submammary fold, the crease underneath the breast, with no scars on the breast itself. But if the nipples are to be moved upwards, as they are in breast reductions, an incision is necessary around the nipple and areola. (Harkness and Farran 1996: 197)

Readers of such descriptions are left with the dual emphasis postoperative results of more manageable (as in the "new" ability to wear bathing suits and low cut neck lines), though visibly marked, breasts.

Significantly, the surgical techniques themselves serve as proof of breast reduction's reconstructive status. Technological change and market demand offer further evidence of the instability of the cosmetic/reconstructive divide. The classic anchor scars associated with breast reduction surgery—the punishment, as it were, for defacing one's body—are not a necessary off-shoot of the surgery after all. New techniques greatly reduce postoperative scarring. Most notable among these new methods are liposuction-based techniques, which promise substantial reductions not only in postoperative scarring but also decreases in the use of anesthetic, length of operation, and recovery time and increased precision of postoperative symmetry of the breasts (Lorenzo 2001). These innovations give rise to the question: if breast reduction surgery can address physical pain as well as produce normative aesthetic results, is it still reconstructive surgery? To acknowledge the physical and aesthetic elements means acknowledging that breast reduction surgery is either *both* reconstructive *and* cosmetic or something else altogether. As Sharleen astutely suggests in her contribution to the epigraphs that open this article, breasts are "different." This critical difference is not simply relative to other parts of one's body but between one person's breast(s) and another's. Regardless of the continued surgical refinement of the procedure, distinctions between reconstructive and cosmetic, between physical, emotional, and aesthetic are dubious and misleading given their inherent interconnectedness.

These connections are also inherent in the most established of surgical breast reduction techniques. As described by Elizabeth Haiken, the "inferior pecticle technique" involves significant cutting and postoperative scarring:

> The surgeon makes two C-shaped horizontal incisions, underneath the breast and the areola, and two vertical incisions running between the horizontal ones. He [*sic*] removes a "wedge" of fat, tissues, and skin, reshapes the breast, and repositions the nipple and areola before closing the incision. The standard scar, after recovery, is anchor-shaped, running vertically from nipple to the curved, horizontal scar, which is normally hidden underneath the breast. (1997: 232)

According to Haiken this procedure has changed very little in the more than 80 years of its modern history. Indeed, according to a recent survey of Canadian plastic surgeons, this method is routinely employed by 65 percent of surgeons (Carr and Freiberg 2003: 3).

A great deal of the existing social comfort with breast reduction surgery and, to a certain extent, its status as a state or insurer funded medical benefit, is due to the fact that the *necessary* postoperative scars offer visible proof that this is not an operation undertaken principally for aesthetic enhancement.[6] Such scarring functions to mitigate the skepticism about women who seek the surgery. Women who choose breast reduction *potentially improve* their appearance, their ability to pursue physical activities, and their self-esteem. Many studies highlight the social and economic benefits accruing to beautiful people (Sullivan 2001). Against such benefits, the surgical scars visibly testify to another form of acceptable suffering and thus rescue breast reduction surgery from the terrain of purely aesthetic surgery. Thus, postoperative scarring secures a measure of *fairness*; a balance of enhancement and suffering with regard to breast reduction surgery.

Instances of postoperative scarring associated with breast reduction surgery are in practice highly variable. Factors such as age at the time of surgery, degree of elasticity of skin, quality and consistency of postoperative care, surgical technique, and ethnic heritage all factor into the severity of the scarring. Persons of African, Hispanic, and Native American heritages are often prone to "keloid" scars. These scars are a "genetically inherited disorder in which scars heal as if they were tumors, growing outside the confines of the original wound or trauma" (DeWire

6 While there can be scarring associated with other cosmetic procedures such as breast augmentation, the surgical techniques of these operations are designed to minimize, hide, or otherwise lessen the possibility of visible scarring.

2003). For this reason plastic surgeons often recommend liposuction-based techniques for breast reductions for their patients of color. Thus the accessibility of breast reduction surgery is limited not only by the existence of public or private insurance funding for the operation, but also by a person's predisposition to scarring and how it relates to their sense of their own allegiance to popular norms of an unblemished, smooth and feminine body. For clearly, according to these norms, women are not undergoing this procedure for vanity's sake. The deliberate, medically assisted, scarring of one's breasts testifies to the unbearability of the physical (and emotional) pain of large breasts.

Breast Reduction Surgery and Cosmetic Surgery

The conceptual divide between reconstructive and cosmetic plastic surgeries is materially grounded in the dynamics of funding and access. In Canada, provincial and territorial health plans cover reconstructive surgery. While the documentation required varies somewhat from province to province, patients seeking government-funded breast reduction surgery must have a referral from a general practitioner to a licensed plastic surgeon that, in turn, makes a diagnosis of breast hypertrophy requiring reduction mammaplasty/breast reduction surgery. In the United States and Britain a similar path of medical diagnosis is required by private insurance firms before they will agree to cover the cost of the operation. Whether publicly or privately funded, the denial of access is dictated by medical and bureaucratic assessments of whether an individual's desire for the surgery is too cosmetically motivated, is a substitute for weight loss and, though unacknowledged in any literature on the subject, whether or not the desired outcome reasonably promotes the dictates of normative femininity.[7]

The discursive effects of these funding arrangements were quite evident in interviewees' narratives of breast reduction surgery. Specifically, interviewees drew on the cultural resources of popular understandings of "cosmetic" surgeries (Gimlin 2007) in order to distance themselves (their experiences and motivations) from other, less legitimate, forms of medicalized bodily intervention. I encountered these narrative strategies as a result of reading the growing body of feminist scholarship on cosmetic surgery and pondering the (almost complete) lack of engagement with the popularity of breast reduction surgery, I began to wonder about the significance of this absence and how it might relate to or reflect women's experiences with breast reduction surgery. In order to consider these connections, interviewees were asked: "Can you describe the relationship between breast reduction surgery and cosmetic surgery?"

7 For example, the province of Quebec currently requires a minimum weight for tissue removed in reduction mammaplasty (250 grams per breast). Removals of lesser weights are not considered "medically necessary" and are not covered through the provincial health insurance plan: http://www.breasthealthonline.org/cgi-bin/mwf/topic_show.pl?tid=84681.

There was a lot of confusion when participants were encouraged to distinguish between their understandings of what constituted cosmetic and plastic surgeries. While most had a clear idea of what operations and procedures were generally considered cosmetic, they often had difficulty distinguishing the benefits of breast reduction surgery from those cosmetic procedures. This excerpt from Sharleen's interview exemplifies these difficulties:

> *D.N.*: So, when you think of cosmetic surgery and plastic surgery is there a difference or are they the same thing?
>
> *S.A.*: Um, very similar … When I think of cosmetic I think of people doing things to enhance themselves. Plastics would be repairing the scar on your arm … to make it look nicer … I guess that probably makes it similar doesn't it? When I think cosmetic, I think oh, tucks and … [i]njections to make lips puffy or, you know. That's mostly what I think of as cosmetic even, I guess, at the same time as I think of [breast reduction surgery as] cosmetic but more as plastic surgery. I don't know why. It's just totally different, eh?
>
> *D.N.*: So where would breast reduction surgery fit or is it someplace else?
>
> *S.A.*: [pause] I don't know. I never thought of that … when I think of my surgery I think of it as a surgery, not as cosmetic … I would never tell anyone I had cosmetic surgery.

Sharleen's confusion demonstrates that she is conversant with the slippery distinctions between cosmetic, aesthetic, reconstructive, and plastic surgeries. Simultaneously, her insistence that she would never identify herself as having had cosmetic surgery also indicates an understanding and adherence to the norms of femininity. She knows what efforts to manage femininity can be unproblematically acknowledged (Bordo 1990: 90).

The critical distinction between cosmetic and breast reduction surgery, for Sharleen, is that cosmetic surgery improves self-esteem through improving appearance—for example, collagen injections, lifts and tucks—whereas breast reduction surgery improves physical symptoms such as shoulder pain, also resulting in improved self-esteem. Similarly, Deb, another interview subject, notes that cosmetic surgery is about "superficial change" and "fitting the status quo." Her operation benefited her because "I wasn't able to breathe, I wasn't able to exercise." For Deb, the distinction between breast reduction and cosmetic surgery lies in the fact that, "there are more factors … in a breast reduction, more than just cosmetic …" Sharleen and others who have had the surgery believe that the benefits of the operation exceed those of cosmetic surgeries and procedures. More specifically, these women find that the benefits of breast reduction surgery are more legitimate than those of cosmetic surgeries. Such assertions are "central to their experiences of the practice, in that they not only reflect those experiences but also help constitute them as well" (Gimlin 2007).

Interviewees' attempts to explain the distinctions between breast reduction surgery and cosmetic surgery, however, often collapsed under the weight of similarities across any such distinctions. Deb found qualifying the relationship "difficult":

> … in some ways [breast reduction surgery] is more medical … more than just a superficial change … [I]t did a lot for me emotionally … I would [not] have lost weight had I not got a breast reduction and that makes me feel better. Which I guess is kind of superficial but … it's not about fitting the status quo.

Interestingly, three interviewees explicitly offered rationalizations of their surgeries that downplayed its cosmetic features. Emma noted, "I think I have consciously *not* considered it to be cosmetic surgery." Similarly, Annie says, "I think that I've put some energy into thinking about […] that it's not plastic surgery. When really, it *is* plastic surgery." Sharleen likewise responds, "When I think of my surgery I think of it as a surgery and not cosmetic."

Many interviewees found that their impression of the surgery had changed since they were first preparing for it. For some, these changes in perspective were influenced by popular representations of cosmetic surgery.

> *Leah*: … I've seen some shows lately talking about plastic surgery and I've just been more conscious of my operation and wondering where it falls … it's made me think differently about women who have plastic surgery … I know how I felt when people looked at me like I was … a tramp or something because I had big breasts … And … women with small breasts … are they going through anything different … when they have what we call cosmetic surgeries?

Self-esteem is a troubled terrain when situating breast reduction surgery in relation to cosmetic surgery. Surgeons and patients alike attest that the extent and visibility of postoperative scarring with traditional methods of reduction mammaplasty is not always ideal. The relationship between this scarring and issues of self-esteem is critically implicated in larger questions about this surgical relationship and femininity. A few of the participants mentioned less than total acceptance of their postoperative scarring. Emma, for one, has contemplated corrective surgery, "I … looked into having a procedure where they would lighten the scarring … I had an appointment that my MD had arranged … but one of the reasons why I didn't go is because I really felt like *that* would be cosmetic …" Here, she hits a conceptual line concerning what, and how much, she can do to feel better about her body without having to consider the intervention a cosmetic procedure. While it is clearly a conflicted value, a similarity in these excerpts suggests acceptance of improved self-esteem as an ancillary or bonus result of the operation (but not as its primary goal) is central to the surgery's situation as reconstructive. To the extent that normalization is a project of prevailing social discourses, it is not possible to separate breast reduction surgery or plastic surgery in general from this context. Just as importantly however, potential breast reduction patients and those who study this surgery need to acknowledge the interplay of the physical, emotional, and cosmetic/aesthetic elements of this medical body modification (Petro 1997). The material situation of breast reduction surgery highlights the necessary embeddedness of aesthetic considerations in "reconstructive" plastic surgeries.

Conclusion

We can learn a lot about contemporary understandings of gender and health through an analysis of the delivery of breast reduction surgery. In particular, breast reduction surgery demonstrates the precariousness of the commonly accepted cosmetic/reconstructive divide with the use of plastic surgical technologies. This divide elides its own dependence on notions of normalcy and gendered embodiments. The lack of interrogation of the boundaries of the cosmetic/reconstructive divide, by feminists and other scholars, unwittingly participates in the entrenchment of normative notions of femininity. The acceptance of this divide is only one aspect of society's unwillingness to accept scarred and/or differently proportioned female bodies.

Social and cultural understandings of the gendered aesthetics of normalcy are the fundamental structuring forces of a personal sense of gendered embodiment. The field of plastic surgery and the taken-for-grantedness of the cosmetic/reconstructive divide are, in part, features of the production of these normalcies and the identities they support. The commonsense acceptance of this divide illustrates how bodies become products of social knowledge in their everyday engagements with social institutions and emerge "as object[s] of processes of discipline and normalization" (Davis 1997: 3).

In examining the contours of the accepted divide from the perspective of breast reduction surgery, we are compelled to differently consider the boundaries of the cosmetic and the reconstructive. While these distinctions are always bounded by the particular unity of body and subjectivity of the person upon whom such procedures are enacted, meanings of embodied practices necessarily shift through time and context. What was undertaken as reconstructive in one context may have more in common with understandings of cosmetic in another. By looking at the uneasy middle ground of this divide, where breast reduction surgery is most certainly situated, nuances of the disciplining effects of gendered normalcies become evident as do productive directions for future feminist scholarship.

References

American Society of Plastic and Reconstructive Surgeons. 2002. "Breast Reduction." The Plastic Surgery Information Service. October 21. Available at: http://www.plasticsurgery.org/surgery/reconstructive/breast_reduction/breast_reduction.cfm#1.

American Society of Plastic Surgeons. 2008. "What is Reconstructive Surgery?" Available at: http://www.plasticsurgery.org/Patients_and_Consumers/Procedures/Reconstructive_Procedures.html.

Bermant, Michael. No date. "Breast Reduction—The Problem with Large Breasts." Available at: http://www.plasticsurgery4u.com/procedure_folder/breast_reduction.html.

Bordo, Susan. 1990. "Reading the Slender Body," in *Body Politics: Women and the Discourses of Science*, edited by M. Jacobus, E. Fox Keller, and S. Shuttleworth. New York: Routledge, 83–112.

Bordo, Susan. 1999. *Twilight Zones: The Hidden Life of Cultural Images from Plato to O.J.* Berkeley: University of California Press.

Brumberg, Joan Jacobs. 1998. *The Body Project: An Intimate History of American Girls*. New York: Vintage Books.

Carr, Michele M. and Freiberg, Arnis. 2003. "Canadian survey of reduction mammaplasty techniques." *The Canadian Journal of Plastic Surgery*. Available at: http://webserver.pulsus.com/PLASTICS/o304/carr ed.htm.

"Cosmetic Surgery Jumps 50 Percent: Liposuction and Breast Augmentation Top Procedures." February 15. Available at: http://www.drsutkin.com/plasticsurgery/stats.html.

Davis, Kathy. 1995. *Reshaping the Female Body: The Dilemma of Cosmetic Surgery*. New York: Routledge.

Davis, Kathy. 1997. "Embodying Theory: Beyond Modernist and Postmodernist Readings on the Body," in *Embodied Practices: Feminist Perspectives on the Body*, edited by Kathy Davis. London: Sage Publications, 1–23.

Davis, Kathy. 2003. "Surgical Passing: or Why Michael Jackson's Nose Makes 'Us' Uneasy." *Feminist Theory*, 4(1), 73–92.

DeWire, Thomas M., Sr. 2003. "Breast Surgery in African American Women." April 27. Available at: http://www.advanced-art.com/Breast-Aug-Afr-Am.htm.

False Creek Surgical Centre. 2008. National Surgery.Com website, October 15. Available at: http://www.nationalsurgery.com/FCSC/index.php.

Furman, Frida. 1997. *Facing the Mirror: Older Women and Beauty Shop Culture*. New York: Routledge.

Gilman, Sander L. 1999. *Making the Body Beautiful: A Cultural History of Aesthetic Surgery*. Princeton, NJ: Princeton University Press.

Gimlin, Debra. 2002. *Body Work: Beauty and Self-Image in American Culture*. Berkeley: University of California Press.

Gimlin, Debra. 2007. "Accounting for Cosmetic Surgery in the USA and Great Britain: A Cross-cultural Analysis of Women's Narratives." *Body & Society*, 13(1), 41–60.

Haiken, Elizabeth. 1999. *Venus Envy: A History of Cosmetic Surgery*. Baltimore, MD: The Johns Hopkins University Press.

Harkness, Libby and Farran, Sandra. 1996. *Everything You Need to Know About Cosmetic Surgery*. Toronto: Key Porter Books.

Lorber, Judith. 1997. *Gender and the Social Construction of Illness*, 2nd ed. Walnut Creek, CA: Altamira Press.

Lorenzo, Robin Merrill. 2001. "Sleek vs. Stacked, Part Two: The Minimal Scar Breast Reduction." April 27. Available at: http://canoe.talksurgery.com/consumer/new/new00000071_1.html.

Morgan, Kathryn Pauly. 1991. "Women and the Knife: Cosmetic Surgery and the Colonization of Women's Bodies." *Hypatia: A Journal of Feminist Philosophy*, 6(3), 25–53.

National Clearinghouse of Plastic Surgery Statistics. 2001. "2001 Reconstructive Surgery Trends." Available at: http://www.plasticsurgery.org/medicatr/rectrends2001.cfm.

Petro, Jane A. 1997. "Breast Surgery, the Surgeon's Perspective," in *The Lesbian Health Book: Caring for Ourselves*, edited by Jocelyn White and Marissa Martinez. Seattle, WA: Seal Press, 41–55.

Plastic Surgery Information Service. 2000. "Breast Reduction/Reduction Mammaplasty." October. Available at: http://www.plasticsurgery.org/surgery/brstred.htm.

SurgiCare. 2008. "Breast Reduction Surgery." October. Available at: http://www.surgicare.co.uk/cosmetic-surgery/breast-reduction.aspx.

Sullivan, Deborah A. 2001. *Cosmetic Surgery: The Cutting Edge of Commercial Medicine in America*. New Brunswick, NJ: Rutgers University Press.

Wolf, Naomi. 1990. *The Beauty Myth*. Toronto: Random House.

Young, Iris Marion. 1990. "Breasted Experience: The Look and the Feeling," in *Throwing Like a Girl and Other Essays in Feminist Philosophy and Social Theory*. Bloomington: Indiana University Press, 189–209.

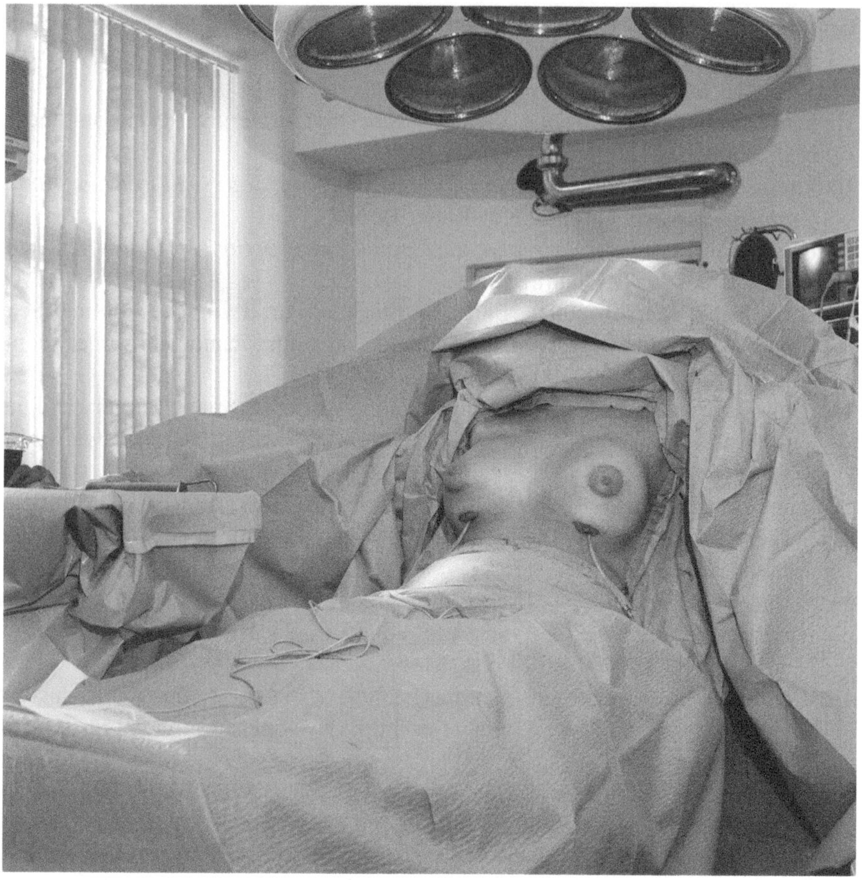

Figure 14.1 "Untitled 1" from the series "Plastic Surgery" 2004
Source: © Jenny Nordquist

Chapter 14
Farewell My Lovelies

Diana Sweeney

I never grew breasts. Tall and skinny, my teenage years were spent jealously watching my friends' breasts grow into things of beauty. At 13 I was told not to worry. To placate me, my mother bought me a bra, tiny and padded. The ambitiously named "training bra" was testament to the inevitability of breasts and for a while I believed in its magic. I stuffed the empty cups with tissues and wore it relentlessly until, at around 16, I gave up hope and went bra-less in defiance.

At 20 I was told I was lucky. Older women, deformed from years of carrying enormous bosoms, would envy my freedom. But younger women, whose breasts were large enough to warrant stares, seemed unconcerned at gravity's promise. And why not? I would have traded places with them in a heartbeat.

It was a "trade" I eventually made, undergoing breast augmentation after the birth of my second child. I had small Dow Corning silicone gel implants inserted through a tiny incision in the armpit, placed under the breast tissue but on top of the muscle. The small implant size was recommended by my plastic surgeon as being in keeping with my build. He also cautioned against large implants as being highly problematic. It was a relatively easy decision, guided by the expert to what, on balance, seemed an informed choice.

However, I was hardly informed. I had done the minimal amount of shopping around, consulting just two surgeons. The first had little to say in favor of breast augmentation and seemed less than happy with the operations he had performed. He used my consultation time to list the problems associated with the various implants on the market.[1] He critiqued three basic types. Silicone gel implants were the most popular but he preferred to not use them due to suspected problems with silicone. Saline implants overcame the silicone problem but they were less life-like to the touch. Also, due to the impossibility of matching the implant saline to the body's tissue salt, saline implants were vulnerable to water loss. This loss could be countered by the use of a valve—a small protuberance visible outside the body

1 These criticisms are as explained to me by the surgeon. They are by no means definitive and are included here not as a factual account of implants but as a personal reference point. As regards the silicone gel implants, there is still much debate. For example, while the decade-long class action suit against Dow Corning demonstrated a case against silicone gel implants, plastic surgeon Dr. Kourosh Tavakoli (based in Double Bay, Sydney) endorses their use, believing there is no conclusive evidence linking the use of silicone implants to disease.

and situated beside each breast—which enabled the surgeon to "top up" the saline. While I tried to get my head around the idea of a valve, he calmly explained the benefits of valved implants for pregnant women. These included deflation during pregnancy and lactation, and re-inflation once lactation had ceased. In this respect he viewed the valved implant as restorative.

A third type of implant (which he had used with disastrous results) was surrounded by an outer layer of cortisone-impregnated foam, an innovation designed to prevent the formation of scar tissue. When scar tissue contracts around the implant it forms what is commonly known as an encapsulation (or capsular contracture). Encapsulation is the most common complication of breast implants and affects both feeling and appearance. The breasts feel overly firm or hard and are often uncomfortable. Their appearance becomes rounded and outlined and easily distinguishable as fake.[2] Even mild encapsulation affects appearance, evidenced by a discernable lack of softness and movement and natural cleavage. This usually presents as either a wide flat gap between small breasts or a distinct separation between larger breasts. Encapsulation is an undesirable outcome, which the foam shield hoped to counteract. Unfortunately the foam either disintegrated or became overzealous, breaking down breast tissue.[3]

I believed then, and still do now, that in sharing the fearful aspects of breast augmentation, the first surgeon was attempting to dissuade me. Sadly, he had no argument outside his contempt for inferior implants. For example, he made no attempt to assure me that my breasts, while small, were perfectly fine.[4] In fairness to him the fineness of my breasts never occurred to me either. Plus, I wasn't shopping for an opinion, but a technician; someone I could trust to do the job. Thus I ignored his warnings and found a second surgeon who was relaxed, cheerful, and positive.

Like the first, surgeon no. 2 made no inquiries as to why I wanted to increase my breast size. Small breasts, it seemed, required no explanation. However, the size of my breasts apparently needed verifying because, midway through the consultation—and in a strangely intimate move—surgeon no. 2 rose from his desk, walked behind me, and cupped a hand around one of my (clothed)

2 Photo evidence of encapsulated breasts can be found at http://cosmeticsurgeryoz.com under the heading, "Breast Augmentation vs Boob Jobs." Dr. Darryl Hodgkinson distinguishes successful breast augmentation surgery as that which has produced a natural result and the "boob job" as that which has not. To make his point, he critiques breasts that show all the hallmarks of encapsulation, however he ignores this diagnosis and infers instead that they are the result of inferior surgery. To support this position, the photos of the "boob jobs" carry the disclaimer "Dr. Hodgkinson did not perform this surgery," while the pleasing photos on the following pages state "after breast augmentation by Dr. Hodgkinson."

3 In the worst-case scenario, breast tissue broke down to the extent that the implant was visible.

4 See Blum's discussion of the surgeon's inability to acknowledge an individual's less-than-perfect feature/s (2003: 3–5).

breasts. Reassured, he returned to his desk and continued to discuss my options. Eventually he asked me to remove my top and proceeded to conduct a more doctorly appraisal.

During the examination he remarked that he could restore my drooping nipples. Breast-feeding had stretched my nipples and, granted, they drooped as a result, but I had never thought about fixing them. It was a comment that highlighted a flaw, an imperfection that in the surgeon's eyes required attention. Virginia Blum says that plastic surgeons "see the defect from the other side of the room. The defect … hails them, flags them down, implores their assistance. They see, in other words, the need for surgery." According to Blum, such a perspective is fairly common to plastic surgeons and flags "a particular kind of reality populated with bodies requiring correction" (Blum 2003: 6). However, I was reluctant to undergo nipple repositioning. Apart from the risk of loss of sensation, I found it hard to imagine a scalpel slicing into my nipples. My decision was countered by the surgeon's reassurance that, luckily, the implants would partly restore nipple plumpness due to the pressure exerted by a full breast.

My surgeon's nipple comment, seemingly underscored by his belief that there is a logical desire to improve one's appearance, was damaging. The strength of his opinion was such that it caused me to view my nipples as failures. To rectify the problem, I began taping small flesh-toned sticking plasters to the underside of each nipple to hold them in place. I continued this practice even after breast augmentation.

The surgeon's nipple comment aside, the consultation went without a hitch. I was more than happy to place myself in his hands. Problems were not discussed—other than the assurance that most were easily fixed. I felt confident and excited.

Surgery was successful, but the desired result—where the breasts look and feel natural—lasted just seven years. By year eight, my implants had begun to encapsulate. Besides the undesirable effects listed above, encapsulation can affect each breast differently. In my case, as my breasts became firmer they ceased to resemble each other. This may sound strange given that many, if not most, breasts are less than identical pairs. But these changes became significant triggers for me, fueling an anxiety over the longevity and health of my implants. Removal, which had never been a consideration, started to haunt my thoughts. Also adding to my physical and aesthetic discomfort was the increasing amount of information surrounding silicone gel implants. All of it was negative; some of it was terrifying. Yet I had a strong emotional attachment to the implants; they were *my breasts* and, even though the accompanying problems had begun to take center stage, I was reluctant to give them up. For seven sweet years my breasts had been close to perfect. They were soft, comfortable, and natural looking, and I loved them. I felt feminine and womanly, a state of being quite distinct from my previous incarnation as boyish or androgynous.

As encapsulation worked its nasty trick, teasing me with the threat of implant removal, I reassured myself that I was OK. There was a certain familiarity to the feeling (which resembled milk-engorged breasts) and, given that I had handled all the discomforts of breast-feeding, I would handle this too. It was no coincidence that I should compare the experience of motherhood (which I credit as being the motivation behind my breast augmentation surgery). Motherhood had been my introduction to the visual and public markers of womanhood. Pregnancy was a powerful experience on its own, but as an initiation into life within a woman's body it was extraordinary. The whole experience, from the body changes through to the breast-feeding, altered me forever. My first child gave me a taste of what I'd been missing, but my second child enabled me to embrace it completely. I became the new body, refusing to believe it was transitory, and was shocked when my old body returned, unbidden, within days of weaning. I felt devastated. I was almost 30 and had become comfortable in a more womanly skin.

A decade later, I seemed to be facing the same situation. Thus, even as my breasts became firmer and firmer, I suspended logic rather than confront what was happening. However, as fate would have it, someone bumped into me, sharply knocking into one of my breasts.

I might add that I was highly protective of my breasts by this stage. Encapsulation had changed them into a pair of Dr Hodgkinson's despised boob jobs.[5] My breasts were overly firm and often felt tight and uncomfortable. This meant that I avoided anything that might cause them (and me) stress. I didn't like them to be touched and avoided sleeping on my stomach. I virtually eliminated all arm stretching exercises. I even kept my arms in a protective brace-type stance when walking in crowds. So, the bumping incident came as quite a shock. It was accompanied by a slight popping sound, after which the breast seemed softer, more pliable. I spent a number of days inspecting the breast, wondering whether the change was real or imaginary, doubting whether I had heard a sound. Eventually I had no choice but to call my surgeon.

I was advised to have a mammogram. This was an extraordinarily stressful procedure performed by a woman with no experience or knowledge of implants. It was rough and brutal and I cried through the entire ordeal. Adding to my distress was the fear that the procedure itself was enough to place the implants at risk. The results were inconclusive which meant I had to fly to Sydney for further tests. I had another mammogram (this time performed by a woman familiar with my circumstances), an X-ray, and an ultrasound. The tests confirmed that one implant had ruptured.

My surgeon was quite upbeat delivering the news. His positivity, the attribute that had once held such appeal, now seemed offensive and out of step with the situation. He told me that even though there was a rupture, it did not present a problem (to him?). His exact words were: "We'll just whip'm out." In other scenarios, such as a change of breast size or shape, implants can be removed and replacement implants inserted during the same operation. But ruptures are messy. Best, he advised, to allow a number of months of recovery time. Then, if I wanted, I could return for another set. I declined. I'd had enough.

5 See Note 2.

Given the age of my implants, I was to have both removed, not just the damaged one. However, his reference to my implants as "old" really struck me. I was under the impression that, had there been no problems, I would have kept them for the rest of my life. In hindsight it is an appalling thought, but at the time it seemed logical. I was never informed otherwise.[6] But this raises the obvious question: Why was I not informed? Why are recipients of other forms of surgery that involve the introduction of an artificial part—hip replacement surgery for instance—warned about the life of the prosthesis? If implants warrant replacing at some point in the future, shouldn't I have been told?[7] But I didn't ask this question. I simply waited politely while he booked me in for surgery. All things considered, I believed I was lucky to have enjoyed a good result for seven years and, from what I have learned since, extremely fortunate to have refused "treatment" for encapsulation. (Treatment consists of the breasts being squeezed until the encapsulated tissue breaks. This is often painful and requires some women to have it performed under anesthetic. Moreover, it is a dangerous—some say negligent—procedure because of the risk of damage to the implant membrane.)

I had the implants removed just prior to my fortieth birthday. They had been part of my body for a decade. Surgery was complicated. Besides the rupture, both implants were sticky, a result of the silicone gel oozing through the implant membrane. This required the surgeon to scrape all traces of silicone from the affected breast tissue. Apparently sticky implants are not uncommon, yet they are not accounted for in any litigation proceedings against Dow Corning. The condition is undetectable other than through surgical means and, prior to surgery, I was not warned of the possibility. Recovery was painful, slow, upsetting. Full recovery left large scars under the breast line and the right breast smaller than the left due to extra breast tissue removal. Parts of the right breast remain numb and uncomfortable.

When it comes to the body, the line between the virtual and the actual is a fine one.[8] My grandmother's false teeth, for example, which she removed and placed in a glass beside the bed each night, were an integral part of her body. As kids we considered them nana's teeth as opposed to nana's false teeth. Besides, occasionally we left our teeth in a glass beside the bed; lost baby teeth for fairies to collect in the night. Teeth, it seemed, were always on a journey. As an adult, my perfectly straight white teeth are testament to the demands of the journey—one

6 I checked with a friend who had breast augmentation surgery the year after me. She has had a further two operations, the most recent in 2000, but has never been advised that this was to be expected.

7 The website http://cosmeticsurgeryoz.com warns prospective breast surgery patients to expect to undergo more than one procedure and is quite clear in stating that implants don't last forever.

8 See Dagmar Reinhardt's discussion of the congruence of the virtual and the actual (2005: 51).

quite different to the course nana's teeth took, albeit similar in some respects. In my forties (a few years after the removal of my breast implants) I embarked on a regime of dental work that included 18 months of braces followed by the removal of all gray amalgam fillings. Each cavity was filled with a new hard white plastic. Teeth that were adversely weakened by the amalgam removal process (which was fairly disruptive, occasionally causing a tooth to fracture) were replaced with crowns. The work is ongoing due to the age of my teeth, which require seemingly endless rounds of maintenance. The point I am making is that, even after all this work, my teeth remain wholly mine, both physically (because the replacement work is bonded and cannot be removed) and emotionally (because even the fillings and crowns feel as organic as the original). I am able to make sense of the process; moreover, my senses make sense of the process, reaffirming the ownership and congruence of my teeth. Emotionally, aesthetically, and physically, any similarity to nana's prosthetic teeth seems virtual in an intellectual sense, rather than actual.

I raise the comparison between nana's teeth and my own to draw forth the question of authenticity. If teeth that have been straightened, fixed, crowned, bridged, and whitened retain a claim to authenticity, what makes nana's false teeth any less authentic? After all, hers were equally a fashionable cosmetic alternative to deterioration—at the time. Is the fact that they can be removed from the body the context that brands them false? Never mind that they were part of her life for seven decades, does their lifelessness outside the body dismiss them as imitations, unfashionable markers of another age? Is the ability to remove the prosthesis from the body the context where falseness sits?[9] And if so, what then are the differences distinguishing the real and the fake, the actual and the virtual, when we're talking about breasts? For example, in my experience, the breast implant prostheses, while housed within my body, staked a claim for authenticity, a claim that was supported by their natural form and shape, their softness and pliability. Conversely, the authenticity of my breasts dissipated as they began to encapsulate. The hated visual cues heralded by encapsulation outed me as a breast implant recipient and I began to feel as though my own claim to authenticity was being revoked. The prosthesis-as-obvious renders not only the whole breast false, but the person with it. Encapsulated breasts became my grandmother's false teeth: funny, entertaining, a point of ridicule. False teeth, falling from their embarrassed owner's mouth and captured and shown on programs such as *Funniest Home Videos* are little different from the "plastic surgery gone wrong" articles in women's magazines. Thus, the anxiety inherent in coping with encapsulation is not only founded upon the aesthetic, but is underpinned by the threat to one's own sense of authenticity. Little wonder that implant removal, while emotionally and physically draining, was such a resounding relief.

9 I deliberately envisage the prosthesis as false. This is a limited view compared to Vivian Sobchack's detailed analysis of her experiences as a prosthesis user (2004: 205–25).

As an adolescent, my first experience of body authenticity must have been a confusing one. While authentic bodies all around me were growing breasts, my body was not. At least my mother had the foresight to buy me a bra, lest I be the only one in my group without one. The training bra, besides authenticating me to my peers, was an introduction, at 12 years old, to a world of appearances. Brassieres of the 1960s were highly functional and my tiny, plain, white, minimally padded training device emulated this trend. It staked its claim for authenticity, not by what it was (which was a pretence) but by what it purported *not* to be. The training bra did not say "woman." Instead it, rather politely, announced the blossoming girl. The pretence, however, was deeply felt by me, the wearer; a guilty secret that accompanied every tissue-filled wear, always fearful that my ruse would be discovered. Similarly, decades later when encapsulation betrayed my breasts as fake, I felt fearful that I would likewise be perceived as such.

I had twice been bothered by the "fake"; as a young girl and again as a woman in her late thirties. Both experiences rendered me uncomfortable and stressed. Yet I had coped magnificently in between, in a profession which many would say is the epitome of fake. I began modeling in 1975, at age 20. Tall, blonde, and thin, my Twiggy-ish figure[10] was a natural clotheshorse and I began to appear regularly in *Cleo*, *Cosmopolitan*, and *Vogue*. However, the glamorous side of modeling—the magazines and catwalk shows—accounted for only a fraction of my work. Mostly I worked for Grace Bros, David Jones, Sportscraft, Pattons Wool, and Osti, to name a few. All these jobs would find me donning a flesh-tone bra with foam inserts, and for shots that required me to be bra-less I had flesh-tone foam falsies (with "nipples" sewn into the fabric). However, the difference between this and my training bra days was that this time everyone knew. I had no desire to disguise the real me from my work colleagues. This meant that even though I was photographed with "breasts" I never felt inauthentic. Authenticity, in this instance, was reconfigured to mean honesty. As long as I was honest with the people I worked with, I no longer resembled the frightened adolescent. Plus, by utilizing one of the most basic elements of the industry—the fake—my padded bra and falsies became coded to reflect the plethora of practices the industry called upon to manipulate the image.

I modeled at a time (1975–90) when the emphasis on body perfection was not as intense as it is today.[11] I was one of the thinnest models at that time and, while it occasionally worked against me, people accepted that that was who I was. My padded bra was simply an accessory—for which I never apologized. And while I concede that my padded bra no doubt worked as a daily reminder that breasts were

10 British model Twiggy's stick-like (hence the name) androgynous body paved the way for models like me.

11 Cyndi Tebbel (2000) blames media images of the thin "ideal" for creating a culture of body hatred. Her criticism is all the more poignant given she was fired from her position as editor of *New Woman* magazine for putting a less than thin woman on the cover. She notes, also, the insanity of expecting models to have tiny bodies but large breasts.

an expected feature of a woman's body, I dispute the conclusion that modeling enticed me towards breast augmentation. As I've said already, this pressure only surfaced once I'd experienced the joy of breasts during pregnancy and breast-feeding. However, if my reasons for choosing breast augmentation surgery fall primarily outside the pressures of modeling, I must mention something that counters my claim that modeling was ostensibly pressure free.

A year following breast augmentation I had eye surgery. Skin was removed from above and below each eye. I wanted *all* the lines and wrinkles removed, but my surgeon (the same one who performed the breast augmentation) was cautious; the removal of too much skin could result in the bottom lid being pulled away from the eyeball. The operation could also cause nerve damage. Thus he advised a small section be removed from the bottom lid and suggested the removal of loose skin from the upper lid. The eye surgery was most definitely the result of my profession. At 30, I was working with girls half my age. They were young and wrinkle free with time-to-go-to-the-gym bodies. I felt old, had stretch marks from two pregnancies, and was often tired from the demands of work, travel,[12] and parenting. Few models, even those my age, had families, so the atmosphere at work was sometimes alienating. And even though I was the "old" married woman with children, I never made the transition into young mum roles. I was told repeatedly that I looked "modelly" as opposed to "mumsy." So, yes, modeling definitely had its pressures.

Very few people knew of my eye surgery. I told only immediate family and two friends. All were sworn to secrecy. In contrast, I told everyone about my breast surgery. Of course, in a profession such as modeling it would have been impossible to hide brand new breasts, so I had little choice but to be candid. As for the eye operation, the surgeon's caution meant that the difference was virtually undetectable. At 30, I wanted to look 20, so the result was disappointing and did little to boost my self-confidence at work. By 35 I found myself in the midst of a mid-life crisis and quit modeling, believing it to be the source of my distress.

I had made a promise to myself, following the eye surgery, that I would never put myself under the plastic surgeon's knife again. This may sound strange given that I had no regrets following my breast augmentation the preceding year, but eye surgery left me feeling battered. With two black eyes I looked (and felt) like the victim of domestic violence—which the secrecy surrounding the surgery only served to compound. The fact that I had chosen this course of action meant I confronted the extremes of my vanity. The bruising and swelling took two weeks to completely disappear. There was no scarring under the eye and a fine scar-line in the fold of the upper lid. In hindsight, the operation should not have been performed. The minimal amount of skin that was removed from the bottom lid meant there was little discernable difference in my appearance. The skin that was removed from the upper lid was, in all probability, unnecessary. The lid was

12 I commuted from Byron Bay to Sydney, Melbourne, and Brisbane between 1981 and 1990.

neither hooded nor loose. The result left me unable to close my eyes when sleeping for approximately two years.

At 53, I am modeling again. Funnily, it was at the insistence of an old modeling buddy who has resumed his career after a similar absence. He called one afternoon and suggested I give it a go. When I resisted he assured me it was different now. And he was right; I'm only called when they're looking for a woman in her fifties. Another difference is that, while casting calls in my past were highly competitive affairs, these castings are relaxed and enjoyable. The other women are warm and welcoming, we come in all shapes and sizes and no one seems to care (our measurements are a source of laughter rather than competition) and we pass the time talking about our children, grandchildren, and how far we've traveled to get to the casting. It is, without question, liberating.

Plastic surgery seems, and is, a lifetime away. I would still like to have actual bra-filling breasts but I am more than happy in my own skin. I was lucky to experience breasts—safely while breast-feeding, then expensively through surgery—and even luckier to come through the latter experience unscathed. As for my promise never to go under the knife again, apart from implant removal surgery which was a necessity, I have never forgotten it, or the thoughts that compelled it.

References

Blum, V. L. 2003. *Flesh Wounds: The Culture of Cosmetic Surgery*. Los Angeles: University of California Press.

Reinhardt, D. 2005. "Surface Strategies and Constructive Line: Preferential Planes, Contour, Phenomenal Body in the Work of Bacon, Chalayan, Kawakubo." *COLLOQUY: Text, Theory, Critique*, No. 9. Available at: http://colloquy.monash.edu.au/issue009/reinhardt.pdf.

Sobchack, V. 2004. *Carnal Thoughts: Embodiment and Moving Image Culture*. Los Angeles: University of California Press.

Tavakoli, K. 2006. "A Few Facts on Silicone." February 17. Available at: http://cosmeticsurgeryaustralia.com.

Tebbel, C. 2000. *Body Snatchers: How the Media Shapes Women*. Sydney: Finch.

Index

Aalten, Anna, 37
Aboudib, J. H., 159
Adams, A., 134, 135, 142
Adler, Alfred, 5
Aesthetic citizenship, 163
Agar, Nicholas, 119, 120
Ageism *see* Elderly people, marginalization of; Middle-aged men; Middle-aged women
Agency
  as action, 39-40, 63
  agency/structure debate, 39
  as constitution of historical subjects, 63
  cultural and social constraints, 24-25, 27, 36, 42, 199
  and discursive production of subjects, 100-1, 103-4, 106, 114, 183
  historical constraints, 36
  ideological mystification as constraint to, 13, 36, 40, 58
  intentionality, 39
  and magazines, 100, 102, 104-5, 107-10, 113
  material constraints and opportunities to, 24-25, 27, 113
  and practical knowledge, expertise, 39, 103
  racism as constraint to, 38, 199
  as self-creation, 56
  and self-knowledge, 40
  situated by power relations, 39, 56
  as sociological concept, 39
  and specialized knowledge, 25
  and TV makeovers, 111-14
Akin, Susan, 55
Aldrich, Robert, 80
Allotey, P., 134, 135
Alter, G. J., 134
American College of Obstetrics and Gynecology, 134
Annas, George, 122
Appropriation, feminist, of expertise and technology, 63-65, 120
Ardener, S., 133
Art, cosmetic surgery as, 6, 91
Ashton, Madeline, 88
ASPS (American Society for Plastic Surgeons), 4n, 225
Assimilation, 193
Atkinson, Michael, 12-13, 37
Atlas, James, 79
Attwood, F., 141
Authenticity, 23-24, 31, 118, 121, 124, 128, 244-45

Baartman, Saartjie, 201
Baby Jane (film character), 80, 94
Bacall, Lauren, 92
Ballard, J.G., 86, 88
Balsamo, Anne, 70, 71
Banderas, Antonio, 109
Banet-Weiser, Sarah, 118
Bankard, B., 173
Banks, Ingrid, 44
Banks, Tyra, 197n
Barker-Benfield, G.J., 54
Bartky, Sandra, 35, 63, 142, 154
Bassenezi, C., 165
Baudrillard, Jean, 91
Beauty, 56, 65, 117, 121, 142, 154, 178-79
  in Brazil, 166
  in gay men, 213, 219, 222
  in magazines, 102
Beauty pageants, 19, 55, 59n, 60
Beauty practices, 35, 37
Beauty products, 29-30
Béhague, D., 161
Belo, Vicky, 172
Bergen, Candice, 86, 89
Berger, John, 57

Berman, Jennifer, 135
Bermant, Michael, 229
Bhalla, Nita, 68
Biehl, J., 153, 156, 163
Biological determinism, 120
Biomedicine, 67, 71, 160-61
Biotechnology, 117, 119, 122
Blank, J., 133
Blum, Virginia, 134, 140, 173, 174, 184-85, 241
Boasten, Michelle, 67
Botox, 2, 10, 11, 15, 29, 32, 122, 181-83, 186, 220
 as moral actor, 182-83
Body
 as artifact, 119
 body-as-text metaphor, 6n
 feminine practices of, 37
 historical imaginaries of, 21
 materiality of, 7, 45, 79, 137
 mechanical metaphor, 21
 as product of social knowledge, 235
 as raw material, 22, 58, 174
 as site of agency, 54
 as site of challenge, 53
 as social construct, 119-20
Bostrom, Nick, 119
Black market, 6. *see also* Techniques: illegal or unsupervised
Blepharoplasty. *see* Eye-lid surgery
Bordo, Susan, 2, 7, 63n, 71, 93, 118-21, 123, 136, 154, 163, 226, 233
 debate with Davis, 35, 37-38, 40-42, 45
Bowlby, R., 140
Bras, 245
Brazil
 and aesthetic medicine, 159-62
 and capitalism, 153, 166-67
 and class relations, 153-57, 160-61, 163-64, 166
 competitive logic in, 166
 consumer culture in, 166
 cosmetic surgery industry in, 9, 153-67
 and democracy, 153
 and health care, 153-64
 medical tourism in, 14
 and reproduction management, 60-62
 and young patients, 165
Breast augmentation, 1, 3, 13, 25, 52, 57, 158, 176, 180-81, 225, 239-44, 246
Breast reconstruction (post-mastectomy), 15
Breast reduction, 13, 164, 225-35
Brooks, Abigail, 134, 70
Brown, Sarah, 68
Brownell, Susan, 14
Burana, Lily, 28
Burr, V., 136
Butler, Judith, 63-64

Caetano, A., 160, 161
Cairnie, Allie, 11
Caldeira, T., 153
Canada. *see* National contexts
Capitalism, 177, 200. *see also* Consumer culture
Carr, Michele, 231
Carranza, Maria, 161
Carrey, Jim, 88
Cassell, Joan, 174, 177, 186
Castells, M., 160, 165
Castle, D. J., 141
Celebrity, 6, 8, 101
Cesarean section, 135, 159-61
Chancer, Lynn, 37
Chase, C., 133n
Cher, 22, 29, 45
Chernin, K., 154
Childbirth, 135, 139, 159-62
China. *see* National contexts
Choice. *see* Freedom of choice; Agency
Clarke, Adele, 67, 71
Class
 in Brazil, 153-57, 160-61, 163-64, 166
 depoliticization of, 121
 and gender, 100, 114
 middle-class norms, 43, 166
 surgery recipient distribution by, 113
 working class, marginalization of, 43
 see also Economic inequality
Commodification
 of beauty, 61
 of body, 65-67, 70
 of cosmetic surgery, 8, 14
Compulsion
 patterns of, 53

surgical, 91
Connell, John, 14
Consumer culture, 24, 27, 185
and capitalism, 27
Consumer demand, 177, 230
Consumer power, 62
Corey, Jeff, 67
Corinne, T., 133
Corman, Roger, 83
Costs, financial, of cosmetic surgery, 51-52, 86, 90, 155
Crawford, Joan, 84
Credit companies. *see* Financing of cosmetic surgery
Creighton, S., 134, 137, 140, 141
Crouch, N. S., 137
Crum, Howard, 172
Cultural criticism, 31, 39, 41-42
"Cultural dope", 23, 35, 39, 40
"Cultural plastic", 21
Culture
power of images, 24, 38
systemic nature of, 23
Western beauty culture, 38, 42, 45, 53
Cuomo, Chris, 203
Cuvier (anatomist), 201

D'Amico, Richard, 4n
Davis, Bette, 84
Davis, Kathy, 2, 4, 7, 8, 11, 70, 102, 136, 143, 157, 173, 186, 192, 195-6, 203-4, 235
debate with Bordo, 24-25, 28
Davis, S. W., 134, 135, 138, 139, 140, 143
de Alencar Felicio, Y., 134
Death, 84. *see also* Risks and dangers of surgery
de Beauvoir, Simone, 84
de Certeau, M., 166
Defect, self-perception of body as, 25-28, 36, 38
de Haro, F., 134
Dein, Edward, 83
Dellinger, Kirsten, 37
Denizart, H., 165
Dental surgery, 15, 244
Derek, Bo, 57
Desire 122, 129, 143, 163, 175
discursive organization of, 25
and fetish, 162
production of, 136, 154
as realized by technology, 87, 89
reduction to neediness, 94
Desmond, Norma (film character), 80
Dewire, Thomas, 231
Diaspora, 192
Difference
commodification of, 43
embodied, erasure of, 44-46
proliferation of, 120
Disability, 43
Disciplinary power and practices, 56, 125, 154, 180, 235. *see also* Foucauldian critique
Dittman, M., 141
Divine, 125
Dodson, B., 133
Douglas, Mary, 108
Dow Corning, 239n, 243
Downie, A., 161
Drugs
company profit motive, 28
HIV medication, 213-16, 221
imported and non-approved, 175
Prozac, 28
steroids, 126
Valium, 86
Dysmorphia, body, 5
Dull, Diana, 10, 11
Dunaway, Faye, 29

Eating disorders, 37
Economic inequality 22, 43
and access to cosmetic surgery, 30, 113
and access to health care, 30
in Brazil, 153-57, 160-61, 163-64
and nutrition, 30
Elderly people, marginalization of, 43, 80, 83-85, 93-94
Elective surgery, 59-60
Embodied experience, 36, 45, 79, 122, 197, 235
Empowerment, cosmetic surgery as, 38, 92, 104, 107, 133, 219, 222
Encapsulation, 181, 240-45
Ensler, E., 133

Equality discourse, 44-45
Eroticism
in Brazil, 164-65
and HIV, 219
pathologization of, 53
women's, 8, 174
Eroticization
of cosmetic surgery, 89, 176
Essén, B., 135
Essentialism, 117, 120, 122, 124, 126-27, 129
Ethnic Cosmetic Surgery (ECS), 191-204
Ethnicity
African, 191, 201-02, 231
Asian, 194-202
ethnic belonging, 192
European, 202
Hispanic, 231
Native American, 231
surgery recipient distribution by, 3-4, 113, 153
see also National contexts
Ethnocentrism, 193, 198
Etcoff, Nancy, 67, 70
Eugenio (doctor), 155-56
Exoticism, 153, 203
Extropians, 119
Eye-lid surgery, 10, 13, 14, 22, 45, 52, 57, 176, 192-94, 196-202, 246

Face-lift, 3, 52, 86
Facial lipoatrophy, 209-23
Facial surgery (in men with HIV), 11, 209-14, 216-17, 220-22
recipient narratives, 209-11, 216-23
Farran, Sandra, 230
Faveret, F., 156
Featherstone, M., 139, 141
Feiner, Susan, 14
Femininity
in Brazil, 164, 167
"Femininity Politics", 63
and inferiority, discourses of, 36, 38, 42, 60
and magazines, 105-7, 110, 113, 140
male-feminine identity, 12
naturalness stereotype, 2, 9, 117, 121-29
normative ideal of, 6, 24, 37, 40, 61, 63-64, 66, 117, 121, 158, 227-28, 232-33, 235, 242
production and regulation of, 35
Feminism
activist, 120
agency feminism, 38
constructionist 142-43
corporeal, 71
cyberfeminism, 71
feminist fascism, 61n
and justification of body alteration, 29
left, 36
liberal, 61n
multicultural, 199
post-feminism, 37, 120
post-modern, 7, 21, 24, 31, 118
radical, 8, 63, 195
second-wave, 30, 133
Feminist critique of cosmetic surgery
and breast reduction, 232
as consciousness raising, 23
deconstruction of feminine representations, 37, 129
disciplinary perspectives, 2
early critique, 1, 6-8
economic analysis, 15
and ethnography, 4
and ethnic cosmetic surgery, 194-203
and men's facial surgery, 212-13
as political action, 63-64
Fetishism, 162
of body, 50
of face, 91
Few, Julius, 202
Figueira, S., 165
Film
fantasy, 87-90
horror, 83-85, 94
representation of cosmetic surgery, 81, 83, 88-89
representation of men, 87
representation of women, 8, 80-85, 86-89
special effects, 82-83, 87-89
Financing of cosmetic surgery, 155. *see also* Insurance, medical
Firestone, Shulamith, 120

Fitness craze, 37
Foucault, Michel (and Foucauldian critique), 24, 37, 56, 104, 119, 125, 154, 162, 180
Frankel, Martha, 22
Frankenburg, Ruth, 203
Fraser, Suzanne, 138, 140, 143, 174n1
Freedom of choice, 7, 13-14, 22-23, 37-39, 54-56, 142-43, 166, 183, 195, 197
  see also Agency
Freiberg, Arnis, 231
Freud, Sigmund, 85
Freyre, G., 164
Froes (doctor), 165n1
Frueh, J., 133, 134, 139
Fukuyama, Francis, 122-23
Functionalist critique, 35n3

Geertz, Clifford, 102
Geldof, Bob, 106-7
Gender: "Age of Gender," 3-4
  constitution through class discourse, 100, 114
  normative discourses of, 227-28
  performatives, 63-65, 120, 128
  politics, progress model of, 100
  surgeon distribution by, 3, 4n, 174n1
  surgery recipient distribution by, 3-4, 26, 52, 113, 158
  see also Femininity; Masculinity
Genital mutilation, 60n, 135
Genital surgery. *see* Vaginal surgery
Gerike, Ann, 79
Giddens, Anthony, 40
Gilman, Sander, 3, 4, 14, 118, 140, 157, 192, 201-02, 226
Gimlin, Debra, 4, 67, 230, 231, 234
Giraldo, F., 134
Globalization, 14
Goering, Sara, 68, 71, 197
Goin, J., 173
Goin, M., 173
Goldenberg, M., 165
Goldstein, D., 164
Goldwyn, Robert, 175
Gonzalez, C., 134
Good Face Project, 210-13
Goodman, Ellen, 49
Goodman, M. 23, 134
Green, F. J., 134, 135, 138, 140, 141, 142
Greer, G., 102
Gregg, J., 163
Griffin, Anthony C., 191
Griffin, Susan, 57n
Griffiths, Melanie, 29, 109
Grosz, Elizabeth, 71
Grover, S., 134
Guilloff, E., 134
Gurley, G., 134

Haddad, B., 134
Haertsch, Peter, 180
Häggström-Nordin, E., 140
Haiken, Elizabeth, 3, 5, 70, 140, 157, 177-78, 185, 192-93, 196, 203, 212, 229, 231
Hall, Kim, 203
Hanshard, M., 164
Hanson, U., 140
Harkness, Libby, 230
Harris, John, 119
Hartley, Paddy, 3
Hartsock, Nancy, 63
Haug, Frigga, 58
Hausman, Bernice, 43
Hawn, Goldie, 29
Haworth, Randal, 26
Hawthorne, Susan, 71
Health care
  in Brazil, 10, 153-64
  bureaucratic structure of, 10, 232
  in Canada, 13, 232
  diversion of resources, 15
  and HIV, 214, 216-17, 219, 221
  in Netherlands, 157
  in United Kingdom, 232
  in United States of America, 232
  see also Insurance, medical
Helström, L., 141
Hepburn, Audrey, 86
Hermaphrodism, 126
Heterosexuality
  and desire, 175
  social construction as norm, 53-57, 70-71, 228

Heyes, Cressida, 5, 10, 70, 112-13, 118, 121
Hicks, Karen, 135
Hirschfeld, Magnus, 201
Hirshson, Paul, 52
HIV metabolic syndrome /AIDS, 209-23
  psychological effects, 213-14, 217-19, 222
Hoagland, Sarah Lucia, 66
Hodgkinson, Darryl, 240n1
Hoefflin, Steven, 67
Holliday, Ruth, 11, 120
Homogenization. *see* Normalization
Homosexuality
  gay culture and community, 211, 222
  marginalization of, 43, 53, 126, 222
  and stereotyped effeminacy, 13
Honigman, R. J., 141
Hopkins, K., 161
Human nature, as moral ground, 122, 124, 126-27, 129
Humanist critique, 193
Hurwitz, Dennis, 68-69
Huss-Ashmore, Rebecca, 184

Immortality, 91
Individualism, 27, 38, 44, 143
  methodological, 39
Industrial society, Western, 54, 57
Inferiority complex, 5
Insurance, medical, 228, 231-32
  and HIV treatments, 214, 216-17, 219, 221
International Research (company), 32-33

Jackson, Michael, 6, 22, 44, 203
Jagger, E., 141
Jahoda, S., 135
Japan. *see* National contexts
Jaspers, Karl, 42n
Jeffreys, Sheila, 195, 134, 140, 154
Johnsdotter, S., 135
Jones, Meredith, 10, 70, 71, 111-12
Jordan, J. W., 134, 139, 140
Juran, Nathan, 83

Kapelovitz, Dan, 71
Kass, Leon, 121-124, 126-27
Kaw, Eugenia, 194-203
Kitzinger, S., 135, 142
Klein, Renate, 71
Klinge, Ineke, 37
Knives, 54, 123
Korea, South. *see* National contexts
Kramer, Peter, 25
Kristeva, J., 139
Kuczynski, Alex, 5, 14, 29, 70, 71, 120, 173, 175
Kulick, Don, 6, 164

Labor, 112
Lakoff, Robin Tolmach, 57
Lam, Samuel, 67
Laqueur, T., 136
Lauer, Matt, 33
Lawsuits, 177, 239, 243
Lee, Sharon Heijin, 14
Legislation, 110
Leibovich, Lori, 70
Lemack, G. E., 141
Lerche Davis, J., 177
Levine, Ronald, 49
Liao, L.-M., 134, 137, 140, 141
Liberal democracy, 102-3
Libertarianism, 117, 119, 121
Libidinal economy, 163
Liposuction, 3, 6, 11, 50, 52, 159, 176, 221, 230, 232
Little, Margaret, 71
Lizardi, Tina, 22
Lloyd, J., 137
Lopez, Jennifer, 203
Lorber, Judith, 229
Lorenc, Paul, 120
Lorenzo, Robin Merrill, 230
Louis-Sylvestre, C., 134
Luciana (doctor), 165
Luhrman, Baz, 29
Lupton, Deborah, 108
Lury, Celia, 43

MacCannell, Dean, 35
MacCannell, Juliet Flower, 35
McCaughey, Bobbi, 30
McCurdy, John Jr., 67
McDowell, L., 113

MacFarquhar, Larissa, 87, 89, 92
McLish, Rachel, 21
MacNair, P., 135
McNamara, K. R., 134, 135
McNulty, T. A., 173
Madonna, 49
Magazines 21, 22, 26, 28, 30, 43, 72, 81, 85, 99-115, 140, 245
 representation and constitution of subjects in, 100-1, 104-8, 110
Mammogram, 242
Marketing of cosmetic surgery, 182
 to lower income people, 14
 see also Media
Martine, G., 160
Malpractice, 108
Manderson, L., 134, 135, 136, 139
Markovic, Mihailo, 50
Marx, Karl (and Marxist critique), 24, 35n3, 154, 162
Masculinity
 and gay men, 211-12, 217, 219
 discursive construction of, 11-13, 25-26, 45, 121, 135
 and magazines, 110
 male-feminine identity, 12
 and social pressure, 25
Masks, 89, 221
Massive weight loss (MWL), 173
Materiality of the body, 7, 45, 79, 137
Matthews, Gwyneth Ferguson, 59n
Mayer, Vicki, 15
Meade, T., 160
Media
 and demand for surgery, 164
 and construction of women's self-image, 5, 8, 23, 25-28, 37, 93, 179, 185
 and gender stereotypes, 9
 representation of cosmetic surgery in, 9, 43, 234
 and surgery information dissemination, 176
 see also Film; Television; Websites
Melamed, Elissa, 79, 84
Micromastia, 25
Middle-aged men
 aging with HIV, 213, 215-20, 222-23
 self-image of, 26, 55
Middle-aged women
 in Brazil, 166
 demonization of, 8, 82-84, 93
 self-image of, 8, 29, 80-81, 83, 85, 93-94, 123, 183, 246
Miklos, J. R., 134
Minto, C. L., 137, 141
Modeling, 245-47
Moore, R. D., 134
Moral relativism, 127n5
Morgan, Kathryn, 2, 8, 11, 15, 35, 122-23, 163, 221, 228
Motherhood, 8, 53, 154, 162-63, 166-67, 242, 246
Motive, surgeons, 28
 profit as, 35
Motive, surgery recipients, 28, 36, 49, 55, 62, 67, 101, 105-7, 109, 112, 195, 239, 246
 financial gain as, 106, 113
 romantic success as, 24, 35, 55, 57, 67, 105-6, 109, 111.
 see also Professional pressure
Multiculturalism, 164
 as aesthetic ideal, 43-44
Mutilation, cosmetic surgery as, 195-96
Mutilation, Self-, as resistance, 65

Narrative self-understandings and justification
 by recipients of cosmetic surgery, 4-7, 10, 12, 36, 38, 40-43, 54, 62, 68-70, 81, 86, 158, 162, 174, 183-85, 193, 195, 199, 225-26, 230, 232-34, 239-47
 by recipients of facial surgery (men with HIV), 209-11, 216-23
 by surgeons, 10, 43, 177-80, 182, 184-85
Nash, Karen, 68
Nasrulla, Amber, 67
National contexts (cosmetic surgery)
 Brazil, 10, 153-67
 Canada, 13, 232
 China, 66n
 Japan, 22
 Korea, South, 14

Netherlands, 157
Thailand, 67-70
United Kingdom, 232
United States of America, 232
Naturalness, as body ideal, 2, 9, 31, 60, 117, 121-29, 198
see also Femininity
Negrin, Llewellyn, 70, 120
Neoliberalism, 14-15, 71, 143
Netherlands. *see* National contexts
Nilsson, B., 141
Nip and tuck, 52
Normalness, as body ideal
among men with HIV, 213, 219, 223
among women, 28, 36-37, 43-44, 61, 226-27, 229, 235
Nose job, 52, 57

Obesity, 30n1
marginalization of obese people, 43
Obsessional neurosis, 85
O'Connell, Brian, 14
O'Connor, E., 173
Odunze, Millicent, 202
Olesen, Marie B. V., 70
Olesen, R. Merrel, 70
Oliveira, P. J., 156
Ordinary. *see* Normalness
Orlan, 6, 91
Ormrod, S., 183
Orr, D., 135

Padmore, Catherine, 197
Palmer, Francis, 179-80
Paniel, B.J., 134
Paradoxes of surgery choice, 56-61
Pardo, J., 134
Parker, R., 160, 166
Parody, 64
Parthenogenesis, 174
Pathologization
of bodies, 60-61, 180
of surgery recipients, 1, 9, 104, 124, 133, 136-40, 175, 184, 226
Patriarchy, 4, 53-54, 58, 62-63, 65, 85, 176, 178, 200
in Brazil, 10, 164-66
Penile enhancement, 26, 109
Perfection, as body ideal, 26, 35, 43, 53, 60, 142, 245
Petro, Jane, 173, 235
Phillips, K. A., 141
Pitanguy, Ivo, 153, 156, 157, 159n5, 164, 172
Pitts-Taylor, Victoria, 5, 71
Pizzini, F., 135
Plástica. see Brazil, cosmetic surgery industry
Political protest, surgery as, 67
Popular culture. *see* Media
Portwood-Stacer, Laura, 118
Positivism, 159-60
Poststructuralist critique, 38, 100, 103
Potter, J., 100, 160, 161
Powell, Michael, 177
Power, colonizing forms of, 58-59
Pregnancy, 242, 246
Preventive procedures, 26, 165
Price, Katie, 1
Princess Margaret, 86n
Pringle, Rosemary, 105n
Prochazka, Tony, 179n
Professional pressure, 24-25, 55, 66, 105, 107, 113, 200, 246
Psychoanalysis, 85
Public debate, 41

Racial psychology, 192
Racism
internalized, 10, 14, 193, 198, 202-3
racial marginalization and normalization, 22, 43-45, 57, 65, 121, 128, 191-93, 195-97, 200-4
as structure of inequality, 38
see also Whiteness, normative
Rankin, C., 154
Ransley, P. G., 141
Rational choice, 59, 108, 143
Raymond, Janice, 195
Real, conception of, 50, 90-91, 138, 244-45
Reese, Vail, 90
Regina, Ana, 156
Restylane, 2, 11, 15, 174
Ribeiro, C., 158
Ricci, P.A., 134
Ricoeur, Paul, 42

Rights discourse, 158-59, 163, 165
Risks and dangers of surgery, 41, 50-52, 62, 90, 92, 108-9, 111-12, 137n6, 181, 239-41, 243, 246
  discourses of, 139
  inadequate information on, 36, 243
Roberts, Tom, 68
Robinson, A., 135
Roiphe, Katie, 37
Rooks, Noliwe, 44
Rose, Nikolas, 102-4, 111, 114
Rosen, Christine, 70, 177
Rosen, Trix, 21
Rosenberg, David, 202
Rossellini, Isabella, 88-90
Rouzier, R., 134
Royal Australian and New Zealand College of Obstetricians and Gynaecologists, 134
Rubin, Gayle, 178
Ruzek, S. B., 133

Sachs, Michael Evan, 179n
Sacks, A. Chasby, 179n
Saharso, Sawitri, 37
Sandberg, J., 147
Sarandon, Susan, 29
Sarwer, D. B., 141
Scarring, 11, 163, 227, 230-32, 234, 240, 243
Scheper-Hughes, Nancy, 160
Scherr, Raquel, 57
Schroeder, Curtis, 67
Schult, John, 67
Schwarzenegger, Arnold, 21
Sedgwick, Eve, 178
Self, practices of the, 106
Self-determination. *see* Agency
Sexism, 43
  as structure of inequality, 38
Sexual consumption, 141
Sheldon, S., 135
Sherwin, Susan, 54
Silence, 87, 89, 92
Silicone, 3, 6, 164, 165. *see also* Breast augmentation
Silver, Harold, 62
Singer, Natasha, 6
Slenderness, 37
Smith, Dorothy, 25
Smith, Liz, 29
Sobchack, Vivian, 2, 8, 68, 70, 244n
Sola, V., 134
Sontag, Susan, 80
Spindler, Amy, 26
Spinoza, 187
Spitzack, Carole, 1-2, 70, 171, 175-76, 180-81, 183-84
Starlin, Janet, 90
Statistics, cosmetic surgery, 92, 134n, 225, 231
  see also Gender; Ethnicity
Stepan, N., 160
Sterilization, 160-61
Stock, Gregory, 119, 120
Streisand, Barbara, 81, 82, 85, 91, 92, 93
Structural determinism, 39, 197
Suffering
  cosmetic surgery as solution to, 35, 40-41, 112-13, 184, 229-30, 232-33
  personal histories of, 36, 45
  post-surgery, 231, 243
Sullivan, Deborah, 67, 226-28, 231
Sullivan, N., 134, 135, 140, 203
Sullivan, Toni, 50
Supernatural, 125-26
Surgeons, cosmetic
  as artists, 10, 22, 62, 173, 175, 178-80
  as authority figures, 43, 185
  as butchers, 186
  as caregivers, 56, 174
  and ethnic cosmetic surgery, 191, 200-1
  as experts, 2, 10, 53-54, 57, 180
  as fathers/creators, 172
  as healers, 72, 177
  and HIV, 215
  as lovers, 174-78
  and media trends, 185-86
  as middlemen, 182
  post-WW1, 178
  and power networks, 185-86
  protection of professional territory, 10
  as Pygmalion figures, 171-74, 186
  relationship with patient/client, 2, 6, 171-87

as risk-takers, 175
savior fantasy of, 28
as technicians, 13, 181, 240
unlicensed or unqualified, 6
see also Motives, surgeons
Surgery
illegal or unsupervised, 6
post-WW1, 3, 212
reconstructive/medical vs. cosmetic distinction, 3, 13, 15, 59, 155-57, 159, 161, 209-10, 212, 220, 223, 225-35
"rogue" techniques, 6

Tait, Sue, 118, 121, 124
Talwar, P. K., 173
Tavakoli, Kourosh, 239n
Taylor, Elizabeth, 57
Taylor, Jacqueline Sanchez, 120
Tebbel, Cyndi, 245n11
Technologization of women's bodies, 59-63, 66-67, 70, 91
Technology, neutral, 44
Teeth, 243-44
Television
makeovers, 2, 9, 15, 31, 60, 66n, 71, 111-14, 117-130, 191, 203
news personalities, 29, 33, 82
talk shows, 23, 197
Thailand. *see* National contexts
Thatcher, Margaret, 184
Tiefer, L., 133, 134, 136
Tools, surgical, 51, 54
Tourism, medical, 1, 8
in Brazil, 14
emerging markets, 14
in Thailand, 67-70
Tracy, E. E., 134
Transcendence, Self-, 56, 58, 63, 111, 119-22, 128-29, 142, 184, 198
Transformation, Self-. *see* Transcendence, Self-
Transhumanists, 119
Transvestites, 164n1, 165n14
Travolta, John, 22
Turner, Leigh, 172
Twiggy, 245
Tydén, T., 140

Ugliness, 64, 219, 221
United Kingdom. *see* National contexts
United States of America. *see* National contexts
United States Food and Drug Administration, 175
United States President's Council on Bioethics, 121, 126, 128
Ussher, J., 104n

Vaginal surgery, 69, 133-43
in Brazil, 162
and psychology, 140-43
Value, production of, 111
Vanity, 99, 111-13, 219-22, 232
Van Susterin, Greta, 29
Victimhood, 104, 109-10
Violence, 176
Voluntarism, 119-21, 124

Waldby, Catherine, 68
Walsh, F., 141
Warren, Mary Anne, 61n
Websites
of dermatologists, 90
educational, 142
Google, 134, 136
of surgeons, 9, 11, 69, 133-44, 179-80, 229, 240n1
Wikipedia, 134
YouTube, 1
Weber, B., 112
Wei, Zhang, 66
Weldon, Fay, 62
West, Candace, 10, 11
Wetherell, M., 100
Wexler, Patricia, 174
Whiteness, normative, 10-11, 22, 43, 45, 54, 57, 128, 191, 197-200, 203
WHO, 161
Wildenstein, Jocelyn, 6
Wilder, Billy, 80
Wildish, Toni, 1-2, 6-7, 9
Wilkinson, S., 135, 138, 139, 142
Williams, Christine, 37
Williams, Jim, 50
William, John, 50
Williams, Linda, 83-84

Williams, Tennessee, 88
Willis, Paul, 167
Winfrey, Oprah, 14, 30n1, 118
Winnicott, D.W., 5n
Winslet, Kate, 121
Wolf, Naomi, 35, 37, 70, 154
Wollstonecraft, Mary, 55
Woodhouse, C. R. J., 141
Woodward, Kathleen, 87, 90

Xu, Gary, 14

Yalom, Marilyn, 202n
Yates, Paula, 106-7
Young, Iris Marion, 35, 43, 71
Youth, construction of meanings of, 26, 50, 58, 61, 65, 79, 83-84, 88, 123, 138

Zane, Kathleen, 14, 198-99
Zemeckis, Robert, 87
Zimmern, P. E., 141